The Handbook of
Pediatric Audiology

The
HANDBOOK
of
PEDIATRIC
AUDIOLOGY

Sanford E. Gerber, Editor

With a Foreword by Aram Glorig, M.D.

Gallaudet University Press
Washington, D.C.

Gallaudet University Press
Washington, D.C. 20002

http://gupress.gallaudet.edu

Printed in the United States of America

15 14 13 12 11 10 09 08   4 5 6 7 8 9 10 11

Library of Congress Cataloging-in-Publication Data

The handbook of pediatric audiology / Sanford E. Gerber, editor:
with a foreword by Aram Gorig.
p. cm.
ISBN-13: 978-1-56368-109-7, ISBN-10: 1-56368-109-9 (pbk.) (alk. paper)
ISBN 1-56368-037-8 (hc) (alk. paper)
1. Hearing disorders in children. I. Gerber, Sanford E.
RF291.5.C45H26   1996
618.92'0978—dc20   95-44871
CIP

Many things can wait, the child cannot. Now is the time his bones are being formed, his blood is being made, his mind is being developed. To him we cannot say tomorrow, his name is today.

Gabriela Mistral
CHILEAN POET

About the Editor

SANFORD E. GERBER is emeritus professor of audiology in the department of Speech and Hearing Sciences at the University of California, Santa Barbara. Since retiring from the University of California, he has been serving as chair and visiting professor of the department of Communication Disorders at Eastern Washington University and as adjunct professor of Speech and Hearing Sciences at Washington State University. Dr. Gerber is a Fellow of the American Speech-Language-Hearing Association, a Fellow and past president of the Society for Ear, Nose, and Throat Advances in Children, and an Associate Fellow of the American Academy of Otolaryngology–Head and Neck Surgery. He is president of the Pan American Society of Audiology and a former member of the executive committee of the International Society of Audiology. Dr. Gerber served for five years as chair of the national Joint Committee on Infant Hearing and was president of the International Congress of Audiology in 1984. He has been a Fulbright scholar at Southampton University in England and a visiting professor at the University of Nebraska and Dalhousie University in Halifax, Nova Scotia. He is the author or coauthor of ten books, most of them in pediatric audiology, and of more than one hundred journal articles.

Contents

Foreword

PEDIATRIC audiology, in which I have always had a keen interest, is a relatively new addition to audiology as a profession. Having qualified for the pediatric boards in 1941, I became probably the first pediatric audiologist in the United States and practiced for a year before joining the army in 1942. I am also board qualified in otolaryngology, have practiced only otology since 1947, and was certified by ASHA in audiology in 1948.

It gives me much pleasure to prepare a foreword for this book. Dr. Gerber is especially competent to edit such a needed volume. It will surely eliminate the large gap that now exists in this extremely important specialty. Dr. Gerber should be commended for taking on the dual task of selecting these highly qualified authors to summarize the present knowledge and of coordinating the material into a well-organized volume. The list of specialists is quite impressive, and I can think of no one better to present their contributions.

I am indeed delighted to read this volume.

Aram Glorig, M.D.

Preface

IN 1965, when I moved to Santa Barbara, a local otolaryngologist introduced me to a group of people who conducted a monthly infant hearing screening program in the community. This was my introduction to pediatric audiology. Until that time, I had no more experience with children than producing a few of my own. Since then, I have done little else professionally than pediatric audiology. My entire career (now thirty years long) has been devoted to the youngest among us. The newborn nursery and well-baby clinic have been my main laboratories. The babies have been my teachers, and good teachers they are indeed. I continue to be amazed at the things they do and to be instructed by their behavioral capacities. Human infants are truly precocious.

However, not all of us are able to be quite so precocious so early in life. Endogenous and exogenous factors sometimes get in the way; social and economic events occasionally intrude. Nevertheless, as humans and as professionals, we assume an obligation to remove these and other barriers to full development.

Every child has a right to be the best, and it behooves us to help. Over the years, I have learned many ways to help, and science continues to find more.

As professionals, we are driven by two forces in pediatric audiology—genuine caring for the children and technology. Back in 1965, we knew nothing about the auditory brainstem response and rather little about the other auditory evoked potentials. Only recently have we learned about the otoacoustic emissions. Cochlear implants did not exist in 1965. However, we were able to identify hearing loss in infants. How did we do it? We made noises at babies and endeavored to learn what noises served as stimuli and how babies demonstrated that fact.

Moreover, we learned that it is all right to put hearing aids on babies, if we do it wisely. The youngest child who was fitted with aids in our clinic was seven weeks old at the time. I mention this not because it is remarkable but because it is not; I have known still younger children with hearing aids. I have tried to teach all my students that no infant is too young to be diagnosed and that it is never too soon to start treatment. The time to begin treatment is immediately.

My dear friend and colleague, Jeff Danhauer, gets the credit for conceptualizing this handbook. He observed that our respected colleague, Jack Katz, has made a brilliant contribution to the profession with his *Handbook of Clinical Audiology* but that there is no handbook of *pediatric* audiology. Because I am an old-timer in the baby hearing business, Jeff thought I was the one to do it. So I contacted my favorite editor, Ivey Pittle Wallace at Gallaudet University Press, and solicited her opinion. Ivey and her colleagues liked the idea, and here we are.

There is an African proverb that says it takes a whole village to raise a child. All our thanks should go to the "villagers" who have contributed to this volume. They are people who I believe are experts. Among them are dear old friends: Aram Glorig, a genuine patriarch in pediatric audiology; George Mencher; Maurice Mendel; Harris Nober; and Bob Ruben. They are here because they truly are authorities in pediatric audiology. I also sought out newer friends because of their expertise. I even had the pleasure of inviting a former student, Judy Brimacombe, to join the group because of her knowledge and experience. This is a teacher's reward. Still, I am the editor and hope that I have not harmed anyone's prose.

This volume is intended to be a handbook—not a textbook—and is written for the professional and the advanced student. It offers advice to practitioners in the hope that babies will benefit from what we have done here.

The organization of the book allows readers to work through or across the content. Every chapter (where appropriate) is organized according to the age of the child. Thus, one might look up information about infants (for example, five to twelve months of age) in each chapter. Or one might choose to read an entire chapter on immittance or cochlear implants, for example.

As professionals, we must remind ourselves that most people who have a hearing loss are not deaf and that most people who are deaf were not born that way. Their audiological, habilitative, rehabilitative, and educational needs differ. It is our responsibility to recognize and address these differences.

The first three chapters of this book define the condition of hearing loss for us in terms of pathology. In an attempt to explain the origins of hearing loss, we begin with a chapter about epidemiology. What are the causes? How widespread are they? How many people are affected? At what ages? Y.P. Kapur, the current president of Hearing International, answers these questions for us with considerable expertise.

Frank Katz is one of those pediatricians who recognizes that children, even very little ones, may have communicative problems and understands that some of them have hearing losses. He also acknowledges that the hearing loss is only one part of the child. Concomitant problems may exist, but may not be related to the hearing loss. In the second chapter, Dr. Katz addresses the concerns of the practicing pediatrician when communicative development or function is questioned. Fortunately for these babies, Dr. Katz is not of the "let's wait and see what happens" school of pediatrics.

Otorhinolaryngology is an integral part of audiological care. Robert Ruben is arguably the most erudite scientist among the world's otolaryngologists. I know no otolaryngologist who cares more about children's communication capabilities or is more skillful in dealing with them. Bob Ruben is at once clinician, teacher, scholar, and writer of premier ability, as chapter 3 attests.

Chapters 4 through 9 address matters of diagnosis. The ultimate issue that concerns us is infants' communicative behavior. Allan Diefendorf, chair of the national Joint Committee on Infant Hearing, and Judy Gravel are the authorities on what it is that babies should naturally do—and on what it means when they don't (chapter 4).

As humans, our ability to hear speech is vital to the development of normal communicative behavior. Jane Madell tells us in chapter 5 how to assess this ability in children. Dr. Madell has published extensively (and wisely) on this topic.

Beginning with chapter 6, we see how technology is being used to assess middle ear and other pathologies. Otitis media is the most common disease of childhood. This and other pathologies of the acoustic conduction system are far more common in children than are sensory hearing impairments.* We have a variety of procedures to assess middle ear function; cumulatively they are called immittance (chapter 6). Shlomo Silman and his colleague Carol Silverman are among the acknowledged specialists in these methods. Their recent joint book on diagnosis and Silman's older book on the acoustic reflex are evidence of their experience.

Pathology is not limited to the middle ear; it may be cochlear, retrocochlear, or a combination of these. At about the time of my birth, Davis and Derbyshire demonstrated that the electrical activity of the living brain is modified by acoustic events and that these modifications are measurable. The evaluation of these events is called electric response audiometry (ERA). The electric responses that emanate from the brainstem are now known as the auditory brainstem response (ABR). Today, the ABR is the most powerful tool in the armamentarium of the pediatric audiologist. Chapter 7 covers the use of ABR to evaluate the electric responses of the auditory system from the cochlea through the cortex. Herb Gould and Maurice Mendel are among the leading students of this phenomenon and its applications among the very young.

Less than two decades ago, David Kemp explicated the fact that the cochlea makes sound. The cochlea's otoacoustic emissions have become the topic of extensive research and clinical application (chapter 8). One of my new friends, Brenda Lonsbury-Martin, is a leader among those engaged in the understanding and application of this phenomenon, and that is why I asked her to contribute.

---

*The reader should be aware that the terms OME (otitis media with effusion) and MEE (middle ear effusion) are used interchangeably throughout this volume.

Ultimately, the ear is not the organ of hearing. The ear is a sophisticated transducer to pass acoustical information to the brain, where we may make sense of it. We call this central auditory processing, and we now know that many people (including many children) have central auditory processing difficulties. I am reminded of Isabel Rapin's description of children who should be educated as though they are deaf. Gail Chermak's work has been devoted to understanding this process and its occasional disruption. In chapter 9, she explains how to assess it.

When all the assessment has been done, we must constructively use the knowledge gained. More accurately, we must assist the children whose hearing we have measured. Chapters 10 and 11 focus on the use of technology for treatment. We can indeed put hearing aids on children at any age. Doing this well, correctly, and early requires great care, skill, and experience. Dale Robinson and Francis Eldis have the skill and experience, and they share them with us in chapter 10.

As I have mentioned, cochlear implants didn't exist when I started in the baby business. The first implants were the single-channel House implants—so named because they were developed at the House Ear Institute in Los Angeles. These were implanted in adults with various degrees of success. Then came the multiple-channel implants, which raised the question of using them in children—a highly controversial issue. The Deaf community (those people who use American Sign Language as their primary means of communication) argues that providing cochlear implants to the very young denies these children their identity, and they have a point. Many questions remain, however: How do we determine which children are good candidates for cochlear implants? What is the best age? Do the implants work? How do we know? To address these difficult questions (chapter 11), I turned to two people who deal with them every day, Judy Brimacombe and Anne Beiter.

Whether parents choose sign language, oral communication, hearing aids, cochlear implants, or any combination of these, deaf and hard of hearing children must still go to school. Harris Nober has walked the line between clinical audiology and the education of deaf children for a long time. He walks it again for us in chapter 12 to explain how audiologists can best advise the teachers of deaf and hard of hearing children. He also offers suggestions for how audiologists can assist these teachers in helping the children.

In addition to our knowledge, efforts, scholarship, and clinical skill, deaf and hard of hearing children and their families need our counsel. Counsel, in this sense, means more than the giving of information, important as that is. No hearing parents expect to have a deaf child. George Mencher confronts this matter in chapter 13 and provides insights regarding what we can tell parents when the unexpected happens.

Finally, all the knowledge contained in this volume is quite meaningless unless we can deliver the services to the children. Our British colleagues, Adrian

Davis and Jane Sancho, have pointed out that it is useless to have screening (diagnostic) and habilitation programs without the means of putting children in touch with them. Chapter 14, by Evelyn Cherow, deals with how to do just this. Ms. Cherow, who has been with ASHA since 1981, is responsible for national policy development affecting the delivery of audiology services.

The purpose of this book is to provide the collected expertise to clinicians for their practical use. In this sense, we are consultants to the practitioners. Acknowledging that our readers already know how to do the procedures described, we intend to advise on when, under what circumstances, and for whom they should be applied. If we succeed, all of us will have become better practitioners.

I would like to acknowledge my gratitude to a trio of undergraduates who labored with me on this book. Kerry McGinnis arranged, edited, rearranged, and listed all the tables and figures. Lisa Gutierrez and Alicia Mariscal assembled the extensive bibliography. Without them, this book would be nowhere finished by this writing.

Sanford E. Gerber   Spokane, 1995

REFERENCES

Davis, A., and J. Sancho. 1988. Screening for hearing impairment in children: A review of current practice in the United Kingdom. In *International perspectives on communication disorders*, ed. S.E. Gerber and G.T. Mencher. Washington, D.C.: Gallaudet University Press.

Katz, J., ed. 1994. *Handbook of clinical audiology.* 4th ed. Baltimore: Williams and Wilkins.

Kemp, D. 1978. Stimulated acoustic emissions from within the human auditory system. *Journal of the Acoustical Society of America* 64:1386–1391.

Rapin, I. 1983. The child neurologist's contribution to the care of children with hearing loss. In *The multiply handicapped hearing impaired child*, ed. G.T. Mencher and S.E. Gerber. New York: Grune and Stratton.

Contributors

Judith A. Brimacombe, M.A.
Vice President of Clinical and Regulatory
  Affairs
Cochlear Corporation

Anne L. Beiter, M.S.
Clinical Services Manager
Cochlear Corporation

Gail D. Chermak, Ph.D.
Professor and Chair
Department of Speech and Hearing Sciences
Washington State University

Evelyn Cherow, M.A.
Director, Audiology Division
Professional Practices Department
American Speech-Language-Hearing
  Association

Allan O. Diefendorf, Ph.D.
Associate Professor and Director
Audiology and Speech-Language Pathology
Department of Otolaryngology–Head and
  Neck Surgery
James Whitcomb Riley Hospital for Children
Indiana University

Frances Eldis, Ph.D.
Communications Disorders
Children's Hospital of Michigan

Sanford E. Gerber, Ph.D.
Emeritus Professor of Audiology
Department of Speech and Hearing Sciences
University of California, Santa Barbara
and
Chair and Visiting Professor
Department of Communication Disorders
Eastern Washington University

Aram Glorig, M.D.
House Ear Clinic, Inc.

Herbert J. Gould, Ph.D.
Associate Professor
School of Audiology and Speech Pathology
University of Memphis
Memphis Speech and Hearing Center

Judith S. Gravel, Ph.D.
Director of Audiology
Associate Professor of Otolaryngology
Albert Einstein College of Medicine

Yash Pal Kapur, M.D.
Professor Emeritus
Department of Surgery
Michigan State University

Franklin R. Katz, M.D.
Children's Medical Group
Thousand Oaks, CA

Brenda L. Lonsbury-Martin, Ph.D.
Professor and Director of Research
University of Miami Ear Institute
University of Miami School of Medicine

Jane R. Madell, Ph.D.
Director of Communicative Disorders
Long Island College Hospital
and
Professor of Clinical Otolaryngology
State University of New York Medical Center

Glen K. Martin, Ph.D.
Co-director of Research
University of Miami Ear Institute
and
Professor, Departments of Otolaryngology,
Cell Biology, and Anatomy
University of Miami School of Medicine

Margaret J. McCoy, M.A., CCC-A
Chief Research Audiologist
University of Miami Ear Institute
University of Miami School of Medicine

George T. Mencher, Ph.D.
Director, Nova Scotia Hearing and Speech
   Clinic
and
Professor of Audiology
School of Human Communication Disorders
Dalhousie University

Maurice I. Mendel, Ph.D.
Professor and Dean
School of Audiology and Speech Pathology
University of Memphis
Memphis Speech and Hearing Center

E. Harris Nober, Ph.D.
Professor of Audiology
Department of Communicative Disorders
University of Massachusetts

Dale Robinson, Ph.D.
Associate Professor of Audiology
Department of Audiology
School of Medicine
Wayne State University

Robert J. Ruben, M.D.
Professor and Chair
Department of Otolaryngology
and
Professor of Pediatrics
Albert Einstein College of Medicine,
Yeshiva University, and
Montefiore Medical Center

Shlomo Silman, Ph.D.
Professor of Audiology
Brooklyn College, CUNY
and
Professor of Speech and Hearing Sciences
   Doctoral Program
Graduate School and University Center,
   CUNY

Carol A. Silverman, Ph.D.
Professor of Communication Sciences
Hunter College, CUNY
and
Professor, Speech and Hearing Sciences Doc-
   toral Program
Graduate School and University Center,
   CUNY

Martin L. Whitehead, Ph.D.
Assistant Professor
University of Miami Ear Institute
Department of Otolaryngology
University of Miami School of Medicine

The Handbook of
Pediatric Audiology

1

Epidemiology of Childhood Hearing Loss

Yash Pal Kapur

EPIDEMIOLOGY is the study of the distribution and determinants of human disease in populations. The primary objective of epidemiology is to use this information to prevent human disease. A review of the literature shows severe lack of epidemiologically representative data on hearing impairment and deafness in various settings. We remain largely ignorant of the epidemiological patterns of childhood hearing loss. Available epidemiological studies, with few exceptions, show inconsistencies of method and classification of hearing loss. Deficiencies include (a) definition of the disease; (b) agreement on terminology; (c) validity of the diagnosis; and (d) comparability of the data.

This lack of information became clear when the World Health Organization (WHO) in Geneva was being persuaded to become involved in the problem of hearing impairment and deafness. In 1985, a resolution (WHA39-19) was prepared by the General Assembly of the WHO, requesting the Director-General of the WHO to investigate and submit a report. This report was to assess the extent, causes, and consequences of deafness and hearing impairment worldwide and to make proposals for strengthening services for their prevention and treatment. The Director-General—in his report to the 39th WHO General Assembly, Seventy Ninth Session EB 79/10 (WHO 1986)—outlined two major deficiencies that accounted for the lack of action in this area. These were (1) a lack of public awareness of the problems of deafness and hearing impairment and (2) a lack of appropriate and reliable information regarding most of their epidemiological aspects.

A Division for the Prevention of Deafness and Hearing Impairment was established at the WHO headquarters in Geneva in June of 1991. One of its first activities was to stress the need for epidemiological data on the magnitude and causes of hearing loss. The Division emphasized the need for conducting such studies using comparable methods and standard examination forms (WHO

3

PDH 91.1 June 1991). Protocols conforming to these criteria have been developed by the World Health Organization and are now available. As a result, epidemiological studies are currently underway in many different countries.

CONGENITAL HEARING LOSS

THE definition of congenital hearing loss is not well delineated. Usually, hearing loss in the first two years of life is accepted as congenital hearing loss. The problem of identification and evaluation of hearing loss at this age, due to the difficulty in ascribing the etiology of hearing loss in individual cases, has resulted in a lack of exact prevalence data of congenital hearing loss. It is estimated that an average of 40% of cases with childhood sensorineural hearing loss are undiagnosed with respect to etiology; most of those with unknown etiology are congenital (Parving 1992). Many studies have shown that children with congenital or early acquired hearing loss are identified only after a delay (Kankkunen 1982; Newton 1985; Parving 1991). Parving (1984) has pointed out that, in the industrialized world, only between 50 and 63% of children with hearing loss were identified by the age of three. Early detection of congenital or early acquired hearing loss remains a serious and unsolved problem, and auditory screening methods have largely failed to perceive them. In the developing countries, the average age of assessment of congenital or early acquired hearing loss can be between six and eight years of age.

A review (Davidson, Hyde, and Alberti 1989) of studies on prevalence estimates of sensorineural hearing loss in children is given in Table 1.1. The table shows the author, the country in which the study took place, age of children, methods of testing, hearing levels, and prevalence per 1000.

Schein and Delk's (1974) estimate included the incidence of prelingual deafness (before the age of three years) to be one per 1000 live births. Below nine years, the rate was 2.3 per 1000 live births. Several other studies evaluating children ranging from birth through six years of age give prevalence rates between 0.9 per 1000 and 1.7 per 1000 (Feinmesser, Tell, and Levi 1982; Kankkunen 1982; Martin 1982; Thringer et al. 1984). Studies from West Africa indicate that 2.2 per 1000 children under ten years of age displayed profound hearing loss (McPherson and Holborow 1985). In India, studies in urban areas showed the rate to be two per 1000 under five years of age and 4.2 per 1000 in children under fifteen years (Pal et al. 1974). A study on the prevalence and etiology of hearing impairment was conducted by the Indian Council of Medical Research in New Delhi in 1983. It encompassed four centers in different parts of India and was conducted in both rural and urban populations. It demonstrated that 0.8% of hearing impairment was due to congenital sensorineural hearing impairment.

From 10 to 26% of hearing loss in children is congenital (i.e., at birth or early childhood). Congenital hearing loss can be due to acquired (nongenetic) or

Table 1.1. Prevalence of Hearing Loss in Childhood

First author	Date	Country	Age of subjects	Method of testing	Hearing level	Prevalence per 1000
Schein	1974	USA	≤ 3 years	questionnaire	'deaf'	1.0
			≤ 19 years		'deaf'	2.3
Pal	1974	India	≤ 5 years	distraction or	60 dB	2.0
			≤ 15 years	pure tone	60 dB	4.2
Feinmesser	1982	Israel	5 years	modified Ewing Stycar test	55 dB	1.7
				or play	70 dB	1.3
Kankkunen	1982	Finland	6 years	VRA = visual reinforcement, respiration, or play	50 dB	1.3
Martin	1982	UK	8 years	questionnaire and review of medical records	50 dB	1.0
		Belgium				0.74
		Denmark				1.48
		France				0.56
		Ireland				0.92
		Italy				0.92
		Netherlands				0.91
						0.93
Upfold	1982	Australia	7–17 years	pure tone	60 dB	1.1
					90 dB	0.48
Parving	1983	Denmark	2–12 years	pure tone, ERA or ECoG	35 dB	1.4
					55 dB	0.92
					75 dB	0.60
Thringer	1984	Sweden	≤ 5 years	play	40 dB	1.4
					60 dB	0.9
McPherson	1985	West Africa	≤10 years	distraction, play or pure tone	70 dB	2.7
					95 dB	2.2

Source: from Davidson, Hyde, and Alberti 1989.

to genetic causes; it can be attributed to prenatal, perinatal, or postnatal causes. The major causes are tabulated in Table 1.2.

Infectious Causes

Maternal *rubella* has decreased dramatically in the western world, thanks to widespread immunization. This infection continues to be a problem in the developing countries, however. Hearing loss is the single most common abnormality resulting from congenital rubella. When sensorineural hearing loss is the sole manifestation, a link to rubella is difficult to confirm and depends upon maternal history and laboratory tests (Ruben and Rapin 1988). Rubella infection can be subclinical, and defects may not develop until later in life.

Cytomegalovirus (CMV) is a member of the herpes group of viruses. It may affect a child by intrauterine infection, at birth, or postnatally via infected breast

Table 1.2. Major Causes of Congenital Hearing Loss

Nongenetic Congenital
1. Prenatal
   Infections of mother*
   Viral
   Protozoal
   Spirochital
   Ototoxic Toxicity
   Metabolic Disorders
2. Perinatal
   Traumatic Delivery
   Anoxia
   Hyperbilirubinemia
   Prematurity
   Infection
3. Postnatal Causes of Early Childhood Hearing Loss
   Infection
   Ototoxic medications
   Trauma
   Others

Genetic Congenital
1. Hearing Loss Alone
2. Hearing Loss as part of a syndrome
3. Delayed Hearing Loss
   Hearing Loss Alone (e.g., otosclerosis)
   Hearing Loss as part of a syndrome (e.g., Usher or Alport)

---

* Incidence of the following TORCH infections in the mother can lead to congenital hearing loss:
1. Viral infection
   Rubella
   Cytomegalovirus
2. Protozoal infection
   Toxoplasmosis
3. Spirochital Infection
   Syphilis

milk or saliva. Natal and postnatal infections are usually asymptomatic. Intrauterine infection is asymptomatic at birth in 95% of cases; nevertheless, 10 to 20% of these develop progressive hearing impairment (Alford, Stagno, and Pass 1980). It is estimated that congenital CMV infection occurs in 0.5 to 2.7% of births in the United States, so it may be responsible for 0.5 to five cases of hearing defect per 1000 births (Catlin 1985). It appears from at least one study (Johnson et al. 1986) that postnatal CMV after the age of three weeks does not result in hearing impairment. The extent of the problem in the developing world is probably higher than in industrialized countries, but, because the disease is usually asymptomatic in adults, assessment of the prevalence rate is difficult.

Toxoplasmosis Gondi is a protozoan parasite common in animals. The infection is prevalent worldwide. In the United States, it occurs in one per 1000 to 3000 births. About 90% of the cases are asymptomatic at birth. Sensorineural hearing loss occurs in 15% of the cases. The onset of the loss is delayed and is progressive (Wilson et al. 1980).

Congenital syphilis occurs in one in 10,000 live births in the United States. A resurgence of the disease may be occurring (Hoekelman et al. 1992). According to the Centers for Disease Control of the U.S. Public Health Service, the number of reported congenital syphilis cases jumped from 160 in 1981 to 2,867 in 1990 (Shimizu 1992). The sensorineural hearing loss that results from congenital syphilis has delayed expression, occurs in 30 to 40% of cases, and occurs at eight to nine years of age. It is usually bilateral and profound (Sando, Suehiro, and Wood 1983). Auditory impairment may not be present at birth.

Ototoxicity

Ototoxicity has long been recognized as an undesirable side effect of medical treatment; as new and more potent therapeutic agents are developed, the list of ototoxic drugs continues to grow. In the United States, the national Joint Committee on Infant Hearing has added ototoxicity to its list of high-risk conditions (1994). Ototoxic drugs—particularly the new generation of aminoglycosides, potent diuretics, and cis-platinum (an anticancer drug)—are responsible for many cases of congenital hearing loss. In previous years, the effects of ototoxic agents on the ear were known only after the hearing loss had occurred. Now studies have shown that knowledge of the early signs and symptoms can lead to modification of the disease or withdrawal of the drug. Audiometric monitoring in susceptible patients contributes to the prevention of hearing loss. The damage is mainly dose related. High fever, kidney disease, advanced age, and concomitant use of other aminoglycosides and loop diuretics are additional risk factors. Hearing loss may be delayed and detected weeks or even months after cessation of therapy. In most prospective studies, the incidence of aminoglycoside ototoxicity is about 10%. It is still higher when cis-platinum is used (Rybak and Matz 1988). Although the use of ototoxic drugs is not a serious problem in developed countries, information on the occurrence of ototoxic hearing loss in developing countries is alarming. A 1992 report from the Beijing Institute of Otorhinolaryngology in China reveals that deafness caused by ototoxic drugs rose from 0.1% in 1954 to 0.78% in 1960, 28.4% in 1979, to 30, 50, or even 70% in some regions of China in more recent years. Isolated reports from India also indicate a shocking increase in hearing loss from indiscriminate use of ototoxic drugs during the prenatal, perinatal, and postnatal phases. Better physician education and public information are needed.

Metabolic Causes

Hypothyroid hearing loss is seen in cretinism and is usually a mixed sensorineural loss that occurs in 50 to 60% of affected persons. The loss may be stable or progressive. Endemic cretinism is due to severe iodine deficiency over several generations and is accompanied by goiter and mental retardation. Changes have been identified in the middle and inner ears (Meyerhoff and Liston 1991). Pendred syndrome, of course, is an example of a genetic deafness accompanied by goiter.

Perinatal Conditions

Erythroblastosis Fetalis

Erythroblastosis fetalis is a haemolytic disease caused by Rh-incompatibility between mother and fetus. Jaundice due to hyperbilirubinemia is the clinical symptom. Bilirubin is toxic to cochlear nuclei and the central auditory pathways (deVries, Lary, and Dubowitz 1985). The prophylactic use of Rh-immunoglobulin has almost eliminated the problem in the western world. Phototherapy and exchange transfusions have decreased the number of hearing-impaired children worldwide.

Prematurity

Sensorineural hearing loss occurs in approximately 10% of infants with a low birth weight, which is defined as birth weight less than 1.50 kilograms (3.3 pounds) (Ruben and Rozycki 1970). The chance of being deaf is twenty times greater for a premature child than for a child with normal weight.

Other Conditions

Several other conditions can cause sensorineural hearing loss during the perinatal phase. These include birth trauma and anoxia. A variety of sequelae have been associated with anoxia (hypoxia and asphyxia, for example), including those affecting language, cognitive development, neuromotor ability, and vision (Gerber 1990).

Postnatal Infection and Early Childhood Hearing Loss

Meningitis

Bacterial meningitis is a leading cause of acquired sensorineural hearing loss. In the western world, it accounts for between 3 and 10% of severe to profound sensorineural hearing loss (Newton 1985; Parving 1991). Among the cases of deafness attributed to acquired postnatal causes, the incidence of bacterial meningitis is even higher. The incidence of hearing impairment as a sequela of bacterial meningitis ranges from 5 to 30% of survivors (Nadol 1980; Newton 1985).

In West Africa—in a "meningitis belt" that extends into the northern part (Nigeria)—meningococcal, pneumonococcal, and viral meningitis were considered responsible for 18% of the cases of postnatal acquired deafness (McPherson and Holborow 1985). The incidence of meningococcal meningitis has increased worldwide over the last ten years and continues to be responsible for many cases of deafness.

Most meningitic hearing losses are bilateral and produce a severe irreversible loss. Many patients suffer a temporary or partial hearing loss that may not be detected unless they undergo a hearing evaluation. The three major bacteria responsible for meningitis in children are *Haemophilus influenzae*, *Neisseria meningitidis*, and *Diplococcus pneumoniae*. Viral infections such as meningitis and measles are also present worldwide.

Measles

Measles is a major cause of morbidity and mortality in young children in the developing world. Immunization against measles is an integral part of the Expanded Program of Immunization (EPI). Morbidity and mortality can be even higher in children suffering from malnutrition (Henderson 1981).

Otitis media is a common complication of measles infection. Otitis media was once considered to be a result of secondary bacterial infection, but Bordley and Kapur (1977) showed that otitis media is due to a primary viral invasion of the middle ear. Sensorineural hearing loss can occur due to damage to the cochlear and vestibular system (Lindsay and Hemenway 1954).

The hearing loss in measles is usually symmetrical and bilateral, and higher frequencies are affected more than lower ones. Since the introduction of the measles vaccine in the United States, the incidence of hearing loss associated with the virus has been reduced dramatically.

Mumps

Hearing loss associated with the mumps virus infection has been reported in 5 to 25% of all infections. Half of these were transient losses. Persistent defects occur in 5% of cases (Baloh 1982). Hearing loss usually occurs at the end of parotitis but can occur without any evidence of a parotidal swelling (Everberg 1957). In 80% of cases, hearing loss is unilateral. Temporal bone studies by Smith and Gussen (1976) showed severe atrophy of the cochlea and stria vascularis.

Others

There are many other causes of sensorineural hearing loss in children. The most common are those related to the use of ototoxic drugs, head injury, and noise trauma.

Ototoxic medications (described under prenatal causes) continue to be a problem for all human beings, including young children. These medications include the aminoglycoside group of antibiotics. Many of these medications are life-saving and have to be administered, but use of several audiometric and, where possible, vestibular studies to monitor the effect of these drugs will be useful in evaluation of therapy. Monitoring of blood levels of the aminoglycoside and of renal function can reduce the ototoxicity. Shimizu (1992) pointed out that there has been an upsurge in the numbers of young children with sensori-neural hearing loss due to ototoxic chemotherapy for malignancies such as leukemia and neuroblastoma.

Genetic Congenital Hearing Loss

In several etiological studies of congenital deafness, it was estimated that 52% of cases were genetically caused (Fraser 1976). Estimates of the incidence of genetic hearing loss in Great Britain, Germany, and the United States are in the range of one in twenty to one in 6000 live births (Steele 1981). Such a wide range of esti-mated frequency depicts the difficulty in making an accurate diagnosis of the condition at birth or in early infancy. Also, the differences among various statis-tical surveys stem from the variation in populations studied and methods used. Reviewing these estimates, Gerber (1990) determined that they range around 43% of the total prevalence of congenital deafness.

Genetic hearing loss may be expressed at birth or be delayed to childhood or even adulthood. It may occur alone or be part of a syndrome manifesting hear-ing loss. Konigsmark (1969) identified more than seventy different types of hearing loss, many of them part of a syndrome. Grundfast and Lalwani (1992) list at least 200 different syndromes known to include hearing loss.

The patterns of inheritance in isolated hearing loss are: (1) autosomal re-cessive genes (70 to 80%); (2) autosomal dominant genes (20 to 30%); and (3) X-linked genes (1 to 3%).

In recessive inherited hearing loss, other family members are unlikely to be affected, especially in a small sibship family. The presence of consanguinity sup-ports this type of inheritance. A study of the causes of hearing loss in South India showed that 24% of the 1,250 cases studied were suspected to have recessive hereditary hearing loss (Indian Council of Medical Research 1983). Among par-ents of children with hereditary deafness in a school for the deaf, the consan-guinity rate was 56%. This was attributed to consanguineous marriages in South India and was higher than the general rate of 33% found in the state of Madras, South India (Kapur 1983). Consanguineous marriages are widely prac-ticed in Muslim countries worldwide and in Africa.

Delayed Expression of Nonsyndromic Genetic Hearing Loss

Autosomal Dominant

Otosclerosis. With 40% expression, otosclerosis is a common progressive dis-ease of the otic capsule. Histologically, there is spongiosis followed by sclerosis of the temporal bone. It can be manifested as low frequency conductive loss, mixed hearing loss, or sensorineural hearing loss. Fixation of the stapes results in a conductive loss; advanced otosclerosis results in mixed loss or sensorineural hearing loss. The cause for the sensorineural hearing loss is not clear. Asymptomatic patients with histological evidence of otosclerosis represent nonpenetrant cases.

Delayed Expression of Syndromic Hearing Loss

The two most common syndromes in which hearing loss becomes manifest in later life are *Usher syndrome* and *Alport syndrome.*

Usher syndrome is generally an autosomal recessive disorder. In some families, it is noticed to be X-linked dominant. Usher syndrome is characterized by retinitis pigmentosa and moderate to severe sensorineural hearing loss. It is estimated to cause 6 to 10% of congenital sensorineural hearing loss. Hearing loss precedes the visual symptoms (Fraser 1976).

Alport syndrome generally occurs via an autosomal dominant transmission. The syndrome is characterized by sensorineural hearing loss accompanied by progressive renal disease and eye abnormalities. Hearing loss is bilateral and occurs in 40 to 60% of cases. Males are affected more often than females. The hearing loss begins by ten years of age and is progressive (Preus and Fraser 1971). If untreated, affected males frequently die by the third decade of life (Ruben 1983).

SUMMARY

BECAUSE sensorineural hearing loss is often inherited, the relative importance of this condition is bound to increase, especially as defects due to other diseases decrease with advancement of medical care. With new developments in genetics and gene mapping, identification of genetic hearing loss is becoming more critical. Genes that cause several types of hereditary sensorineural hearing loss have already been identified (Grundfast and Lalwani 1992); these include, inter alia, Usher syndrome and Waardenburg syndrome.

Early identification of genetic hearing impairment will improve management of the child's hearing loss and—particularly in syndromic hearing loss—make genetic counseling available to the family of the affected child and other family members who are at risk of producing offspring with hearing loss. Prevention remains the primary means of reducing the high incidence of genetic hearing loss. This can be done only through counseling of high risk individuals.

REFERENCES

Alford, C.A., S. Stagno, and R.F. Pass. 1980. Natural history of perinatal cytomegaloviral infection. In *Perinatal infections*, ed. K. Elliot, M. O'Connor, and J. Whelan. Amsterdam: Excerpta Medica.

Baloh, R.W. 1982. Hearing loss. In *Cecil textbook of medicine* 16th ed., Ed. by J.B. Wyngarden and L.H. Smith. Philadelphia: W.B. Saunders Co.

Beijing Institute of Otorhinolaryngology 1992. *Statistics of ototoxic drugs in China.* A report submitted to the World Health Organization. Beijing: Beijing Institute of Otorhinolaryngology.

Bordley, J., and Y.P. Kapur. 1977. Histopathologic changes in the temporal bone resulting from measles infection. *Archives of Otolaryngology* 103:162–168.

Catlin, F.I. 1985. Prevention of hearing impairment from infection and ototoxic drugs. *Archives of Otolaryngology* 111:377–384.

Davidson, J., M.L. Hyde, and P.W. Alberti. 1989. Epidemiologic patterns in childhood hearing loss: A review. *International Journal of Pediatric Otorhinolaryngology* 17:239–266.

deVries, L.S., S. Lary, and L.M.S. Dubowitz. 1985. Relationship of serum bilirubin levels to ototoxicity and deafness in high risk low birth weight infants. *Pediatrics* 76:351–354.

Everberg, G. 1957. Deafness in mumps. *Acta Oto-Laryngologica* 48:397–403.

Feinmesser, M., L. Tell, and H. Levi. 1982. Follow-up of 40,000 infants screened for hearing defect. *Audiology* 21:197–203.

Fraser, G.R. 1976. *The causes of profound deafness in childhood.* Baltimore: Johns Hopkins University Press.

Gerber, S.E. 1990. Review of a high risk register for congenital or early-onset deafness. *British Journal of Audiology* 24:347–356.

Grundfast, K.M., and A.K. Lalwani. 1992. Practical approach to diagnosis and management of hereditary hearing impairment (HHI). *ENT Journal* 71:479–493.

Henderson, R.H. 1981. Vaccine-preventable diseases: The role of the immunization services. In *Disability prevention: The global challenge*, ed. Sir John Wilson. Oxford: Oxford University Press.

Hoekelman, R., S.B. Friedman, N.M. Nelson, and H.M. Seidel. 1992. *Primary pediatric care.* 2d ed. St. Louis: Mosby Year Book.

Indian Council of Medical Research. 1983. *Collaborative study on prevalence and etiology of hearing impairment.* New Delhi: Indian Council of Medical Research.

Johnson, S.J., H. Hosford-Dunn, S. Paryani, A. Yeager, and N. Malachowski. 1986. Prevalence of sensorineural hearing loss in premature and sick term infants with perinatally acquired cytomegalovirus infection. *Ear and Hearing* 7:325–327.

Kankkunen, A. 1982. Preschool children with impaired hearing in Göteborg. 1964–1980. *Acta Oto-Laryngologica* (Suppl. 391) 14:1–124.

Kapur, Y.P. 1983. The principal causes of acute conditions: Deafness. In *Disability prevention: The global challenge*, ed. Sir John Wilson. Oxford: Oxford University Press.

Konigsmark, B.W. 1969. Hereditary deafness in man. *New England Journal of Medicine* 281:713–720, 774–778, 827–832.

Lindsay, J.R., and W.G. Hemenway. 1954. Inner ear pathology due to measles. *Annals of Otology, Rhinology, and Laryngology* 263:754–771.

Martin, J.A.M. 1982. Aetiological factors relating to childhood deafness in the European community. *Audiology* 21:149–158.

McPherson, B., and C.A. Holborow. 1985. A study of deafness in West Africa: The Gambian hearing health project. *International Journal of Pediatric Otorhinolaryngology* 10:115–135.

Meyerhoff, W.L., and S.L. Liston. 1991. Metabolic hearing loss. In *Otolaryngology*, 3d ed., ed. M.M. Paparella et al. Philadelphia: W.B. Saunders Co.

Nadol, J.B. 1980. Hearing loss as a sequela of meningitis. *Laryngoscope* 88:739–755.

Newton, V.E. 1985. Etiology of sensorineural hearing loss in young children. *Journal of Otology and Laryngology* (Suppl. 10):1–57.

Pal, J., H.L. Bhatia, B.G. Prasad, D. Dyal, and P.C. Jain. 1974. Deafness among the urban community: An epidemiological study at Lucknow UP, India. *Indian Journal of Medical Research* 62:857–868.

Parving, A. 1983. Epidemiology of hearing loss and aetiological diagnosis of hearing impairment in childhood. *International Journal of Pediatric Otorhinolaryngology* 5:151–165.

———. 1984. Early detection and identification of congenital/early acquired disability. Who takes the initiative? *International Journal of Pediatric Otorhinolaryngology* 7:107–117.

———. 1991. Detection of infants with congenitally acquired hearing disability. *Acta Oto-Laryngologica* (Suppl. 482):111–116.

———. 1992. Pediatric audiologic medicine: A strategy for a regular department. *Journal of Audiological Medicine* 1:99–111.

Preus, M., and G.C. Fraser. 1971. Genetics of hereditary nephropathy with deafness: Alport's syndrome. *Clinical Genetics* 2:331–333.

Ruben, R.J. 1983. Diseases of the inner ear and sensorineural deafness. In *Pediatric otolaryngology*, Vol. 1, ed. by C.D. Bluestone and S.E. Stool. Philadelphia: W.B. Saunders Co.

Ruben, R.J., and I. Rapin. 1988. Management of the hearing-impaired deaf infant and child. In *Otologic medicine and surgery*, ed. by P.W. Alberti and R.J. Ruben. New York: Churchill Livingstone, Inc.

Ruben, R.J., and D.L. Rozycki. 1970. Clinical aspects of genetic deafness. *Annals of Otology, Rhinology, and Laryngology* 80:255–263.

Rybak, L.P., and G.J. Matz. 1988. Ototoxicity. In *Otologic medicine and surgery*, ed. P.W. Alberti and R.J. Ruben. New York: Churchill Livingstone, Inc.

Sando, I., S. Suehiro, and R.P. Wood. 1983. Congenital anomalies of the external and middle ear. In *Pediatric otolaryngology*, ed. C.D. Bluestone and S.E. Stool. Philadelphia: W.B. Saunders Co.

Schein, J.D., and M.T. Delk. 1974. *The deaf population of the United States*. Washington, D.C.: National Association of the Deaf.

Shimizu, H. 1992. Carhart Memorial Lecture: 1991. Childhood hearing impairment: Issues and thoughts on diagnostic approaches. *American Auditory Society Bulletin* 17:15–37.

Smith, G.A., and R.A. Gussen. 1976. Inner ear pathology following mump infection: Report of a case in an adult. *Archives of Otolaryngology* 102:108–111.

Steele, M.W. 1981. Genetics of congenital deafness. *Pediatric Clinics of North America* 28:973–980.

Thringer, K., A. Kankkunen, G. Lidén, and A. Niklasson. 1984. Perinatal risk factors in the etiology of hearing loss in preschool children. *Developmental Medicine and Child Neurology* 26:799–807.

Upfold, L.J., and J. Isepy. 1982. Childhood deafness in Australia. *Medical Journal of Australia* 2:323–326.

Wilson, C.B., J.S. Remington, S. Stagno, and D.W. Reynolds. 1980. Development of adverse sequelae in children born with subclinical congenital toxoplasma infection. *Pediatrics* 66:767–774.

World Health Organization. 1985. WHA39-19.

———. 1986. *Prevention of deafness and hearing impairment.* Report by the Director General of the 79th Session, EB 79/10. Geneva: World Health Organization.

———. 1991. *Report of the informal working group on prevention of deafness and hearing impairment programme planning.* Geneva: World Health Organization.

2

Pediatrics

Franklin A. Katz

STOP, LOOK, AND LISTEN

Stop

MEDICINE in the United States is changing radically. All referrals will eventually come through gatekeepers: a family practitioner, general pediatrician, or general internist. They are called gatekeepers because they control the flow of health services to patients. In order to become gatekeepers, medical subspecialists are enrolling in courses offered by their specialty organizations. About 10% of medical services offered today use a managed care structure. Every newly proposed medical model employs the gatekeeper concept (Kutnik 1993). All healthcare providers—including audiologists, speech-language pathologists, and physician specialists—will one day be dependent on primary care referral. As health professionals who work with children, we must expand our role if we are to prosper or survive. Referrals from nongatekeepers will not be authorized, and we will not be paid by the new health system.

Look

Evaluate your gatekeepers' interest in and experience and knowledge of your field as well as theirs. Experience with developmentally disadvantaged and disabled children varies greatly from physician to physician. The more you know about your associates' backgrounds, the more you can understand their biases. Stress your own professional skills, interests, and strengths. Stress the cost effectiveness as well as the importance of your early evaluations and interventions. You must foster an atmosphere that allows professional dialog. The pediatrician is typically receptive to this process of education and cross-proselytizing. Your value to any generalist dealing with children will greatly increase if you develop skills that allow you to cross comfortably into areas of screening and early diagnosis as well as prescribed treatment.

Listen

Pediatric literature and training have remained constant on only one point through the decades. The pediatrician is a child advocate in both medical and nonmedical issues. We are taught to think about our patient as an individual, a member of a family and of a large community of children. This community may be as small as the local school yard or school district or as large as the entire world. During the twentieth century, pediatricians have led the medical community in establishing successful public health programs for the prevention and treatment of infectious, genetic, and oncologic diseases. Most of the diseases rampant during the first fifty years of this century are now significant only in a historical context. Office visits and hospital admissions to pediatric facilities have decreased dramatically during the last few years. New trainees are spending more time in perinatal, neonatal, intensive care, adolescent, and developmental medicine and counseling. We are defining new curricula and new ways to help a child reach full adult potential.

Your professional energy is needed now. Generalists at all levels need to be made aware of your skills, intellect, personal interests, and your sincere passion and concern for the welfare of children. It will be well worth your effort to promote such an awareness.

EXCHANGING INSIGHTS WITH THE GATEKEEPERS

APPROXIMATELY two of every 1000 to 1500 children under six years of age are said to have permanent bilateral hearing loss of at least 50 dB. Walking in your "gatekeeper's shoes" may provide insight into the reason for the outrageous delay in many referrals for audiologic diagnosis. Most identified children clearly needed earlier diagnoses and intervention, but it is difficult to be the first to tell parents that their child may not hear or see perfectly. The younger the child, the more difficult the clinical determination, and the less forgiving the family will be for any anxiety suffered from your possible miscall. However, parental concern frequently precedes formal identification by a full year (Matkin 1984). Pediatricians are said to have difficulty recognizing even profound deafness because they so rarely see it and because they have not been taught the importance of early intervention. It is a shame that most physicians never deal with chronically disabled children or meet audiologists, speech-language pathologists, or other clinicians during or after their training. Physicians have to be educated about what can be done and why early identification is important. They have to overcome the attitude that saying a child will outgrow something is cost effective. Sometimes it is, but sometimes it is not.

We have been taught techniques that are considered cost effective. Yet we have no measure of the true cost to the individual or to society. Are we asking the right questions? How can we measure the effect on a family of an irritable or poorly developing child? How can we justify classifying partial deafness as "minimal" or fluctuating hearing impairment as not significant? We have information that strongly suggests just the opposite. The term "minimal" subtly decreases our need to remediate.

Furthermore, why are we still using primarily adult terminology of dysfunction in pediatric audiology? Our young patients are not just small adults. We use different standards for children in everything from blood values to blood pressure and vision screening. Screening techniques suggested by all our major professional organizations are frequently done improperly and have cut-off points that are insensitive to subtle changes. We are afraid to include too many children who may not develop obvious problems from their auditory dysfunction. We have taken a giant step backward to homeopathic practices, which treat a symptom, not the cause of a problem. For instance, "It is probably incorrect to consider asymptomatic middle ear effusion as a disease. The diseases associated with asymptomatic otitis media, such as hearing loss and impaired language development, seem to be correct targets of screening" (Bluestone et al. 1986). The attitude of the gatekeepers, the healthcare insurance industry, schools, and the public regarding the true cost of dysfunction needs to be reevaluated. The public needs to be educated about the potential risks to their children.

CLUES TO DIAGNOSIS AND RISK ASSESSMENT

Interview

THE interview can be an extremely sensitive tool for identifying problems in all age-groups. It is an art form that is cost effective and uniquely yours. "No two people can be interviewed in exactly the same way; no two patients with the same disorder present the same history" (Green and Richmond 1992), and no two skillful professionals conduct an interview in the same way. Listen to the family history and carefully observe the caregivers as well as their reactions to your questions. I find questionnaires helpful when I take the time to go over the questions with the caregiver or patient.

The physician uses primarily three types of interview: the traditional history and physical that are typical for hospitalized patients, the expanded one, and your own unique one. Your expanding interest should guide you to question areas that you may not have considered otherwise. Over time, your own personalized multidimensional interview will evolve.

The clues to early, accurate, and subtle diagnoses are usually encountered in the history. The normal range of the nature of these clues is very wide and extremely subjective, especially in our youngest patients. Listen carefully to the information given to you by the child, the child's parents, and other caregivers. Observe their responses to each other as well as their actual words. In addition, teenagers have special needs and are best interviewed without a parent present.

Initially, the teenager may not tell you anything significant and may even feed you misinformation. Leave extra time after the interview (and after you have established a rapport) to obtain the most significant history from them.

The usual interview begins with a sensitive, probing, general evaluation of the child's family and caregivers. What is their general attitude? In what terms is the child described? What were their early concerns and problems? What are their concerns now? Do they suspect hearing impairment? Do the adults support each other and the child? Can they openly discuss family characteristics? Any characteristic found on both sides of the family—especially family history of childhood hearing impairment—may be significant to a child's general development and to the parents' hopes and fears about their offspring. This can be true even if the characteristic is within the range of usual normal. For instance, "funny-looking children" from funny-looking parents might not be abnormal—or the whole family might be abnormal. You must decide. In any event, unattractive children are not given as much positive attention in school from their teachers or their peers. They are prone to function significantly below their potential. They are "at risk" children.

The interview is a time to trade information and assess attitudes. Let the parents share your experiences so that they can better understand your concern and your eventual conclusions. The history they relate to you must be evaluated carefully. Why are they focused on certain areas and not on others? What secondary family games are being played? What do they expect from you? Your assessment of the temperament of the involved parties can be exceptionally rewarding.

What of the infant's temperament and why should you care (Carey 1982)? Your assessment of the children and their ability to adapt to the environment can be crucial to them and to your evaluation. A parent can be an under- or an over-responder for the infant. Most parents respond normally and concordantly with their infant's needs. Your perception of their infant's need for stimulation can help them modify their behavior and better understand their baby.

Parents are always pleased to find out that their offspring has inborn behavioral characteristics. This is especially true if they have a difficult infant. Nonconcordance between caretaker and child could place the child at risk for later social or emotional problems. This idea of goodness of fit between parent and child is important. You must assess your relationship with the parents and the referring physician before tendering any advice. It will influence your decision when to suggest a diagnostic or treatment program and to whom. The physicians may want all advice filtering through them. This is especially important if several professionals are in contact with the caregivers. Parents listen to the professional whom they choose to hear. Outrageous distortions and denial are frequent in emotionally-loaded situations involving a sick or disabled infant or child. An over-responding parent or grandparent who distorts or amplifies your advice or your input can emotionally injure the child, one of the other family members, or your reputation. Even positive and well-considered advice can have negative side effects. I frequently act as a funnel for information from different health professionals. It's a difficult job. The same diagnosis or word in one discipline may mean something different in another discipline.

Family History

The child's family history and parents' medical history and knowledge of their environmental exposure to infections or mutagenic agents are helpful nonspecific screening tools. Of course, a family history of deafness from any cause should alert you. Genetic hearing loss does not need to be expressed at birth. Otosclerosis, presbycusis, Cockayne and Alport syndromes—although not congenital (present at birth)—remain genetic in origin (Davidson, Hyde, and Alberti 1989). Waardenburg and Leopard syndromes, which can involve pigment changes of the hair or skin, are the most common integumentary-system-related deafness. Retinitis pigmentosa involves progressive eye, vestibular, and sensorineural changes. Pendred syndrome and endocrinopathies primarily involving the thyroid are well described (Fraser 1976). Children with mucopolysaccharide diseases (MPS) can develop intracellular storage of acid mucopolysaccharides and develop a progressive conductive loss due to ossicular dysfunction (Wallace, Prutting, and Gerber 1990). Neurodegenerative diseases (such as Tay-Sachs) and metabolic diseases (such as Wilson disease) have associated hearing loss. Benign hematuria as well as progressive renal insufficiency (Alport syndrome) have associated sensorineural hearing loss in the middle and high frequencies in later years.

Biologists are predicting that they will be able to obtain "flaws that are prediagnostic of disease . . . in fifteen or twenty years when DNA can be extracted from every newborn infant's blood sample" (Jaroff 1992). Today, intrauterine diagnosis using fetal tissue, chorionic villus samples, or amniotic fluid samples are widely used. There are screening methods for various metabolic diseases that may affect hearing (PKU, aminoacidopathies), endocrine disorders (thyroid), and blood diseases (sickle cell, thallasemia). These few tests are very specific but very narrow. Specific preclinical, early diagnosis from a few spots of newborn blood has become the standard in most states. It costs less to screen than to treat or institutionalize later.

What do we do with the information, and can we keep the results privileged? A Pandora's box of ethical questions regarding everything from termination of pregnancy to invasion of privacy has been opened. The immunobiologists and geneticists of this and the next century need accurate clinical information and need to know what we believe is important. Clinicians will have to help codify the many subtle differences found in groups and individuals. We have orphan genes and microorganisms looking for defined conditions. Yes, it's like "pin the tail on the donkey," and we have to supply the donkey! The history can be a nonspecific, cost effective, reliable screening tool in the hands of a trained sensitive observer: your hands. It's available to you now and most certainly will define the direction of future inquiry.

RETHINKING THE HIGH-RISK LABEL

I WOULD like to relabel the high risk infants and call them the highest risk infants. The highest risk infant is the one who is most likely to develop brain damage in general and sensorineural hearing loss in particular. The criteria for this group usually include familial deafness; prematurity (<1500 grams); severe newborn depression; use of ototoxic drugs for more than five days; severe hyper-bilirubinemia; congenital anomalies of the ear, head, and neck; bacterial meningitis; congenital infections (e.g., CMV, toxoplasmosis, herpes, rubella); mechanical ventilation for ten days or more; or known stigmata associated with specific syndromes (Joint Committee on Infant Hearing 1994). Unfortunately, the usual criteria for highest risk do not include the vast majority of "high risk" or the not quite as definable "at risk" group. We must synthesize a great deal of information and soft data from the interview, the family history, and the personal history of the parents and a developing child. It is our job to find and help these potentially vulnerable children. Keep an open mind and reasonable records so that you can cross-validate your observations over a period of time. You don't want to miss an opportunity to intervene early and help the child, nor do you want to cause undue alarm. Do the best you can, and—most of all—do no harm.

In the Beginning

Maternal Factors

Both parents are important, but the maternal condition is obviously more related to the infant's intrauterine development. Maternal factors specific to the pregnancy or an unrelated illness, infection, exposure to toxins, past health, morbid habits, or even age (<17 years or >38 years) can influence the outcome of the infant. A history of previous dysmature infants, genetic problems, interrupted pregnancy, or newborn catastrophes resulting in asphyxia or trauma can be significant. Previous infertility problems or a previous seriously ill child may cause difficulty for the parents in properly relating to their new infant. Maternal health problems specific to the pregnancy include hypertension for any reason, vaginal bleeding, premature rupture of the membranes, or large fibroids that might interfere with the blood supply to the infant. These can interfere with the child's growth and development no matter what the genetic potential.

Intrauterine growth retardation (IUGR) should alert you to possible problems later. Intrauterine growth retardation for any reason—including multiple gestation, postterm pregnancy, poly- or oligohydramnios (too much or too little amniotic fluid), and problems with the umbilical cord (prolapsed)—is always significant. But the effect may not be obvious. Chronic medical diseases (e.g., diabetes, renal disease, asthma with hypoxemia, collagen disorders, malabsorption syndromes) can be problems for the infant. Many of these problems can be prevented by good prenatal identification and care of the parent.

Malnutrition is a significant problem today and will increase over the decades. Because protein-calorie-deprived mothers have poor placentas, intrauterine growth retardation is common. Direct studies of brain DNA show both fewer brain cells and impaired brain cell growth in the malnourished infant. Defects of number or size can cause distortion of normal relationships. This may result in subtle and gross anatomical defects that arise *after* the period of undernutrition. Dendritic networks are 28% less extensive in rats that recovered from undernutrition in early life (McConnell and Berry 1981). There are large populations of vulnerable microneurons in the cerebellum, hippocampus, and olfactory areas that proliferate relatively late in development (Rodier 1980). The brain cells cited in the 1960s as being reduced in number by early undernutrition would include such microneuronal cell populations. The central auditory system, of course, is affected.

Proper diet will increase both the number and size of brain cells in subsequent generations. The present Women-Infants-Children (WIC) program in this country offers free food to pregnant women and free milk to all children. How easy it is to change once we refuse to accept suboptimal as a norm. Parabiosis, or transfusion of one twin to another, can cause significant differences in organ size. The smaller anemic twin should be considered a small-for-date infant. These twin-to-twin intrauterine transfusions tend to cause small and immature, as well as anemic, babies. Both children are high risk infants. Yet, in one study of very low birth weight infants (Hack et al. 1991), many sophisticated observations were made, but hearing was not mentioned. Low birth weight (<1500 g) is a well-established cause of early onset hearing impairment.

Perinatal Infections

Perinatal infections can be important. Parasitic (toxoplasmosis), viral (cytomegalic inclusion, rubella), spirochetal (syphilis), and bacterial infections raise the chance of significant morbidity, especially auditory morbidity. Toxoplasmosis may result in low birthweight infants who are either small (SGA) or appropriate (AGA) for gestational age. Virus diseases, such as cytomegalic inclusion or rubella, can cause IUGR. Syphilis is a cause of prematurity but not of IUGR. Perinatal bacterial infections in the mother or infant can be significant but have widely variable outcomes. I believe that any nervous system infection in an infant, whether from meningitis or an infected myelomeningocele, should be considered significant for later development.

Genetic Factors

Genetic factors, including inadequate sex chromosomes such as female Turner syndrome (X/0 or 45X) and autosomal trisomies, are well known to produce SGA babies. Trisomy 21 infants weigh about 15% less than normal at birth; half weigh less than 2700 grams. Similarly small are infants with trisomies 16/18 and 13/15. Inherited disorders without chromosomal abnormalities (e.g., achondroplastic dwarfs) often produce small-for-date infants who do not have an increased morbidity. These children frequently have hearing impairments. Women who have produced one SGA infant are likely to produce another. Specific screening is imperative if any first-degree relative has a significant screen-able problem. Neural tube defects (e.g., spina bifida cystica), Tay-Sachs syndrome, and others demand an early screening. A family history of congenital or delayed onset sensorineural auditory impairment, even in a distant relative, should be considered relevant and significant since 70 to 80% are autosomal recessive problems.

Other Factors

Mothers who are moderate smokers have double the incidence of SGA infants that nonsmokers have; heavy smokers have three times the incidence. High altitude, x-radiation, certain drugs (aminopterin and antimetabolites), alcohol (fetal alcohol syndrome), hot tubs, and certain illegal drugs can result in SGA infants. Maternal use of narcotics (e.g., cocaine) can result in withdrawal symptoms in the nursery, whereas LSD can cause certain chromosomal and skeletal problems. Legal drugs such as Dilantin (cleft palate), barbiturates (withdrawal), cortisone (clefts, adrenal suppression), estrogen, thyroid suppressants, reserpine, insulin, and so on may cause or contribute to problems. It is my opinion that parents who knowingly, repeatedly expose their child to unnecessary risk are criminals.

Obstetrical Factors

Problems near the time of delivery can be significant. The child has to make remarkable changes to extrauterine life, and not all systems may be ready to adjust during the last transitions of labor. Severe variable decelerations of the fetal monitor strip are caused by hypoxemia (low O_2 in the blood stream); fetal metabolic acidemia (pH <7.20) is a sign of anaerobic metabolism and tissue hypoxia. The latter suggests a much more profound insult to the infant, with known consequences for audition. This child is in the highest risk group. The normal fetal heart rate fluctuates around a base line rate with a rapid return to the baseline after a period of bradycardia or tachycardia. If the infant's heart rate doesn't promptly return to the baseline, then we have a stressed infant with an autonomic imbalance. This is a high risk infant.

Even a baby's position in utero is associated with increased risk. Breech babies have a higher frequency of neurologic abnormalities and motor retardation at one year of age. Many specific syndromes (trisomy, Prader-Willi) have a high incidence of breech deliveries. Even breech babies born via cesarean section are high risk. The opinions regarding the outcome of different cephalic presentations vary. A hard labor for the child may be an easy labor for the mother and vice-versa. Collect your data carefully. Use your senses. Look at the infant and listen to the nursery nurse, the parents, and the delivering physician. Avoid any hint of being judgmental or critical of anybody if you want to get accurate information. In addition, the type of anesthesia and its effect on the infant can be important. A sleepy infant is less likely to bond than a vigorous one. Human companionship during the mother's labor has a direct bearing on maternal behavior. Benefits include a shortened labor, reduced perinatal problems, and heightened aspects of maternal care in the first hours of life. I prefer both regional anesthesia for the mother (epidural) and the presence of helpers in the labor and delivery suite unless the infant is ill.

Newborn

For the last century, the textbooks of pediatrics taught that an infant was perceptually incompetent. The infant was considered deaf at birth and deficient in other areas, including olfaction, taste, touch, and vision. In contrast, research done after 1950 reveals the newborn as a perceptually competent organism. This may also partially explain the abysmal record of delayed audiologic referral by physicians. The average delay between birth and confirmation of significant hearing loss in children in the United States is two and one-half years or more (Bess and Hall 1992). This is clearly unacceptable. The pediatrician carefully follows the orderly acquisition of skills (language, adaptive, personal, motor) as well as the orderly loss of primitive reflexes. A template of expectations is derived from the history as discussed above. The child's genetic and social background are superimposed on other data as a further gauge of expectations. Questionnaires, physical examination, and the parent's feelings guide the pediatrician to early, and sometimes subtle, diagnoses. The standards are subjective, prone to error, and insensitive in certain areas. Any information that we receive from any of our colleagues is greatly appreciated.

All infants should be screened for hearing impairment using otoacoustic emissions, according to a 1993 NIH Consensus Development Panel. It is likely that this will become public law. This may provide you with the opportunity to serve a new part of the hospital and a new medical community. Developmental and other screening might also be mandated. New no-fault malpractice laws are being proposed. More research into subtle problems will undoubtedly be encouraged by their passage.

If the newborn hears a sound by stopping his activity to listen, then, presumably, he hears. Please remember that it is abnormal for a newborn to continue to respond. A neonate should stop responding after repeated stimuli—auditory or visual. A lack of habituation suggests a neurologically-impaired infant. In practice, you will find that the child's temperament and wakefulness will influence your decision as to which child may be abnormal or need further observation. An "at risk" score needs to be developed for all of those "maybe" cases who just aren't quite right. We might judge a child's development potential by using multiple, narrow criteria, such as family history and risk potential. A useful four dimensional scale, the Neonatal Behavioral Assessment Scale (NBAS), used by Brazelton (1973) and others, is an excellent start. It measures motor tone and maturity, interactive processes (consolability, alertness), response to stress (tremulousness, startle), and control of physiologic states (habituation).

You must fully understand the importance of gestational age and newborn maturity. Scales to weigh infants are found everywhere. The risk tables based on weight criteria have been supplemented in most western countries. Criteria for scoring maturity and gestational age should be available in every nursery (Dubowitz, Dubowitz, and Goldberg 1970). Birthweight and gestational age tables show that mortality and morbidity vary with gestation groups among infants with the same birthweight; it also varies with birthweight among those of the same gestation. What does that mean? It means that the genetic predisposition of the infant can be influenced by environmental factors found in the uterus. An infant who is appropriate for gestational age (AGA) is at less risk than the small for gestational age (SGA) or small for date infant or large for gestational age (LGA) infant. Prematurity, when defined simply by weight or by gestation of less than thirty-seven weeks, is not very helpful. In fact, SGA infants with the longest gestation have the highest percentage of severe malformations. The frequency of congenital malformations increases as smallness for gestational age increases.

The most important determinant of a newborn's chances of well-being in later childhood is the degree of immaturity at birth as well as the socioeconomic and educational levels of the parents (Hardy, Drage, and Jackson 1979). The younger, more impoverished, unhealthy, minimally-educated mother consistently had the worst outcomes. Birth control, sex education, and family service programs should therefore be encouraged. The highest incidence of anomalies is found in the low birthweight infant of an older (>35 years) mother. In contrast, the younger group (<18 years) has the highest postneonatal period mortality and morbidity.

Ask the nursery nurse about the baby's Apgar risk scores (Table 2.1), feeding problems, activity, temperature instability, general condition, and attitude of the parents and visitors. Low Apgar scores are clearly associated with impaired

Table 2.1. Apgar Scoring Method in Evaluation of Condition of Newborn Infants

Sign	Score[a]		
	0	1	2
Heart rate	Absent	Slow (< 100)	> 100
Respiratory effort	Absent	Weak cry, hypoventilation	Good, strong cry
Muscle tone	Limp	Some flexion of extremities	Well flexed
Reflex irritability (response to skin stimulation of feet)	No response	Some motion	Cry
Color	Blue, pale	Body pink, extremities blue	Completely pink

Note: The Apgar evaluation is done 60 seconds after complete birth of infant (disregarding the cord and placenta) and again four minutes later.

[a]Score of 10 indicates infant is in the best possible condition.

hearing. Be alert. Any nonroutine test ordered by the physician or nurse could mean an infant at higher risk.

The Apgar risk score is designed to alert nurses so that more intense care can be started immediately on certain infants. It is not a grade of the infant's worth, the parents, or the delivering physician. It is generally more accurate when scored by the nurse than the physician. A low five-minute Apgar or problems at ten minutes correlate with a greater chance of later demonstrable damage to the infant. Be aware that the parents and grandparents frequently misinterpret the significance of this highly publicized number. We should be very cautious in our discussion of the Apgar score. Bonding and long-term maternal anxiety may follow any infant, especially one needing special nursery care or labeled as having an early real, or potential, problem. This long-term maternal anxiety sometimes leads to the "vulnerable child syndrome." The child typically fails to thrive despite an adequate diet and doting parents. Fathers show the same patterns of bonding as do mothers (Parke 1974). The predominant emotion when holding the infant for the first time is indifference. Forty percent feel affection, and this emotion increases over the first week. A malformed infant can result in major family stress, anger, sadness, and anxiety (see chapter 14). Most parents reach a point where they are able to care adequately for their children and cope effectively with feelings of grief, sadness, and anger (Solnit 1961).

Temperature adjustment to the extrauterine environment is carefully followed in most nurseries. Transient temperature instability is frequent. Persistence of abnormal temperature in a normal thermal environment indicates a problem. Follow that infant carefully. Hyperthermia may be seen with drug withdrawal and intracranial or adrenal hemorrhage. Hypothermia may be caused by hypoglycemia, hypoxia, early sepsis, or hypothyroid disease.

Normal term infants can be very active for about the first hour. After that, only 20% of their time is spent awake in active, inactive, or crying states. The infant's cry should be lusty. A feeble, high-pitched, or soft cry suggests a neurologic problem. A hoarse cry might be due to trauma to the hypopharynx or vocal cord paralysis (Gerber, Lynch, and Gibson 1987). Hypothyroid disease is rarely seen in this age-group if the mother is euthyroid. Infants can and do focus on visual and auditory stimuli.

The infant's general muscle tone and posture change dramatically during the first several days. Positions of comfort approximate those assumed in utero. Many deformities are due to constraint and not to congenital abnormalities. Malformations due to morphogenesis can be differentiated from deformities from constraint more easily when you fold the child back into his intrauterine position of comfort. For instance, an abnormal pinna may be due to pressure from an arm, a twin, a fibroid, or other mechanical forces causing deformations. Usually they return spontaneously to normal. About 2% of infants have significant deformities caused by mechanical forces that acted in utero to restrict motion or to create pressure on limbs, spine, thorax, or skull (Smith 1981). The effect of pressure applied to an otherwise normal structure clearly has a different implication from diagnosing a child born with a genetic or dysmorphic problem (Smith 1981). A videotape or picture of the newborn can be very helpful when you are trying to put together the pieces of the diagnostic puzzle years later. Unusual thyroid problems that are associated with deafness (e.g., endemic goiters and Pendred disease) can be diagnosed at birth but are extremely rare.

Gestational age can be assessed from the maternal history, ultrasound measurements of the uterus, x-rays of bone development, and the physical exam of the newborn. Look at the gestation charts in your nursery so that you can better assess which infants you think may be more at risk.

The First 28 Days (The Neonatal Period)

This period in childhood is associated with the highest mortality. The morbidity is more difficult to measure. Morbidity statistics can vary depending upon what is measured and by whom. A significant proportion of central nervous system (CNS) injury resulting in later manifestations of mental retardation, neurologic handicaps, and deafness occur in this period of life. Regionalized neonatal intensive care units are primarily responsible for the reduction of mortality in the past twenty years. Improvement of the survival rate in specific low birthweight gestational age-groups accounts for 85% of this increase. Survival rate is clearly easier to measure than definite or possible morbidity. Thirty percent of infants under 1000 gm and needing ventilator support survive. Severe neurological handicaps (45%), bronchopulmonary dysplasia (75%), and retrolental fibroplasia (20%) occur in these survivors. A 94% follow-up rate on low birth weight (SGA) infants over six years revealed that 9% of 111 infants had hearing loss and 4% were seriously impaired by their sensorineural loss (Abramovich et al. 1979). We measure only major deviations from general, normative data. We are not able to predict which preterm child with transient neurological findings is at risk to develop cognitive delays (D'Eugenio et al. 1993). Our job is to maximize the individual's potential. Since true potential is too subtle for us to measure, we should always aim high. Every professional I know is periodically astounded by a child's unexpected progress.

The Early Years

Many children are said not to hear or pay attention; to talk too loud or too soft; to have chronic otitis, allergies, and school problems. They don't listen, they daydream or fantasize; they play the TV too loud, and on and on. Eighty-five percent of pediatric visits concern middle ear problems (Koch and Dennison 1974). Transient, fluctuating hearing loss that accompanies middle ear disease and variations in normal development have made us all numb. Serous otitis media is the most common cause of hearing loss in children, affecting up to two-thirds of preschool children (Davidson, Hyde, and Alberti 1989). It may be significant to those growing up in linguistically impoverished environments (Allen, Rapin, and Wiznitzer 1988) or with other potential risk factors such as social, emotional, or physical problems. We know that children with prolonged middle-ear effusion (MEE) in infancy may have lower scores on language skill tests later (Northern and Downs 1991). Children of higher socioeconomic status showed the greatest risk for poor performance in later years (Teele et al. 1984). Many physicians and other health professionals have chosen to ignore the obvious. Because we have not intervened, many children have become at risk for language and cognition problems. Auditory confusion, decreased auditory discrimination, attention problems, and appreciation of syntax, receptive vocabulary, processing, and so forth have all been cited. Professionals interested in children have an opportunity to prevent problems. Visual problems of the same magnitude are treated much more aggressively. It's time to educate the professional community and the public about so-called minor problems of hearing.

PREVENTION

Infants

PREVENTION can start early. Infants younger than several months of age are a challenge. The physician's pneumatic otoscope alone is not reliable in early infancy, and we need all the help we can get. A family history can be very useful. Tympanometry is not reliable for screening before six months of age because false normals are frequent (Northern and Downs 1991). The compliance of the ear canal is high. However, an abnormal, flat tympanogram is a significant indicator of middle ear disease. Tympanometry can be very useful in questionable cases in almost any child. Parents should be instructed to look for symptoms of possible ear problems: persistent or extreme irritability, posterior head batting, or head rolling. Remind them that teething is not usually a problem before three months of age.

Infants having early acute, recurrent, or chronic middle ear problems are extremely common. I believe that we can decrease later morbidity by early intervention. Morbidity used to mean mastoiditis, meningitis, and chronic significant infections frequently leading to death or brain damage. These now occur much less frequently and are less significant because we have better treatments than in previous decades. Common secondary problems were ignored. These presumably less significant problems include speech, auditory processing dysfunction, sensory-motor problems, and balance problems, as well as physical and emotional development.

Twenty percent of children seen at well-baby exams have fluid in their ears (Teele et al. 1980). This should not be accepted as normal even though it is common. No child should miss the important windows of speech acquisition at about one year of age or have fluctuating hearing loss. The resultant deficits in expressive language and other skills may not be remediable. Children with uncomfortable middle ears, no matter what the cause, are irritable. Unhappy infants are difficult to live with. They tend to invoke feelings of inadequacy and guilt in today's working parents. I believe that early prevention, identification, and treatment of middle ear disease are crucial if we aim to maximize the child's potential. It is irrational to apply group data to an individual's treatment plan in any except the most general way. I do not know if the otitis is the specific cause of the many problems described or merely associated with them. Pediatric office-based screening of two- to four-year-old children is becoming more common. Some authors report that tympanometry and reflex testing will identify 90 to 95% of significant ear pathology in two- to four-year-old children; pure tone audiometric testing will identify 80%. We must reevaluate the term significant (Bluestone et al. 1986).

Which child should be followed, treated, or ignored? Who has increased risk of frequent, severe, or resultant dysfunction from middle ear problems? Besides the factors mentioned before, all children with cranial, renal, or multiple dysmorphic abnormalities and all developmentally disabled children are at increased risk. Native Americans, Alaskan Eskimos, and other groups also have an increased incidence of middle ear disease. The infection and effusion are apparently more difficult to treat in these groups. Otitis media with effusion (MEE) may cause more functional damage and yet seem less significant in a developmentally disabled child. A minor auditory dysfunction, especially if persistent or recurrent, can be catastrophic and nonremediable in a disabled child. Children with Down syndrome and many other syndromes deserve early intervention including infant stimulation, hearing and speech guidance, antibiotics, and P.E. tubes. Their speech and general development improve remarkably and can be normal. The consensus seems to be that conductive hearing impairment is the most prevalent type, with an incidence that ranges from 2.6% to as much as 60% (Buchanan, Harding, and Hudner 1991). I remember being taught that a child with Down syndrome was dull, poorly responsive, placid, inattentive, and talked funny. That is not what we see after we intervene.

I also suggest that all children at increased statistical risk who have had a history of early and recurrent middle ear effusion start school in the summer. The seasonal incidence of middle ear effusions is well known. These children should have the fall quarter off. This will decrease their exposure to rhinoviruses and to the school problems that result from hay fever and allergies. Antihistamines and decongestants may help the nose, probably do not help the ear, and certainly interfere with concentration, attention, and other subtle functions—no matter what the drug companies tell you.

About one-third of our population suffers from simple allergies. That is a lot of people. Severe, disabling allergies are much less frequent. The infant must be considered at risk if close family members have had ENT surgery for otitis, sinusitis, rhinitis, or allergy hyposensitization. Immediate effective intervention must include prevention. I encourage breast feeding (40% fewer ear infections). Solids should not be added to most infants' diets until after four months of age. Have the mother feed the child in a sitting-up position. Caregivers—including parents, grandparents, and healthcare workers—are strongly advised to avoid exposing the infant to cigarette smoke and respiratory irritants. For instance, they should be advised not to hold the baby on their shoulder if they use shaving lotion, perfume, or hair spray that may remain in their hair or on their neck. Tell them not to expose their infant to feathers or animal hair. Keep the animals away from the air intake of the heating system and away from the infants' sleeping quarters. Grandma's goose down pillow or comforter is off limits especially if it is old. These general rules apply in the child's home and wherever that child is taken for daycare. Advise the parents to put the infant into a home-care situation with six or fewer infants because the incidence of otitis media is much lower.

I advise parents not to use the nasal aspirators they receive from most newborn nurseries. The volume of the aspirator bulb compared to an infant's nose is huge. Most parents cannot gently suck outside their infant's nose. Our primal nose-fiddling, hole-poking instinct overrides common sense. The nostrils get smaller and smaller as they are violently sucked, and the mucosa become edematous.

Regression in speech and motor skills is common in toddlers with chronic or subacute middle ear disease. This regression is obvious to parents if they are taught to observe the child. This type of loss may be reversible, and it is gratifying to see an infant's speech skills accelerate under treatment. Children with chronic otitis sometimes have expressive language skill and other deficits that cannot be remediated by later speech therapy. It is clearly important to protect the infant and small child during periods of language acquisition. Irritability is the presenting symptom in a large majority of infants with significant acute otitis media. That sounds suspiciously like what has been called colic, teething, personality problems, and growing pains of infancy. Many infants develop loose stools as a sign of otitis before being given antibiotics. Some have rare subtle immune deficiency states (IGG1), lazy cilia, or food intolerance. Most do not have a single definable causative problem. Both an increased awareness of the problem by the parents and better tools—such as the halogen light, pneumatic otoscope, and the office tympanometer—in recent decades have allowed earlier and more accurate diagnoses.

Preschool and School Age

Always ask how the child is doing in school and preschool. Does she stand out in any way to a trained, experienced, objective teacher? Does the child have behavior or learning skills problems? A positive history should intensify your focus on this youngster. This child is at risk and has parents who are increasingly motivated to find out why. Any sensory loss is significant to a developing child. The child's acquisition of reality has been modified and distorted. You know instinctively that children with profound or subtle losses are somehow different. All children, no matter what the I.Q. score, develop coping skills and strategies to help themselves.

Children with hearing loss may be sensed by you before you test them. Notice how they relate to their surroundings. Increased visual alertness, touching, behavioral deviations, face watching, and excessive head movement are common. Please don't limit your focus to hearing. Believe it or not, you may be one of the only authorized healthcare professionals to screen a child. It behooves you to know that eye and vision problems abound.

If children have a history of lazy eye or squint, have them tested for vision. You can prevent an all-too-common form of blindness (amblyopia). The eye may look perfectly fine to you during the early advanced stages. Sight is recoverable if the condition is picked up early.

Myopia (nearsightedness) is discovered typically in the preteen and early teen years; yet, some medical plans pay for only preschool screening. School districts are dropping their early childhood screening and rarely screen older children. If both parents are nearsighted, the child should be tested yearly and at the first symptoms of a problem. If one parent is nearsighted, then less frequent screening is acceptable. Many simple eye charts are available for home or office use. You may want to use an illiterate E test, Snellen eye charts, or more elegant equipment. We all have to prepare for coming changes and continually develop new skills.

Specialist physicians are being retrained by their societies and others to do comfortably more general work as a gatekeeper. They will need medically trained professionals who can provide information to streamline their decisions.

The New Epidemic

We know that fluctuating hearing losses can cause deficits in the acquisition of vocabulary, articulation skills, and the ability to receive and express ideas through spoken language (Gottlieb, Zinkus, and Thompson 1979). There are critical periods of language development and, unfortunately, these periods coincide with the time of highest frequency of ear infections. Studies have concluded that deprivation of sound can cause various deficits and that negative middle ear pressure, even with normal hearing for pure tones, can be significant (Cook and Teel 1979). There is a paucity of audiologic data regarding how this occurs. Vision studies seem to indicate that various chemical modifiers may either enhance or impair the formation of memory (and learning) by influencing cerebral metabolism. These modifiers may be present for a finite length of time—perhaps never to return.

Children with learning, attentional, or speech problems appear to have a history of more frequent ear infections. Their verbal scores are depressed and tend to correlate with the number of episodes of otitis media (Kaplan et al. 1973). Reading skills appear to be compromised among children with histories of recurrent middle ear disease (Levine, Carey, and Crocker 1992). This has sparked an upsurge of interest in ear disease by parent groups. Parents of children with learning disabilities or unusual learning patterns have frequently had the same problems and are highly motivated to decrease their child's difficulties.

Forty percent of children with attention deficit disorders (ADD) have a family history of attentional problems. Attentional deficit disorder has been said to occur in about 5% of the population and has been called the hyperkinetic syndrome or minimal brain dysfunction. This diagnosis is now being used generically on increasing numbers of students. Has intolerance of children who are intellectually or socially different increased? Questionnaires that strongly suggest that normal characteristics are deviant are being circulated by parent groups and interested professionals. My own school district now reports that over 15% of students have attentional problems. No lead, toxin, or specific medical reason for this increase has been found.

I was overwhelmed with sadness to hear the almost universal problems that members of the Mensa Society (IQ in the top 2 percentiles of the general population) have had in school. Be aware that the facile misapplication of a diagnosis of ADD or its variants with hyperactivity (ADHD) or oppositional behavior

(ADDO) frequently buries the gifted child or children with sensory or social deficits. We must look beyond the child's immediate behavior and understand why he is acting out. These children develop strategies that grandparents, school teachers, and others may find intolerable. I believe that all children with school problems should be tested for hearing, vision, and psychointellectual abnormalities before any therapy is prescribed.

Children with conductive losses have the most difficulty with selective auditory attention. Surely, strategies can be developed to identify that child at risk and offer aid. Classrooms and teachers need to be evaluated. They are part of the solution, and they may also be part of the problem. We can help by increasing the teacher's awareness of the child's disabilities and explaining why he gets worse when he has a cold or allergy attack. The child's reaction to decongestant medicines, poor sleep, congested ears, or poorly heated classrooms can be discussed. Some children benefit from smaller, quieter classes with fewer visual stimuli. Some may need drug therapy. Others may need corrective lenses, hearing aids, a speech-language pathologist's or an educational therapist's intervention. Many need multiple therapies. Psychopharmacologic drugs are very commonly used. Drugs that affect the inner ear in attempts to solve the problem are rarely used today.

I believe that all identified children and their families develop emotional overlays. They need support and sometimes protection from the system attempting to homogenize their children. This would have included the families of Thomas Edison, Albert Einstein, Winston Churchill, Samuel Clemens, Steven Spielberg, and many others.

We are all child advocates doing the best job we can. I believe that an increasing social awareness about ear disease and its sequelae will inspire a renaissance of research in our fields of interest. I hope that we will collaboratively develop the knowledge and skills to do a better job.

REFERENCES

Abramovich, S.J., S. Gregory, M. Slemick, and A. Stewart. 1979. Hearing loss in very low birth weight infants treated with neonatal intensive care. *Archives of Disorders of Children* 54:421–426.

Allen, D., I. Rapin, and M. Wiznitzer. 1988. Communication disorders of preschool children: The physician's responsibility. *Developmental and Behavioral Pediatrics* 9:164–170.

Bess, F.H., and J.W. Hall III. 1992. *Screening children for auditory dysfunction.* Nashville: The Bill Wilkerson Center Press.

Bluestone, C., et al. 1986. Controversies in screening for middle ear disease and hearing loss in children. *Pediatrics* 77:57–70.

Brazelton, T.B. 1973. *Neonatal behavioral assessment scale.* London: W. Heinemann.

Buchanan, L.H., K.M. Harding, and C.M. Hudner. 1991. Hearing disorder management in Down's syndrome. *Hearing Instruments* 42:12–15.

Carey, W.B. 1982. Validity of parental assessments of development and behavior. *American Journal of Diseases of Children* 136:97–99.

Cook, R.A., and R.W. Teel, Jr. 1979. Negative middle ear pressure and language development. *Clinical Pediatrics* 18:296–297.

D'Eugenio, D.B., T.A. Slagle, B.B. Mettelman, and S.J. Gross. 1993. Developmental outcome of preterm infants with transient neuromotor abnormalities. *American Journal of Diseases of Children* 147:570–574.

Davidson, J., M.L. Hyde, and P.W. Alberti. 1989. Epidemiologic patterns in childhood hearing loss: A review. *International Journal of Pediatric Otorhinolaryngology* 17: 239–266.

Dubowitz, L.M., V. Dubowitz, and C. Goldberg. 1970. Clinical assessment of gestational age in the newborn infant. *Journal of Pediatrics* 77:1–10.

Fraser, G.R. 1976. *The causes of profound deafness in childhood*. Baltimore: Johns Hopkins University Press.

Gerber, S.E., C.J. Lynch, and W.S. Gibson, Jr. 1987. The acoustic characteristics of an infant with unilateral vocal fold paralysis. *International Journal of Pediatric Otorhinolaryngology* 13:1–9.

Gottlieb, M.I., P. Zinkus, and A. Thompson. 1979. Chronic middle ear disease and auditory perceptual deficits. *Clinical Pediatrics* 18:725–732.

Green, M., and J.B. Richmond. 1992. *Pediatric diagnosis: Interpretation of signs and symptoms in different age periods*. 5th ed. Philadelphia: W.B. Saunders Co.

Hack, M., J.D. Horbar, M.H. Malloy, J.E. Tyson, E. Wright, and L. Wright. 1991. Very low birth weight outcomes of the National Institute of Child Health and Human Development neonatal network. *Pediatrics* 87:587–597.

Hardy, J.B., J.F. Drage, and E.C. Jackson. 1979. *The first year of life: The collaborative perinatal project of the National Institute of Neurological and Communication Disorders and Stroke*. Baltimore: Johns Hopkins University Press.

Jaroff, L. 1992. *The new genetics*. Knoxville, TN: Whittle Communications.

Joint Committee on Infant Hearing. 1994 position statement. *Audiology Today* 6:6–9.

Kaplan, G.J., J.K. Fleshman, T.R. Bender, C. Baum, and P.S. Clark. 1973. Long term effects of otitis media: A ten-year cohort study of Alaskan Eskimo children. *Pediatrics* 52: 577–585.

Koch, H., and N.J. Dennison. 1974. *Office visits to pediatricians*. Washington, D.C.: National Center for Health Statistics.

Kutnik, L. 1993. *Surviving the '90s: A primer*. AAP conference, La Jolla, CA.

Levine, M.D., W.B. Carey, and A.C. Crocker. 1992. *Developmental-behavioral pediatrics*. Philadelphia, W.B. Saunders Co.

Matkin, N.D. 1984. Early recognition and referral of hearing impaired children. *Pediatrics in Review* 6:151–156.

McConnell, P., and M. Berry. 1981. The effect of refeeding after neonatal starvation on Purkinje cell dendritic growth in the rat. *Journal of Comparative Neurology* 178:759–772.

National Institutes of Health 1993. *Early identification of hearing impairment in infants and young children*. NIH Consensus Statement 11:1–24. Washington, D.C.: National Institutes of Health.

Northern, J.L., and M.P. Downs. 1991. *Hearing in children*. 4th ed. Baltimore: Williams and Wilkins.

Parke, R. 1974. *Father-infant interaction in maternal attachment and mothering disorders: A roundtable.* Sausalito, CA: Johnson and Johnson Co.

Rodier, P.M. 1980. Chronology of neuron development: Animal studies and their clinical implications. *Developmental Medicine and Child Neurology* 22:525–545.

Smith, D.W. 1981. *Recognizable patterns of human deformation.* Philadelphia: W.B. Saunders Co.

Solnit, S. 1961. Mourning and the birth of a defective child. *Psychoanalytic Study of the Child, Monograph #16.*

Teele, D.W., J.O. Klein, B.A. Rosner, et al. 1980. Epidemiology of otitis media in children. *Annals of Otology, Rhinology, and Laryngology* (Suppl. 68) 89:5–6.

———. 1984. Otitis media with effusion during the first three years of life and development of speech and language. *Pediatrics* 74:282–287.

Wallace, S.P., C.A. Prutting, and S.E. Gerber. 1990. Degeneration of speech, language, and hearing in a patient with mucopolysaccharidosis VII. *International Journal of Pediatric Otorhinolaryngology* 19:97–107.

3

The Pediatric Otolaryngic Assessment of the Child with a Suspected Hearing Loss

Robert J. Ruben

PURPOSE

THE purposes of the pediatric otolaryngic assessment of a child suspected of having a hearing loss or other communicative disorder(s) are many. They include:

1. Determining the cause of the loss;
2. Carrying out indicated intervention(s);
3. Determining which other organ system(s) may be involved;
4. Monitoring the progression of the disorder(s); and
5. Evaluating the effects of the intervention(s).

Methods of carrying out the assessments, except physical examination, are similar for neonates, infants, toddlers, and preschool age children.

The pediatric otolaryngic assessment begins with a detailed history structured to maximize information about communicative disorders in general and hearing function in particular. It is preferable to have objective audiologic data about the child's hearing before the history is obtained.

A behavioral screening audiogram accompanied by a tympanogram (when possible)—including middle ear pressure, the presence or absence of middle ear reflexes, and the volume of the ear canal—is required for patients under six months of age. For those developmentally older than six months of age, it is necessary to have available both an audiometric evaluation of each ear with bone and air conduction and the tympanometric study before the history is taken.

There are instances when the child is unable to complete the initial audiometric evaluation. This in itself is valuable information, for it can reflect the child's development or other social and psychological aspects that may not be readily apparent otherwise.

Observe the child's state of activity as the history is being taken. Spontaneous utterances, the use of language, and the way the child relates to caregivers are all noted. The first question—which is critical—asked by the otolaryngologist is, "Why have you brought the child to be seen?" If the caregiver answers that the child may have a hearing loss, that there may be a delay in speech or language development, or that the child's speech does not seem correct to the caregiver, then we assume that the child has a hearing defect or another communicative disorder—until proven otherwise. The remainder of the evaluation is structured to elicit information concerning such disorders. Normal history and physical examination are compatible with a hearing loss or other communicative disorder(s), and the child must be evaluated by the appropriate objective assessment tools discussed in the other chapters of this handbook.

Initial History

THE history interview is structured to obtain first background and then general information concerning the child, the family, and the environment. The process of deriving this background information allows the otolaryngologist to become familiar with the caregiver and to interpret better the responses to questions. These responses allow the otolaryngologist to interpret accurately what is reported. Some caregivers may enumerate every upper respiratory infection and each temperature elevation, whereas others may mention only casually that the child had meningitis. The details of the *present illness* are drawn out after the otolaryngologist has recorded the background information and, by spending the necessary time, has achieved an understanding of and empathy with the child and family.

The background history begins with an inventory of diseases in the child's family including cancer, heart disease, diabetes, alcoholism, renal disease, and neurological and infectious diseases. Where appropriate, information is obtained about sickle cell disease and other genetically determined hematological disorders.

The caregiver is then asked about infectious diseases the child has had. Several episodes of pneumonia or other infectious disease may indicate an immunological deficiency. These deficiencies can be diagnosed, and knowledge of them will enable the otolaryngologist to provide proper care. A child with ciliary dyskinesia (Kartagener syndrome), for example, will suffer from continual ear infections and require a hearing aid for the restoration of normal hearing in order to enable spoken language development. Tympanostomy tubes are not effective in such cases and, in some instances, may be contraindicated. Children with HIV infections are cared for differently with regard to their hearing problems from those who do not have increased susceptibility to infection.

Injury—especially head trauma—is the next category assessed. There are infants who have had "minor" head trauma resulting in bilateral stapedial footplate subluxation associated with progressive sensorineural hearing loss (SNHL). This portion of the history will note whether the child has sustained a major skull fracture that could be associated with temporal bone fracture or labyrinthine concussion.

The child's operative history is next and includes the age at which procedures were performed and any associated anesthetic complications. The child's hospitalization history is determined: Was the child hospitalized at birth, or has it had other hospitalization? If the child was hospitalized, then the diagnosis, the length of stay, and the name of the hospital are recorded. Hospital records are obtained if there is any suspicion that the child may have been treated with ototoxic medications. These records—especially medication orders and sign-off sheets—are reviewed to ascertain whether the child received no more than the appropriate amounts of ototoxic antibiotics. We also want to know if there was any renal dysfunction; if so, was this compensated for by a reduction of the ototoxic medication? Were blood levels of the ototoxic medication(s) obtained? Were the correct dosages ordered and given as directed? In addition, the nursing notes in a chart will often provide information concerning the child's hearing and language.

REVIEW OF SYSTEMS

THE next portion of the history is the review of the biological systems (Table 3.1). For a child with a suspected hearing loss or other communication disorder, the relevant questions here concern the head, eyes, larynx, pharynx, chest, heart, genitourinary, hemopoietic (formation of blood cells), endocrine, immune, musculoskeletal, and nervous systems. Information concerning the ears is obtained when the present illness information is elicited.

PERSONAL AND SOCIAL HISTORY

THE personal and social history is next. The birthplace of the patient is determined. You may obtain a surprising answer from parents who were in a different and unexpected environment at the time of the child's birth that may have exposed the child to diseases endemic in that part of the world and thus may be related to the suspected hearing loss or communicative disorder.

The caregivers' occupations, which give an indication of their socioeconomic and educational status (SES), are noted. The SES is related to the expected language performance of a child. Children from an average family would be expected to have average linguistic development; children from a family in which the caregivers both have advanced academic degrees should be expected to have linguistic performance above average for their age. Average language

Table 3.1. Review of Systems

Areas of Emphasis for Children with Suspected Hearing Loss or Other Communication Disorder

System	Information to Be Elicited
Head	History of head trauma to include temporal bone fracture.
Eyes	Whether there are any external or internal abnormalities. The child must have a complete ophthalmological examination to determine if there are any changes in the retina that may be compatible with congenital rubella, Usher disease, and so on. Additionally, if the child has a hearing loss or other communication disorder, he or she will be more dependent on vision than others and accordingly must be provided with optimal visual acuity.
Ears	To be ascertained in taking the present illness.
Nose and paranasal sinuses	Breathing patterns and whether there is a history of infections. If so, the possibility of either a structural or humoral defect should be considered. Hyper- or hyponasality is determined. Some hearing–impaired children will be hypernasal.
Mouth and pharynx	Whether there are any congenital abnormalities such as cleft palate. The presence of drooling and the status of the child's chewing and swallowing are noted. If there are abnormalities in this area, these may indicate central nervous system disorder, which may be manifested as abnormalities in speech and articulation. Oral pharyngeal infection may give an indication of immune system abnormality.
Larynx	The presence of hoarseness and whether there has been any history of upper airway obstruction. The quality of the child's voice should be noted.
Chest	The incidence of chest infections is determined.
Cardiac	The presence of congenital malformations is determined. Some of these are associated with specific hearing impairment syndromes such as congenital rubella. There is the rare case of Jervell and Lange Nielsen syndrome, which is characterized by a history of cardiac irregularities and noted by prolonged q-t interval.
Genitourinary	All children who have any malformation of the pinnae and/or the external auditory canal should be screened by ultrasound for urinary tract abnormalities. The history should determine if this has been done. If not, then an ultrasound examination of the urinary tract is obtained. Children with enuresis may have underlying urinary tract disorders. Whether there has been any hematuria should be noted, and if so, a full evaluation should be obtained.
Endocrine	Questions concerning thyroid function will occasionally elicit a family history of goiter or other thyroid abnormality. There will be some children with growth hormone deficiencies, which can be associated with various forms of hearing loss.
Immune system	Specific information as to antibiotics or other medications the child is allergic to must be determined. If the child is said to be allergic, then the form that the allergy takes should be noted. Additionally, the child's allergy history concerning foods and other substances is noted. This information is necessary so that medications can be prescribed. The presence or absence of asthma is noted.
Musculoskeletal	Information concerning the presence of any congenital malformations is sought, especially of the mouth, palate, and limbs.
Central nervous system	The history of epilepsy, including febrile convulsions, is sought. The child's overall development is assessed in this portion of the history. Has the child achieved the proper motor and social development? As age appropriate, does the child feed itself, is it toilet trained, and does it dress itself?

performance in a child who would be expected by reason of the caretakers' SES to be superior may be evidence of a deficit, whether from a hearing loss or other communicative disorder.

PRESENT ILLNESS

THE otolaryngologist, having learned about the child and the family, now obtains information about the present illness (Table 3.2). Its form and content are thus understood in the context of the information already obtained and from the new data that are now acquired.

First, the family history for suspected hearing loss and communicative disorders is determined, since genetics is a major factor in these diseases (see chapter 1). The genetic history is obtained even if there is a presumptive etiological diagnosis, such as meningitis, for one cannot be sure that the presumptive diagnosis is correct; too, there may be more than one problem involved. Thus, a genetic history is taken for all patients. This genetic history begins by noting the number, sex, ages, and health status of siblings, and whether they are affected by a condition similar to the patient's.

Table 3.2. Items for Emphasis in the Present Illness

Area	Emphasis
Family history	Other family members affected with communication disorders History of consanguinity Geographic origin of the families
Prenatal	Congenital infections Abnormalities of pregnancy
Perinatal	Congenital infections Birth weight NICU Ototoxic medications Kernicterus Head trauma Hearing status at birth
Developmental	Changes in hearing: Progressive loss Perilymphatic fistula Congenital/Acquired Genetic/Traumatic Autoimmune disease Changes in language: Regression Hearing loss Language disorder Motor development: Regression Perilymphatic fistula Other
ELM	Benchmark for language development
Final question	"What have I not known to ask?"

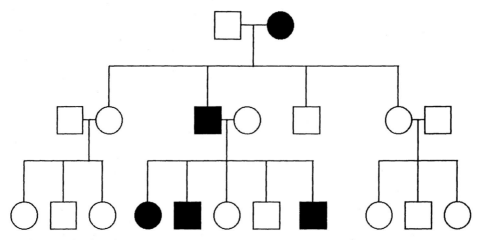

Figure 3.1. A family pedigree

As the genetic history comes to light, a family tree is drawn with the usual symbols: squares for males and circles for females. The parents are asked if they themselves have a similar problem. The family tree is constructed for three generations (as far back as the grandparents) and includes first and second cousins and all children whom the parents may have had by another union (Figure 3.1).

The final question is whether the mother and father are related. Initially, consanguinity is usually denied. Further questioning is directed as to the place of origin of the grandparents or great-grandparents. You may discover that there were common ancestors from a small village from which the patient's forebears emigrated some generations ago, or that there are identical or similar last names in the families of the mother and father—names that originated from the same region, island, district, town, or village. The possibility of cosanguinity is pursued by consultation with older members of the family and family records. If consanguinity is established, then there is greater likelihood of the diagnosis of autosomal recessive disease (Figure 3.2).

Next is child's prenatal history. Specific information concerning maternal infection at the time of pregnancy is recorded as there are still cases of congenital infection including CMV and rubella. Occasionally the mother may have taken a rubella antibody titer at the beginning of the pregnancy; this may have changed from negative to positive during the pregnancy and the information may not have been given to the mother. Congenital rubella is also seen in patients coming from poorer areas of the world.

The perinatal events are noted. These include birth weight, length of labor, complications of delivery, presence of perinatal distress, occurrence of cesarean section (if the last, what were the indications for the cesarean section?). If the child was placed in a Neonatal Intensive Care Unit (NICU), then the details concerning the placement and the course in the NICU are determined. In the NICU,

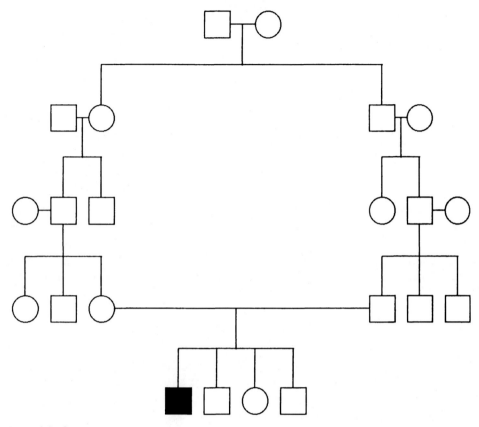

Figure 3.2. Consanguinity

there may have been a sepsis evaluation and treatment with ototoxic antibiotics. If so, or if there is no clear information concerning this, then the records of the NICU hospitalization are obtained and reviewed.

Another perinatal problem is kernicterus, which now rarely results in hearing loss; however, the rarity of the occurrence makes it all the more important for kernicterus to be considered as an etiology of the child's suspected hearing loss or other communicative disorder. Auditory brainstem responses are obtained to determine the physiological integrity of the brainstem's response to sound (see chapter 7). Children with hearing loss as a result of kernicterus may have abnormalities in the interwave latencies of the brain stem response.

Human cytomegalovirus infection (HCMV) may be apparent at birth and manifest itself by low birth weight, petechiae, hepatosplenomegaly, microcephaly, failure to thrive, and positive HCMV cultures. Some children may be congenitally infected but exhibit no symptoms. The diagnosis of asymptomatic congenital HCMV children is made by obtaining an HCMV culture of the child's urine within the first two weeks of life. The asymptomatic congenital HCMV patients often have progressive SNHL (Gerber, Mendel, and Goller 1979). All children with congenital HCMV are at risk for progressive hearing loss and other communicative disorders.

Next we obtain a qualitative description of the receptive and expressive communicative development of the child; a quantitative screen will then constitute the last part of the assessment of the present illness. The initial assessment of the child's expressive and receptive repertory can establish the possibility of progressive disease. The otolaryngologist must try to determine if the child has had hearing and, if so, whether it deteriorated, when this happened, and whether the worsening was associated with otitis media with effusion (OME). Did the hearing return to the pre-OME level? All previous evaluations of the child's hearing or middle ear function (tympanometry) and speech and language development should be reviewed. Often, objective information will be available that can lead to or substantiate a diagnosis of progressive hearing loss.

This information is obtained for all patients as a child with meningitis may have had a hearing loss before the meningitis or a delayed loss following the meningitis; some children with HCMV have progressive losses (Gerber, Mendel, and Goller 1979).

There are two forms of progressive losses in which the hearing loss may sometimes be arrested or, rarely, the hearing partially restored. These occur in cases of children with perilymphatic fistula(e) (PLF) or autoimmune disorders. Perilymphatic fistulae may be genetic (there are twins and brothers and sisters with PLFs), congenital, or acquired (by mild head trauma in an infant or by temporal bone fracture). They may be unilateral or bilateral. The ability to diagnose a PLF in the neonate and the infant depends primarily upon the caregiver's history of an infant who responded to sound for the first few months of life and then responded less or not at all.

In addition, there can be a history of slowing or regression of motor development, which can be a sequela of the abnormal vestibular dysfunction associated with PLF. Older children may graphically describe the vestibular dysfunction as vertigo. Some may also have episodes of severe vomiting that may require hospitalization for fluid replacement. Otitis media with effusion will mask the effects of PLF as the hearing loss from the PLF is mistakenly assumed to be from the OME (Ruben and Yankelowitz 1989). The PLF loss, when measured, is greater than would be expected from OME (>40 dB HL PTA). The OME can be an aid in bringing the child to the point of correct diagnosis.

Besides the worsening of the hearing loss, there may be acute episodes of vestibular symptoms to alert the physician to the problem. These include severe and protracted vomiting with dehydration. Patients have been hospitalized because of the emesis and dehydration when there was no consideration that this was the result of a perilymphatic fistula with an associated OME. These PLFs may present initially as unilateral SNHL. Not until the second ear is affected is the child considered to have a hearing problem; at this point the child undergoes evaluation.

Patients with suspected PLFs are evaluated with a fistula test, and, if results are positive, the PLFs are surgically explored. A negative fistula test does not rule out a PLF. If the fistula test is negative, then a computerized axial tomogram (CAT) is obtained in the sagittal and axial plates to evaluate the osseous structure of the temporal bone. There is some association of an abnormal bony anatomy of the temporal bone, either middle or inner ear, and PLF. If the CAT is abnormal and there is the clinical suggestion of a PLF, then it is reasonable to suspect a PLF; exploration of the more severely affected ear is then indicated.

There are patients with a progressive loss in whom both the fistula test and the temporal bone CAT are normal. If these children do not have HCMV infection or other infections or autoimmune diseases, it is possible that they have a PLF. Any child with an initial history of reasonable hearing development, head trauma, and a subsequent history of hearing loss, defined by audiometric or evoked potential studies, is a child with a probable PLF. It may be associated with major disruption of the oval window and stapedial foot plate and should be surgically explored.

A second treatable cause of progressive sensorineural hearing loss is autoimmune disease(s). This is a group of disorders that is still being defined. Autoimmune disease should be considered if the history is suggestive or if there is documentation of progressive SNHL not associated with PLF or infection. Information concerning the child's allergic history is obtained. Specifically, the otolaryngologist determines whether there are any manifestations of generalized autoimmune disorders such as conjunctivitis, retinitis, arthritis, skin rashes, or gastrointestinal disorders. An occasional child will have one or more of these associated symptoms, but most children do not. The diagnosis depends upon the establishment of an increased titer to inner ear antibodies. The increased inner ear antibody titer is consistent with, but not definitive of, an autoimmune disorder. If the child has a borderline or positive titer, then immunosuppressive therapy is initiated. This therapy has major associated morbidities and should be administered and monitored by a pediatrician who has skills and experience in immune suppression. The otolaryngologist and the audiologist will monitor the hearing of the child so that the pediatrician can be advised as to the effect of the intervention, if any, upon the child's hearing.

LANGUAGE EXAMINATION

THE child's pattern of language development is used to determine what the mode of expressive and receptive communication has been, since some congenitally deaf infants, especially those born into hearing-impaired families, will develop excellent visual communication signs. Children who appear to have adequate hearing and who have not developed language or whose language at first developed but then regressed, must be considered to have intrinsic language disorder(s). The history of some language development to the first or second year of life followed by regression or loss of language is a critical symptom that can be caused by hearing loss or may be associated with autism or other central nervous system dysfunction. These patients need accurate and precise evaluation of their hearing capability.

If the hearing is normal or minimally depressed, then the diagnosis lies in the linguistic domain, and the children are evaluated by the language pathologist and the pediatric neurologist. The language of language-impaired children is more affected by modest hearing losses than that of children who are without language deficiencies. These language-impaired children require close monitoring of their hearing. If there are hearing losses associated with OME or other diseases, then the loss must be corrected to afford the child optimal hearing.

While you are obtaining the present illness data, other items of information will become apparent; the form of the present illness data is therefore structured to take advantage of all the information that is available. Questions are repeated in various ways to confirm what has been said and to elicit more information. Often the two parents or a grandparent may report a different scenario; each version is recorded and evaluated. No one is wrong, for they have all observed the child in their own ways and have their own internal measures about what is expected and what has happened. Some of the most difficult interviews can occur with couples who are becoming or who have been divorced. The otolaryngologist is the patient's advocate and must record and evaluate all the information nonjudgmentally. This may require two separate histories and separate telephone conversations with each parent.

When all the information concerning the present illness has been elicited, an objective and quantitative language screen of expressive and receptive language and speech is administered. There are several tests available, and experience with the Early Language Milestone Scale (ELM) (Coplan 1993; Coplan and Gleason 1982) has shown its utility in an otological setting. The test has good sensitivity and specificity as a screen for patients from birth to 36 months of age and requires only a few minutes to conduct. In our clinics, an ELM is completed for every patient who is seen from newborn to 36 months of age. It gives an objective measure of the child's language and speech development. If the test results indicate delays in receptive or expressive language or in speech development, then further definitive evaluation is carried out by the speech-language pathologist.

The ELM profile obtained at the initial visit serves as a benchmark for all further visits, enabling the effect of interventions to be measured by the outcome of language and speech development. The object of the restoration of hearing in a neonate, infant, toddler, or preschooler is the optimal development of language. The outcome of any intervention is the effect upon the language. As children are treated and cared for, their progress will be assessed with the ELM. If a child is not progressing in language development, then we must consider whether the interventions are effective or whether the diagnosis is correct. The ELM is obtained for oral language as there is no standard for sign language in the ELM. The use of signs can be indicated on the ELM form, and the development of sign language as noted by expressive and receptive signs can be followed.

The final question asked at the end of the present illness examination is: "What have I not known to ask about?" The caregivers have known their children for their entire lives, and the otolaryngologist has known this complex human being for only a few minutes. Often there is a relevant chunk of information that the caregivers have that has not been elucidated by the history. This is to be expected because the history uses a vocabulary that is not familiar to all even though we make every attempt to use terms that will be understood clearly. The final question is also critical when the history is taken through a translator since much of the otolaryngologist's meaning may be lost or changed in translation to another language, including sign language.

PHYSICAL EXAMINATION

THE strategy underlying the physical examination is to obtain as much information as possible from the patient. Crying by an infant may reveal a functioning larynx but does not give much information about the tympanic membrane, tongue control, or ability to communicate. The examination is necessary so that essential information can be obtained from a cooperative child.

There are different techniques for each age. Neonates and infants may sleep. All neonates, infants, and most toddlers should be examined in their caregiver's lap as this is a familiar and calming environment, and the child is not separated from the caregiver.

If the ears are critical to the examination, then the otoscopic examination is carried out first. If the child awakens and begins to cry, the tympanic membranes will become erythematous and will not appear normal. Infants and toddlers who are awake often like to follow the light of the otoscope. Once they have played with the otoscope and perhaps examined their doll (or the examiner) with it, the otoscope becomes a familiar and safe object that is tolerated, and the examination can be completed.

Great care is taken not to hurt the child. This is especially important if there is cerumen in the external canal. Unless it is essential to do so, it should not be removed. Most often a small, normal segment of the tympanic membrane can be seen. If there is no indication of middle ear pathology from the tympanogram, audiogram, or the patient's history, it is usually best to leave the cerumen in place. If the entire external canal or the tympanic membrane needs to be visualized, the cerumen must be removed. The least traumatic method for doing so is usually with a 1:1 water and hydrogen peroxide solution at body temperature so as not to stimulate the vestibular system. Even this will be threatening and disruptive for the infant, toddler, or child. Sometimes the cerumen may have to be removed to complete the audiometric examination, and at other times the

Figure 3.3. Normal landmarks of the normal ear drum as seen when viewing anterior, medially, and posterior. The tympanic membrane is translucent; structures illustrated should be seen.

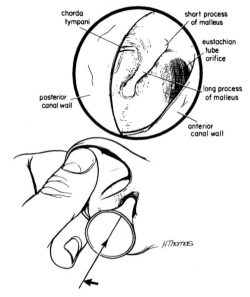

Figure 3.3a. Anterior view

cerumen may account for a conductive loss. In the latter instance, the correction of the conductive loss should be verified by repeating the appropriate portion of the audiogram.

Examination of the ears begins with a visualization of the pinnae and the surrounding area. Are there abnormalities of the pinnae such as brachial cleft sinuses (preauricular pits) or other malformations? These may be associated with congenital middle ear, ossicular malformations, and congenital or progressive conductive loss. They are also associated with urinary tract malformations; thus, if they are observed, ultrasound examination of the urinary tract should be performed. The diameter of the external auditory canal should be noted and the presence of any abnormalities such as fistulae, masses, or dehiscences should be determined.

The tympanic membrane is examined for its normalcy. The normal tympanic membrane is semitransparent, and most of the following structures can be seen through the normal tympanic membrane (Figure 3.3):

1. Cephalad and ventral: the shadow of the eustachian tube orifice;

2. Cephalad two-thirds and in the middle of the tympanic membrane: the umbo of the malleus;

3. Cephalad, dorsal, and almost parallel to the malleus: the long process of the incus;

4. Lateral to the long process of the incus and medial to the umbo of the malleus; perpendicular to both is the chorda tympani;

5. Medial to the long process of the incus are the crurae of the stapes; and

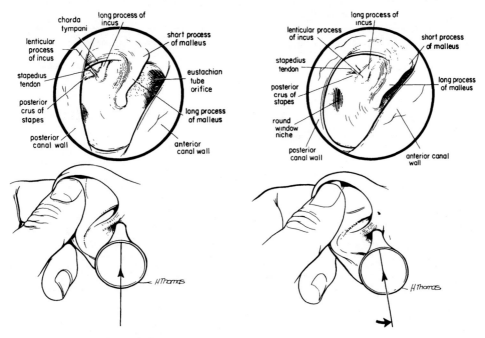

Figure 3.3b. Medial view   Figure 3.3c. Posterior view

6. Caudal and slightly ventral to the long process of the incus and the head of the stapes is the shadow of the round window niche.

An observer who has practiced looking for these landmarks will be able to identify many of them in children with normal middle ears. A child who has been crying will usually have an erythematous tympanic membrane that will not be translucent. The change in the tympanic membrane will decrease the oto-laryngologist's ability to observe the normal landmarks, making diagnosis more difficult. The lack of, or malpositioning of, one or more of these landmarks may be associated with a congenital malformation or an acquired condition such as necrosis of the long process of the incus. The presence of middle ear effusion is seen as distortion in the position of the tympanic membrane and as changes in the color or the translucency of the tympanic membrane.

Pneumatic otoscopy has a limited use. If there is a suspicion of middle ear fluid, the gentle movement of the tympanic membrane with the pneumatic oto-scope may help to support this diagnosis. Younger children poorly tolerate the use of the pneumatic otoscope, and its use may prejudice further examinations.

The remainder of the head and neck is examined (Table 3.3), including the head, hair, external eyes, face, nose, mouth, pharynx, neck, and when indicated, the nasopharynx and larynx. The nasopharynx and larynx are examined with the flexible pediatric laryngoscope. This can be done at any age. Children older than 42 months of age will usually be cooperative if properly anesthetized. This

Table 3.3. Physical Examination

Structure	Technique	Comment
The Child	Sit in caretaker's lap	Relate to child and do not hurt the child as crying will change the examination and make subsequent examinations more difficult.
Pinnae	Direct observation	Abnormalities may be associated with urinary tract malformations.
External Auditory Canal	Direct observation or otoscopy	Abnormalities may be associated with urinary tract malformations.
Cerumen	Direct observation or otoscopy	Removed only if the tympanic membrane is totally occluded and/or there is a need for more information about the tympanic membrane or if the cerumen is thought to be a cause or a contributing factor of the hearing loss. Avoid instruments and use irrigation.
Tympanic membrane	Otoscope or microscope	Make a drawing of the findings and note how many normal structures can be seen. The microscope is useful in looking for mass medial to the tympanic membranes, such as congenital cholesteatoma, and for confirming ossicular abnormalities. The microscope can be used in children over 12 months and in sleeping neonates and infants. Pneumotoscopy can be used to further support the diagnosis of OME, tympanic membrane retraction, and ossicular disruption and is confirmatory of tympanometric findings.
Head	Direct observation, palpation, and a measuring tape	Observe for proper closure of the fontanelle, head size, and general shape.
Hair	Direct observation	Observe for white forelock, which is associated with Waardenburg syndrome, and other hair abnormalities that have a genetic association.
Face	Direct observation	Symmetry for facial nerve function. Note other abnormalities that may indicate a syndrome such as partial paresis, found in Goldenhar or Mobius syndrome. Facial dysmorphology can also suggest such syndromes as Treacher Collins sequence and others.
Eyes	Direct observation	Note the color of the iris, which may suggest Waardenburg syndrome. A conjunctivitis would be compatible with autoimmune disorders. Spontaneous nystagmus may be found with an active perilymphatic fistula. Strabismus should be noted so that it may be corrected. Cataracts associated with congenital rubella can usually be seen by direct inspection.
Nose	Direct inspection of the nares with and without closure of the nostrils and a laryngeal mirror	The use of nasal sounds such as "catch a fish" or "Susie's slippers" in the toddler or preschool child will give information on the possibility of velopharyngeal insufficiency. If the child has hyponasality with these expressions, velopharyngeal insufficiency can be suspected. The child should also be asked to say the letter "m." The child is asked again, this time with his nares gently closed. If there is no change in the sound of the "m," this is consistent with hyponasality. Whether or not the nose and/or the choanae are open is tested with a laryngeal mirror. The mirror is placed about 3 mm below each nostril. On exhalation, the mirror will fog if there is air going through that nostril. If it does not, the nostril may be clogged by mass in the nose, choanae, and/or nasopharynx.

is done with the use of Pontocaine sprayed in the mouth and pharynx and with Pontocaine-impregnated cotinoid strips placed in each nares for five to ten minutes. The examination should be carried out with the endoscope attached to a television recording camera because this will provide a permanent record; an additional advantage is to enable the child to follow and participate in the examination.

Observation of the pharyngeal opening of the eustachian tube, the soft palate, the movements of the pharynx and the larynx are important in children with hearing loss and other communicative disorders. Children with possible articulation defects may also have associated swallowing disorders; the action of the larynx and the cricopharyngeus can also be observed with the flexible laryngoscope. The larynx is observed for its anatomical and physiological integrity.

FURTHER STUDIES: THE "WORK UP"

COMPLETION of the history and physical examination can allow the otolaryngologist to make a differential diagnosis of the cause of the hearing loss or other communication disorder. The need for and sequencing of additional information is predicated upon what is considered in the differential diagnosis. The studies required and their sequencing are individualized for each child. The sequencing of studies is carried out to eliminate the more probable or treatable conditions that may need immediate attention.

Children with progressive or suspected progressive losses are those for whom therapy, surgical (PLF) or medical (autoimmune), may be able to arrest the loss and occasionally to restore hearing. These patients must have the etiology promptly defined. The fistula test is one of the most important for children with progressive loss or those who are suspected of having a PLF. The test should be done in a matter of days; if the fistula test is positive, there is a high likelihood of finding a perilymphatic fistula that must be repaired. The repair of the fistula may stop progression of the loss and, in a few children, restore hearing sensitivity and improve speech discrimination. Because of the critical time factor in working with a fistula, the fistula test is done before many of the other necessary studies.

A second treatable cause of progressive SNHL is autoimmune disease. Antibody titers to inner ear tissue are obtained from children with a suggestive history of autoimmune disease. All of these children will also undergo fistula testing. Almost all children with progressive loss, in whom the fistula test is negative, will have autoimmune antibody studies and a CAT scan of their ears to determine whether there are abnormalities of the bony structure of the middle or inner ear.

All the children with hearing loss or the suggestion of hearing loss as determined from auditory screening will have a complete evaluation of their auditory systems (Gravel 1989). This will include assessment of the external and middle

ear by immitance, which includes a tympanogram, measurement of the middle
ear pressure, middle ear muscle reflex, external canal and middle ear volume,
and, where possible, some measure of eustachian tube function (see chapter 6).
Outer hair cell function is assessed with evoked otoacoustic emissions (chapter 8); eighth nerve and brainstem with the use of auditory evoked brainstem potentials (chapter 7); and the cerebral cortex using the cortical evoked potentials.
The cortical evoked potentials may be further utilized to assess the efficacy of
hearing aids.

The evaluation of the language of infants, toddlers, and preschoolers is essential to the care of children with hearing loss or other communication disorders. The most important outcome measure of the care of hearing loss or other
communicative disorders in the neonate, infant, toddler, and preschooler is the
child's language. The precise and accurate evaluation of the child's language
provides the basis for care of the child. This evaluation provides an initial measure so that the otolaryngologist and all others caring for the child can tell
whether the interventions have been useful in achieving language proficiency.
Although the hearing may be improved, the language may not be improved and
must be monitored periodically.

Language evaluation will also provide additional information necessary for
the care of the child. It may determine the diagnosis, especially in those children
who are found to have normal peripheral hearing. It will also determine which
areas of language are deficient and will dictate the language intervention with
the appropriate therapies available for the different types of language disorders.

Speech evaluations are carried out in all age-appropriate cases. Abnormal
speech is more noticeable to caregivers than is abnormal language. Speech development is of critical importance, yet language development is the more fundamental issue. There may be instances in which resources will not permit both
speech and language interventions; at such times, it is preferable to emphasize
language. Once this is secured, then speech can be attended to.

Table 3.4 presents the strategies and tactics used in obtaining additional information that will aid in the care of the child's hearing loss or other communication disorders. The individuality of patients requires that the evaluation be specifically developed in each case. There is no one recipe that can be unilaterally
applied. Otolaryngologists must use their clinical knowledge to shape an effective and efficient scenario, so that the possibilities for restoration or maintenance
of function, primarily language communication, are optimized for each patient.

CONCLUSION

THE information that has been obtained about each patient must be documented and shared with the caregivers of the child. This can be accomplished through a structured informational conference. The primary caregivers
and other interested parties such as grandparents discuss the findings with the

Table 3.4. "The Work-Up": Assessments

Assessment	Who	When and Why
HEARING ASSESSMENTS		
Tympanometry	All	At first visit and at all hearing evaluations; need to know the status of the middle ear
Behavioral audiogram	Those greater than 6 months of age	At first visit and at all hearing evaluations; establish baseline to monitor for changes
Evoked and/or spontaneous cochlear emissions	Those with or suspected of having sensorineural hearing losses	During the course of the evaluations; will allow for differential of outer hair cell loss
Auditory Brain Stem Evoked Potentials	Those with suspected sensorineural hearing loss and all who do not have reliable behavioral test data. Also those with language disorders.	As soon as possible for cases in which there is not an accurate behavioral assessment and for others during the course of the work-up. The exception is any child with a suspected cerebral angle tumor, such as involved in von Recklinghausen II. Gives an air and bone conduction threshold in children who cannot be tested behaviorally; supplies information that is confirmatory of the behavioral studies; supplies information concerning the neural integrity of the statoacoustic nerve and the brainstem.
Auditory Cortical Evoked Potentials: responses to phonemes	Those with suspected sensorineural hearing losses; with conductive or mixed losses that may require hearing aids (e.g., congenital malformations) and language impaired children	During the course of the work-up or after the hearing aids or other habilitative devices have been used for several months; this will give information on the cortical response to phonemes and the efficacy of the hearing aids or other device.
Audiological assessment of family members	All those suspected of genetic disease	During the course of the work-up; to identify other affected family members, especially younger siblings, and to detect carriers to secure a diagnosis
VESTIBULAR ASSESSMENTS		
Fistula test	All with suspected or documented progressive sensorineural hearing loss	As soon as possible; will be critical in determining whether surgical intervention is to be carried out
Electronystagmographic analysis of vestibular function	All with suspected sensory or neural hearing loss	If not progressive, then during the period of data gathering. Occasionally a positive fistula will be detected. This assessment includes optokinetic, calorics, and rotary chair response; information will be obtained about brainstem integrity and the function of each vestibular labyrinth. Children who have little or abnormal labyrinth function may have delayed motoric development that could be mistaken for mental retardation.
OTHER MEDICAL ASSESSMENTS		
Ophthalmological	All with permanent or probable permanent hearing loss	During the course of the work-up; to determine the visual status and note any ophthalmological stigmata that would be diagnosed (e.g., retinitis pigmentosa)

(continued)

Table 3.4., *continued*

Assessment	Who	When and Why
OTHER MEDICAL ASSESSMENTS, *continued*		
Pediatric neurology	Children with suspected primary language or cognitive disorders; those with other neurological signs or symptoms (e.g., seizures)	During the course of the work-up; those children with normal peripheral hearing should be seen promptly so that a definitive diagnosis can be supported and intervention undertaken.
Genetics	All those with definite genetic history, all who are syndromic, and all for whom an etiology cannot be determined	During the course of the work-up; to provide a confirmation of the genetic disease; provide detailed genetic information and genetic counselling
Pediatric urology	Those with proven or suspected urological abnormalities	After there is information concerning the existence or the probable existence of a urological abnormality; to provide urological diagnosis and care
SPEECH AND LANGUAGE ASSESSMENTS		
Speech and language pathology	All those with hearing losses and/or communication disorders	Those with known hearing loss during the course of the evaluations. Those who have probable normal peripheral hearing should be seen as soon as possible; this evaluation provides a baseline for language and speech; definition of the types of language and speech abnormalities that will determine the type of intervention needed
IMAGING		
Computerized Axial Tomography (CAT) scan	Suspected or known middle or inner ear malformations, candidates for cochlear implants, postmeningitis, progressive losses with negative fistula test, and/or negative autoimmune antibodies	During the course of the work-up. Those with progressive losses may have a CAT after a negative fistula test but before the report of autoimmune antibody is returned. This is especially so in ears that show rapid progressive loss. The children who have had meningitis should be examined within several months after the meningitis for ossification of the labyrinth. All children who are cochlear implant candidates have a CAT before implantation; malformations of the middle ear may not be examined until surgery is considered, which is not until at least 5 or 6 years of age as there is little that can be done with the information in the early years; as time progresses, there will be improvements in the quality of the images (e.g., 3-d virtual images of the bony integrity of the inner and middle ear)
Magnetic Resonance Imaging (MRI)	Children suspected of having neural pathology, such as those with von Recklinghausen II	After the diagnosis of probable neural involvement from a family history and/or an abnormal evoked auditory brainstem response or as indicated from a behavioral audiogram—integrity of the central nervous system including the eighth nerve (acoustic and vestibular portions)

(*continued*)

Table 3.4., *continued*

Assessment	Who	When and Why
IMAGING, continued		
Ultrasound of the genitourinary tract	Children with malformations of the pinnae, external auditory canals, and/or the middle ear	During the course of the work-up—integrity of the genitourinary system
BLOOD AND SERUM STUDIES		
Autoimmune antibodies	Patients with progressive losses when the fistula test is negative or there is a suspicion of autoimmune disease	As soon as possible; probability or possibility of autoimmune disease
TORCH Titers (Toxoplasmosis, rubella, syphilis, cytomegalovirus, herpes)	As indicated from the history and/or the physical examination	During the course of the work-up; enable a diagnosis and give the precise prognosis and information, especially in congenital rubella
Renal function	Patients suspected of parenchymal renal disease from history (e.g., Alport syndrome)	During the course of the work-up; confirm diagnosis and allow for referral and intervention
Immune profile (IgG, IgE, IgA, and white blood cells studies, sedimentation rate, differential, and white blood cell count)	Children suspected of immunological defects, as evidenced by increased number of infections, including meningitis.	During work-up; define the immune status of the child
CULTURES		
Urine for cytomegalovirus	Children with progressive sensory neural loss suspected of CMV infection	During the course of the work-up; to define the possible cause of the progressive loss and possible intervention
OTHER		
Urine analysis	Children suspected of having parenchymal renal disease from history (e.g., Alport syndrome)	During the course of the work-up; enable a diagnosis
Electrocardiogram	Those suspected of cardiac abnormality	During the course of the work-up; to detect treatable conduction defects
Medical records	Patients suspected of having received ototoxic medication	During the course of the work-up; to determine if proper dosage was given
Mouth, palate, and tongue	Direct observation and digital palpation	The presence of drooling can indicate neurological abnormality, which may account for an articulation defect. The mouth is inspected for any masses, clefts of the palate, and bifid uvula, which is associated with the submucosal cleft of *(continued)*

Table 3.4., *continued*

Assessment	Who	When and Why
	OTHER, *continued*	
		the palate. The size of the tonsils is noted to see if they are occluding the airway. The palate is palpated to note if there is dehiscence in the dorsal portion of the bony palate, which would also indicate a submucosal cleft of the palate. The tongue is watched to note if there are any fasciculations, which may be associated with articulatory and other speech deficits.
Larynx	Listening to the vocalizations, auscultation with a stethoscope, and examination with a flexible laryngoscope	The quality of the vocalizations is noted. An observer can hear hoarseness or inappropriate pitches that are indications of intrinsic laryngeal abnormality. A small stethoscope is used to auscultate the larynx. Ordinarily, almost no sounds are heard on inspiration or expiration. A child with intrinsic laryngeal abnormality may have readily aparent inspiratory and/or expiratory sounds on auscultation. The use of the flexible laryngoscope is discussed in the text.
Neck	Direct observation	Branchial clefts and sinus that can occur with middle ear malformation are noted.

people who evaluated the child: the audiologists, speech-language pathologists, otolaryngologists, and other healthcare providers. The conference centers around the findings of the healthcare team, the prescribed therapy for the child, and the possible consequences for the child and the family.

The conference will take time and cannot be rushed. A method that has proven satisfactory is to hold the conference in the evening. At this time the healthcare providers have fewer other duties, all the caregivers may be able to come, and there is little constraint on the time spent in transferring and explaining all the information and responding to questions. A written record of the conference is placed in the child's chart with a copy sent to the caregivers.

REFERENCES

Coplan, J. 1993. *Early language milestone scale.* 2d ed. Austin: Pro-Ed.

Coplan J., and J. Gleason. 1982. Validation of early language milestone scale in high-risk population. *Pediatrics* 70:677.

Gerber, S.E., M.I. Mendel, and M. Goller. 1979. Progressive hearing loss subsequent to congenital cytomegalovirus infection. *Human Communication* 4:231–234.

Gravel, J.S., ed. 1989. Assessing auditory system integrity in high-risk infants and young children. *Seminars in Hearing* 10:213–292.

Ruben, R.J. 1991. Language screening as a factor in the management of the pediatric otolaryngic patient. *Archives of Otolaryngology–Head and Neck Surgery* 117:1021–1025.

Ruben, R.J., and S.M. Yankelowitz. 1989. Spontaneous perilymphatic fistula in children. *American Journal of Otology* 10:198–207.

4

Behavioral Observation and Visual Reinforcement Audiometry

Allan O. Diefendorf and Judith S. Gravel

INTRODUCTION

THE early detection of hearing loss has been emphasized for more than four decades. As a result, the screening of auditory function in infants and young children has received considerable attention during the past thirty years. Test procedures have been investigated in clinical and laboratory settings in an attempt to identify and specify the procedure that could detect hearing loss at the earliest possible age.

In the early 1960s, clinicians were actively pursuing behavioral and electrophysiologic test procedures for identifying hearing loss in infants. Marion Downs and her associates (e.g., Downs and Sterritt 1964, 1967) in Denver were attempting neonatal screening using a method of behavioral observation audiometry called the arousal test. Due to the large number of false positive identifications and the unnecessary parental anxiety that resulted, behavioral screening during the newborn period was not supported. Hallowell Davis and his group (Davis and Onishi 1969; Davis and Zerlin 1966) at the Central Institute for the Deaf were working on a physiologic measure called the late cortical, or V, potential as a vehicle for "objective audiometry." However, for predicting hearing levels in infants, the late V potential was limited because it was so state dependent.

In 1969, the national Joint Committee on Newborn Hearing Screening (now the Joint Committee on Infant Hearing) was formed. It had representatives from the American Academy of Ophthalmology and Otolaryngology, the American Academy of Pediatrics, and the American Speech and Hearing Association. From available clinical reports and laboratory data, the Joint Committee issued the following statement (1972): "In light of the urgent need to detect hearing impairment as early as possible, the Joint Committee urges further investigation of screening methods but discourages routine hearing screening which is not research oriented." Thus, a focus on the importance of early identification of hearing loss was maintained by the Joint Committee; however, the lack of an appropriate test procedure for identifying hearing loss in infants was clearly recognized.

Subsequently, attempts were made to develop, refine, and improve behavioral and electrophysiologic screening procedures. In the behavioral domain, this led to detailed procedures for calibrating the signal precisely (Thompson and Thompson 1972), attempting to calibrate the observer precisely (Mencher et al. 1977; Weber 1969), and attempting to define the state of the neonate (Downs 1976; Eisenberg 1969) as rigorously as possible. More pervasive clinical concerns, however, still centered on the excessive false positive and false negative outcomes from behavioral screening. Concomitantly, the search for more objective methods resulted in attempts to define auditory function based on cardiotachometry (Schulman 1973) and respiration audiometry (Bradford 1975). These physiologic methods, as well as auditory evoked potentials (middle, late, and slow cortical responses), however, were not embraced by clinicians for use with the pediatric population.

An important milestone occurred in 1974 when Hecox and Galambos showed the value of the auditory brainstem response (ABR) for screening auditory sensitivity in newborns. This, of course, set off the modern era of auditory evoked potentials that ultimately revolutionized both hearing screening and assessment in the newborn period and early infancy (see chapter 7).

Advances in behavioral hearing assessment paralleled this progress in auditory electrophysiology. Before about 1974, it was generally believed that only gross behavioral hearing tests could be obtained on infants two years of age and younger. Refinements in methodology began to emerge that capitalized on the interests and abilities of infants. A new view of infants was advanced that recognized infants as active receptors of auditory information who, if given the chance, interact with their acoustic environment. In turn, it became possible to obtain a rather complete behavioral assessment of auditory function in infants six months through two years of age.

Despite advances in behavioral and electrophysiologic evaluation of auditory function throughout the 1970s, the decade of the '80s revealed an alarming statistic. Despite a focus on improved assessment procedures, the average age of identification for severe hearing loss in the United States remained constant at about 2½ years of age (Bergstrom 1984; Stein, Clark, and Kraus 1983; Stein et al. 1990). Lesser degrees of impairment were going undetected even longer. The result was that, for many infants and young children with hearing loss, much of the crucial period for speech and oral language learning was lost.

Consequently, our focus for the 1990s is two-fold. First, our goal is to develop comprehensive early identification programs that are accessible to all newborns, committed to providing appropriate follow-up for all failures, and to the provision of family-centered intervention services in accordance with Part H of the Individuals with Disabilities Education Act (IDEA). Much of this focused energy on early identification will be fostered by the national initiative, "Healthy People 2000," that has established a goal of reducing the average age of identification of hearing loss in children from 2½ years to 12 months (1990). Our second area of focus is to provide in-depth, timely audiologic assessments of infants and young children delineating the type, degree, and pattern of any hearing loss for each ear. Such comprehensive assessment allows appropriate intervention services to be initiated, be they communicative, medical, prosthetic, or educational.

The purpose of this chapter is to focus on behavioral test procedures and provide a framework for their appropriate application. Clearly, for newborns and very young infants (four months and under), the auditory screening procedure of choice will be selected from one or both of two electrophysiologic procedures. These are auditory brainstem response audiometry (see chapter 7) or evoked otoacoustic emissions (see chapter 8). However, both procedures have some inherent limitations for use in assessment. For example, neither procedure easily allows specific frequency-by-intensity threshold information necessary for a complete description of hearing loss. In addition, many problems of these procedures as screening tools (e.g., activity level, length of test, expense) are compounded for older infants. For example, the need for sedation, prolonged test time, and cost associated with the ABR in a follow-up clinic are likely to be questioned in today's healthcare environment. Evoked otoacoustic emissions (EOAEs), while present with normal hearing to mild hearing loss, are obliterated by more severe degrees of sensory impairments. Their value in hearing screening is obvious; however, they may not offer the specificity necessary for delineating many forms of hearing loss.

Fortunately, infants who are at risk for hearing loss and who require follow-up or infants for whom an assessment of hearing is recommended can be tested efficiently and effectively with behavioral test methods. Refinements in behavioral methods coupled with a better understanding of auditory abilities in infants elevates behavioral testing to "first alternative" status for most diagnostic assessments. Indeed, many early identification programs may also incorporate behavioral screening, for example, those that identify acquired permanent or transient hearing loss. Beyond the time, cost, and ease of administration, the most important advantage of behavioral test methods is that they allow infants and young children to demonstrate actively what they perceive. This allows a valid description of their functional hearing abilities. Visual Reinforcement Audiometry (VRA) and Behavioral Observation Audiometry (BOA) are two procedures available to clinicians for use with infants and children of various ages and developmental levels for whom definition of thresholds and auditory responsiveness are necessary for educational (habilitational) planning.

Underlying this chapter is also the authors' belief that testing auditory function in infants and young children is a process driven by professional setting, program goals, and population characteristics. As such, choices in service delivery for screening, assessment, follow-up, and intervention are individually based and family focused. Once our goals, objectives, and supporting rationale are clearly formulated, then the selection of appropriate procedures is greatly simplified.

VISUAL REINFORCEMENT AUDIOMETRY

NORMALLY developing infants make head turns toward a sound source in the first few months of life. This localization response represents a behavioral "window" through which many aspects of auditory behavior can be studied. Although there is an obvious tendency for infants to turn initially toward interesting or novel auditory stimuli, there is a limit to the number of times head turns will occur to repeated stimuli (Moore, Thompson, and Thompson 1975; Moore, Wilson, and Thompson 1977). From a hearing assessment standpoint, habituation of response to repeated stimulus presentations is undesirable because it reduces the number of stimulus trials available for threshold determination.

To overcome the restrictions imposed by habituation, it is possible to approach the behavioral assessment of hearing in infants and young children through an operant conditioning paradigm, specifically, through use of an operant discrimination procedure. In an operant discrimination procedure, the stimulus cues the child that a response will result in reinforcement. Operant behavior is increased by the application of positive reinforcement. Thus, it is possible to increase the rate of response if a positive reinforcer can be identified and used. Since audible signals of the type used in assessing auditory function are known to have little reinforcing value in children (Moore, Thompson, and Thompson 1975; Moore, Wilson, and Thompson 1977), it is best to use a test procedure in which the signal and reinforcer are separate and the signal serves only to cue the youngster that a correct response will result in reinforcement.

The foundation for work on VRA was laid by Suzuki and Ogiba in 1960, and the label was coined in 1969 by Lidén and Kankkunen. The technique was studied and refined at the University of Washington (Moore, Wilson, and Thompson 1977; Wilson 1978; Wilson and Thompson 1984) and has become widely used in clinical practice. Visual reinforcement audiometry has emerged as a valid and reliable procedure for infants and young children, 5½ months through two years of age. In VRA, conditioned head turns (localization of a sound source in a sound field and a conditioned behavior under earphones) are reinforced by an attractive three-dimensional animated toy. The success of VRA is certainly related to the fact that the response (head turn) and reinforcer (animated toy) are well suited to the developmental level of children between these ages.

Operant Behavior

Operant behavior is frequently spoken of as willful or purposeful behavior. A behavioral response elicited by a stimulus is controlled by the consequence of

Table 4.1. Influence of Reinforcement on Operant Behavior

	PRESENT	WITHDRAW
POSITIVE REINFORCEMENT	Increases response probability	Decreases response probability
NEGATIVE REINFORCEMENT	Decreases response probability	Increases response probability

the behavior. Operant behavior is increased or decreased in frequency by the changes it brings about in the organism's environment. The events in an environment may be classified as positive reinforcers, negative reinforcers, and neutral events. Neutral events have little or no specific effect on behavior. Depending on the application of negative or positive reinforcement, the response probability effect can be either increased or decreased (Table 4.1).

In VRA, the frequency of head turn responses is increased because the behavior of head turning results in a pleasurable visual event (positive reinforcement). Visual reinforcement audiometry employs an operant discrimination paradigm in which the auditory test signal serves as a discriminative stimulus. This cues the child that a response (head turn) will produce reinforcement or a desirable event (in this case, the lighting and activation of the toy). *Conditioning* refers to the process of training or shaping the desired behavior.

Personnel and Equipment

Accurate VRA assessment depends in large part on the ability of an examiner to keep an infant appropriately attentive during the stages of operant conditioning and response acquisition (i.e., audiometry). Program choices and budgetary considerations relating to personnel and equipment determine whether testing can be done by one examiner or whether two examiners will be required.

Figures 4.1, 4.2a, and 4.2b show a room arrangement incorporating two examiners. The examiner in the control room has full view of the testing situation and activates the auditory stimulus and visual reinforcer. A second examiner, seated at the infant's side, maintains the infant's head in a midline position by encouraging the child to observe passively or play with colorful, non-noisy toys. The use of two examiners, however, reduces the efficiency of VRA. When limitations exist regarding personnel or when cost considerations preclude the use of two examiners, a remote audiometer switching apparatus or a personal computer puts control of the equipment into the hands of one audiologist who can be in direct contact with the child (see Figure 4.3).

Whether one examiner or two, response behavior is enhanced by an examiner's direct interaction with an infant for maintaining the infant's head in a

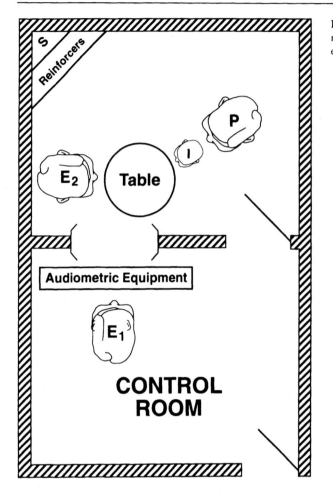

Figure 4.1. VRA procedure: Test room arrangement with two examiners.

S = Speaker
E₁ and E₂ = Examiners
P = Parent
I = Infant

midline position. That is, if the youngster under test shows too much interest in the colorful, non-noisy toys, the potential exists for no response during a signal trial or for elevated response levels due to decreased attention. On the other hand, if the youngster under test shows no interest or is bored with the colorful, non-noisy toys, false responses may occur regularly. When in the test room, an examiner can choose from a variety of toys available and judge when a toy change in either direction (more entertaining or less entertaining) may be necessary to maintain the child's midline position and optimum response state. A single examiner in the control room can use a "centering toy" positioned at midline in the test room for maintaining a child's midline position. However, this

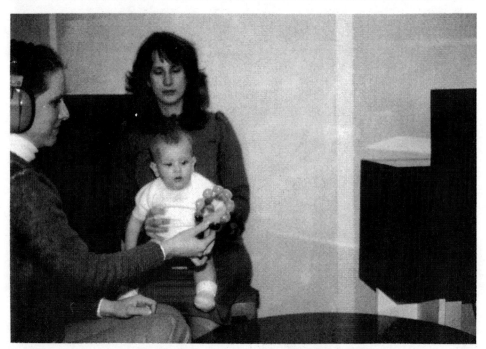

Figure 4.2a. VRA procedure: Assistant maintains the infant's attention at midline.

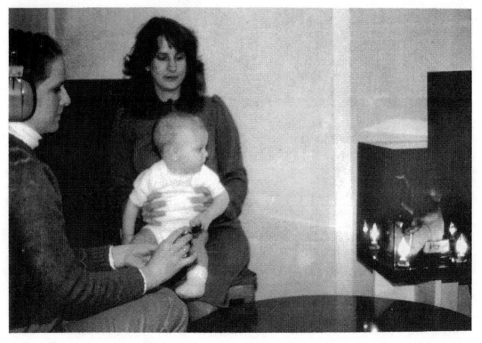

Figure 4.2b. VRA procedure: Head turn response.

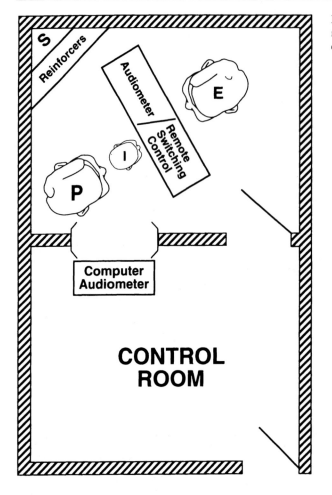

Figure 4.3. VRA procedure: Test room arrangement with one examiner.

S = Speaker
E = Examiner
P = Parent
I = Infant

approach removes the examiner from the test room, creates noisy competition with both the test signal and the novelty of the reinforcer, and eliminates the examiner's ability to control the infant's interest level.

Transducers

Conventionally, estimates of auditory thresholds are obtained using standard earphones (TDH-49 or TDH-50) and bone oscillators (Radioear B-70A) to obtain ear-specific information about hearing loss type, degree, and pattern. The use of a standard earphone and cushion assembly is recommended in pediatric assessment; however, for small heads, soft support padding between the head-band and the top of the head is highly desirable. This allows the assembly to fit comfortably and aligns the earphone diaphragm with the baby's ear canal open-ing. An infant headband or similar padding is used for bone oscillator place-ment. The availability of insert receivers coupled to an appropriately-sized ear tip can also be used with infants. These same transducers are also used during ABR assessment, allowing comparisons of test results. The term *threshold* can be used to describe the responses obtained from infants whenever a psycho-physical procedure, a predetermined step-size, and a specified number of re-sponse reversals are utilized. Infants' thresholds may improve slightly with age, primarily due to changes in attention and motivation. Thresholds may also be influenced by size changes in the external auditory canal and pinnae and inade-quate transducer-coupling effects. The term *minimum auditory response level* (MRL) is used when no prespecified psychophysical procedure is utilized in as-sessment. Minimum auditory response level represents the lowest or "best" re-sponse obtained from the infant for a given stimulus.

Most often, it is the older infant or toddler who may be resistant to the placement of the headset. However, activation of the visual reinforcer or toys in the infant's hands can distract the toddler, and, after several shaping trials, the child forgets about the assembly. When maintaining placement of the assembly is impossible, a drop-back posture includes insert phones or sound field assess-ment. Most infants (more than 80%) and young children, however, can be as-sessed successfully using standard earphones and bone oscillators (Gravel and Traquina 1992). When switching between transducers (for example, from shap-ing in sound field to earphone assessment), a very brief reshaping period is fre-quently necessary. This serves to demonstrate to the baby that, although certain signal properties may have changed, the behavioral response that receives rein-forcement (the head turn) is still the same.

Conditioning in VRA

The first phase of VRA is the conditioning process. Response shaping is critical to the success of the operant procedure. This phase of testing is completely under the examiner's control. Thus, the examiner must be skilled in response training and sensitive to the various stages of response acquisition. Two different approaches that can be attempted in the first phase of VRA are (1) pairing the stimulus with the reinforcer and (2) observing a spontaneous response from the infant followed by reinforcement. Following several training trials, a criterion of several consecutive head turn responses must be met before moving to the second phase of actual test trials (refer to Figure 4.4). Successful completion of training occurs when the infant is making contingent responses and random head turning

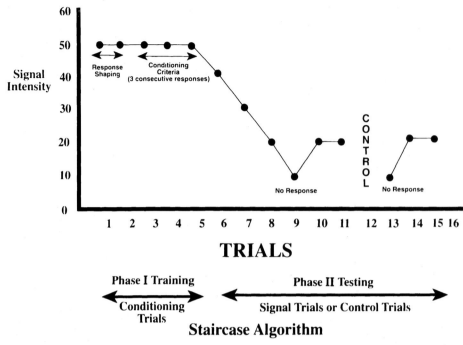

Figure 4.4. Adaptive test procedure with 10 dB step size; threshold (minimum response level) based on the mean of four reversals. In this patient, the MRL was approximately 20 dB HL.

is at a minimum. If criterion is not reached, phase one retraining must occur until criterion is met. The number of training trials needed before phase two trials begin differs among infants. However, the training phase is usually brief.

A spontaneous head turn will not be elicited from children who, because of earphone testing, hearing impairment, or central auditory problems, do not have or have not yet developed auditory localization skills. When training children under earphones or children suspected of hearing loss or other developmental problems in phase one, it is preferable to administer several paired conditioning trials at suprathreshold levels. This strategy will probably be required to teach the head turn response before stage two threshold exploration. Failure to condition rapidly should alert the examiner to a potential calibration or auditory problem or other important factors (physical, cognitive, social) that may affect the child's behavior.

Primus and Thompson (1985) investigated three stimulus conditions (complex noise presented at 50 dB nHL and at 25 dB nHL, and a 1500-Hz warble tone presented at 50 dB nHL) on the conditioning rate in VRA with one-year-old children. These authors concluded that variation in stimulus properties (stimulus type and starting intensity) had no effect on the rate of conditioning in their sample of children. Thirty-two of thirty-six infants satisfied the conditioning criteria (three consecutive correct responses) immediately following two training trials. The remaining four subjects required four training trials (paired presentations of stimulus and reinforcement) before reaching the conditioning criteria. These findings provide evidence that examiners need not compromise signal parameters in the assessment of infants as long as the children condition well to the VRA task.

Thompson and Folsom (1984) compared the effects of two conditioning procedures in VRA with one- and two-year-old children. One conditioning procedure used an initial stimulus presentation of 30-dB HL and only two conditioning trials before threshold exploration. The second procedure used a 60-dB HL initial presentation level and five conditioning trials before threshold exploration. The stimulus was complex noise, filtered to pass frequencies primarily between the 500- and 2000-Hz range. This study revealed no differences between the two conditioning procedures with regard to minimum response levels (discounting conditioning trials). Results from the Primus and Thompson study and the Thompson and Folsom study lead to the inference that signal type or starting intensity has minimal effect on conditioning success or response consistency.

More recent reports by Eilers and colleagues (1991a, b, 1993), Tharpe and Ashmeade (1993), and Widen (1993), however, suggest that starting level does influence the false-alarm rate. The higher the start level, the greater the possibility that false-positive responses may occur as rewarded head turns are first made at higher-than-necessary levels. Widen (1993) has suggested a protocol for assessment that initiates testing at 30-dB HL, increasing the intensity in 20-dB steps until a spontaneous head turn toward the sound source occurs. The spontaneous localization is reinforced, and the threshold search is initiated at this starting level.

A further clinical variation of this basic procedure is used for situations where the infant's hearing status is unknown. If infants do not localize (or show awareness of) the stimulus (usually a 500-Hz narrowband noise) at the highest soundfield presentation level (70–80 dB HL) after two presentations, this mode of stimulus delivery is discontinued. The bone oscillator is placed on the infant's mastoid closer to the reinforcer. The traditional conditioning procedure is initiated, that is, pairing the stimulus with the availability of reinforcement. The stimulus usually selected for bone-conducted conditioning is a 500-Hz narrowband noise presented at 45 dB HL. Thus, the clinician is assured that the discriminative stimulus is salient, although vibrotactilely. If the infant does not ultimately condition, then other developmental problems are suspected.

As always, individual circumstances in hearing assessment may dictate the use of various starting intensities. Given that most infants can be expected to have normal hearing, the most efficient test is one that uses a low starting level. Another test situation that warrants a low starting level (i.e., 30–40 dB HL), however, is when children cannot ultimately be conditioned to respond satisfactorily to the VRA procedure and show only a few spontaneous responses before habituation. In this situation, it is clinically more productive to obtain MRLs to signals of lower intensity levels as opposed to higher intensity levels.

Developmental Considerations

Several studies (Greenberg et al. 1978; Thompson, Wilson, and Moore 1979) have reported the use of VRA on children with Down syndrome and other developmental disabilities, suggesting that developmental age may be a determining factor in VRA success. Widen (1990) evaluated VRA as a function of developmental age in high-risk babies. Clearly, the developmentally mature babies were more often tested successfully. Visual reinforcement audiometry was successful for most infants by five to six months corrected age. Infants' ability to participate in the VRA task was also compared with their mental age score on the Bayley Scales of Infant Development (BSID). When test outcome in VRA was compared to developmental age in a subset of infants, success was achieved approximately 90% of the time in infants with a developmental age of 5½ to 6½ months of age. Therefore, applications of VRA in clinical protocols must consider (a) corrected age adjusted for prematurity rather than chronological age or (b) developmental age when disparities exist between corrected age and the child's developmental status.

Reinforcement

A critical feature of the VRA procedure is that the reward for correct responding must be highly appealing. Maintaining response behavior over repeated trials depends on the child's continued interest in viewing the reinforcement.

Moore, Thompson, and Thompson (1975) investigated the auditory localization behavior of infants 12 to 18 months of age as a function of reinforcement type. They used four conditions: (1) no reinforcement; (2) social reinforcement; (3) simple visual reinforcement (a blinking light); and (4) complex visual reinforcement (a lighted three-dimensional animated toy). The results showed that the complex visual reinforcement resulted in significantly more localization responses than the simple visual reinforcement. The light resulted in significantly more responses than social reinforcement, which in turn resulted in significantly more responses than the nonreinforcement condition. The inference from these data is that visual stimuli do in fact reinforce head turn response behavior, thus reducing the habituation effect to repeated stimulus presentations. In addition, it appears that the type of visual stimulus employed is an important determiner of response behavior. Visual stimuli containing movement, color, and contour appear to be more effective reinforcers than less complex visual stimuli. The strength of the complex visual reinforcer was subsequently shown with normally developing five-month-old infants.

Figure 4.5 shows a reinforcement unit. The plywood tri-cornered display fits into one corner of the test booth and is five feet high. Three separate compartments house three different mechanical toy reinforcers. The toys are brightly colored, highly animated, and most produce noise (such as drumming, barking,

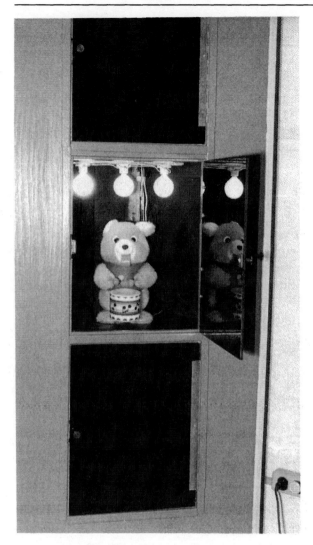

Figure 4.5. A reinforcement unit for visually reinforced audiometry.

cymbal clapping) when activated. Each of the three compartment doors is made of dark, smoked Plexiglas, and the compartment interiors are painted black. A light bulb strip affixed to the ceiling of each compartment brightly illuminates the toy during activation of reinforcement. Thus, when not illuminated, the toys are completely out of the infant's view.

Effects of Novelty

The use of novelty in a reinforcement protocol is an effective technique for improving responses. Besides slowing the decline in response rate, novelty can renew an infant's interest in the clinical task and revive response behavior (Bond 1972; Lipsitt and Werner 1981; Primus and Thompson 1985). Evidence shows that infants and young children attend more to novel versus familiar stimuli and are more willing to respond appropriately to elicit novel stimuli (Caron and Caron 1968, 1969; Lewis and Goldberg 1969; Lipsitt and Werner 1981). The availability of multiple visual reinforcers in VRA enhances novelty and, therefore, the impact of reinforcement. Switching among toy reinforcers enhances reinforcement by increasing novelty and uncertainty. The primary benefit of novel reinforcement in VRA is an increased amount of information about hearing in a single test session. This is an especially valuable advantage when children may be unable to return for multiple visits.

Effects of Reinforcement Schedules

In general, a 100-percent reinforcement schedule (reinforcement for every correct response) results in more rapid conditioning, yet more rapid habituation. Conversely, an intermittent reinforcement schedule produces slower conditioning but also a slower rate of habituation. Consequently, most clinicians recommend a protocol that begins with a 100-percent reinforcement schedule and then gradually shifts to an intermittent reinforcement schedule.

To investigate the influence of reinforcement schedules on the VRA procedure, Primus and Thompson (1985) compared a 100-percent reinforcement schedule to an intermittent reinforcement schedule with two-year-old children. The two reinforcement schedules revealed no differences in the infants' rate of habituation or the number of infant responses during stimulus trials. These findings provide an excellent guideline for reinforcing questionable infant responses. That is, reinforcement should be withheld when clinicians are uncertain about reinforcing delayed or ambiguous head turn responses. The risk of reinforcing a false response is that it may lead to confusion for a child under stimulus control. Moreover, it is important that the reinforcer not be activated during random head turning. These errors in reinforcement must be avoided. Failure to reinforce a correct response, however, does not degrade performance. In this situation, withholding reinforcement is viewed as intermittent reinforcement, which will not interfere with subsequent infant responses.

Threshold Acquisition

During threshold estimation, the examiner brings the infant to the midline position preceding and following a test trial. Throughout testing, two types of trials are presented: Signal trials contain a stimulus; control trials do not. Reinforcement is provided only for correct responding during signal trials.

Following a training procedure, the test phase of VRA begins. Depending on response outcome during the test phase, signal intensity is either attenuated after every "yes" response or increased after every "no" response. An adaptive threshold search is initiated until a stopping criterion is met. For example, stimulus intensity is attenuated in 10-dB steps until the infant makes the first "miss" (no response to a signal trial). A miss is followed by an increase of signal intensity. Two correct responses are followed by a decrease in signal level. After a specific number of reversals, the threshold search is ended. Threshold is then defined as the mean of the reversal points (refer to Figure 4.4).

STOPPING RULES: How many reversals should be required before stopping a threshold search? Too few may sacrifice response accuracy. However, too many may reduce efficiency as well as the number of trials that can be spent obtaining thresholds to other stimuli before an infant tires of testing. Eilers et al. (1991a, b), using computer simulation and infant subjects, suggest that from three to six reversals has little impact on test accuracy. That is, less than a 3-dB difference in threshold was demonstrated across the range of stopping rule conditions (three, four, five, and six reversals for computer simulation and three and six reversals for infant subjects). Thus, beyond three to four reversals, little accuracy is gained. However, these authors demonstrated that stopping rules do have a significant effect on test length. Tests with a three-reversal stopping rule were significantly shorter than those with six reversals. As stopping rules are increased from three to six, there is about a 50% increase in the number of test trials with no improvement in response accuracy. Thus, these results suggest that, by using relatively few reversals to estimate threshold, a staircase algorithm may be shortened without sacrificing accuracy.

CONTROL TRIALS: False positive responses must be monitored by control trials when assessing infant hearing. As mentioned earlier, signal trials (signal presented) and control trials (no signal presented) occur during threshold estimation. Either trial initiates an observation interval of approximately four seconds during which responses are judged. If a head turn response occurs during a signal trial, it is considered a correct detection, and reinforcement is activated. A response occurring during a control trial, however, is considered a false response. Control trials are interspersed with signal trials to examine systematically the infant's false-alarm rate. The assumption is that infants produce a comparable number of incorrect head turns during both signal and control trials. Therefore, it is possible to estimate chance responding (false responses during signal trials) during test trials by monitoring false response rate during control trials.

The purpose of the control trial is to assess the reliability of responses. Test results on any infant who reaches an unacceptable false response rate should be excluded or interpreted with extreme caution. In clinical and research protocols, test results are frequently discounted if false responses during control trials exceed an arbitrary criterion of 20 to 25%. Eilers and coworkers suggest that a 30% false response rate may not be excessive for clinical purposes. However, when a specified criterion is exceeded, clinicians should focus on two factors to rectify clinical outcomes: (1) reconditioning the desired behavior and (2) reexamining the difficulty of keeping the child entertained at a midline position before starting a test trial. Occasionally, overactive parents can bias their children to respond, thereby resulting in excessive false responses. Therefore, parents may need to wear headphones through which music or noise is delivered. Masking the parent is intended to remove observer bias during test sessions.

ASSESSMENT OUTCOMES: Clinical outcomes need not be compromised by using one examiner in VRA. Under these circumstances, the audiologist engages the infant's attention at midline, selects and presents a test signal, varies its presentation intensity as appropriate, judges the infant's behavioral response, and directly activates the reinforcement for correct head turning. We have found that a careful and thoughtful clinician guarding against the same hazards of single-examiner assessment in traditional audiologic assessment (observer bias, response cuing) may obtain reliable and accurate audiograms from infants.

Clinical reports shared among clinicians as well as reports in the literature reveal highly consistent findings from different settings. That is, for normal-hearing infants, thresholds are consistently obtained within a conservative definition of normal hearing (≤ 15 dB HL) and only slightly elevated from adult comparisons. These reports support the accuracy of the VRA procedure in correctly identifying normal hearing, thereby resulting in an impressive test operating characteristic for specificity. More important, however, is the indication that, because the range of normal is tightly grouped, the range of abnormal is appropriately wide. The advantage of a wide range of abnormal is the ability to differentiate various degrees of hearing loss from mild to profound.

Figure 4.6 presents audiograms representative of those that may be obtained from infants on one test day using the visually reinforced head turn procedure. Note that the audiograms resemble those that might be obtained from older children or adults. They provide audiometric information that is specific to frequency, ear, type, degree, symmetry, and configuration of hearing loss. Displayed are the results from infants younger than ten months of age with normal hearing, asymmetric conductive hearing loss secondary to otitis media, and sensorineural hearing loss of various degrees and configurations. Of particular interest with regard to the examples of sensorineural hearing loss is the fact that all audiograms were repeated and VRA accuracy confirmed by play audiometry as these children were seen over the years. Thus, as with specificity, the test-operating characteristic for sensitivity is also impressive. Provided that the child is under stimulus control, VRA provides (with a high degree of confidence) audiometric information necessary for making diagnostic, medical, and management decisions.

Thus, the VRA procedure may be applied successfully to both screening and assessment programs. Indeed, Eilers and colleagues (1991a, b, 1993) and Widen (1990) have shown the efficiency of the VRA procedure in a large, hospital-based infant hearing screening program. The application of VRA for the comprehensive audiologic assessment of infants and young children has been stressed by us and others. The technique is likely the single most important tool available to today's pediatric audiologist.

BEHAVIORAL OBSERVATION AUDIOMETRY (BOA)

IN developing a protocol for the early identification of hearing loss, it is important to recognize that the demographics of sensorineural hearing loss may be shifting toward an increase in the prevalence of milder losses and sloping, high frequency losses. Moreover, more infants with congenital or acquired losses have other neurodevelopmental disabilities in addition to hearing impairment. To respond appropriately to this trend, our auditory test procedures must

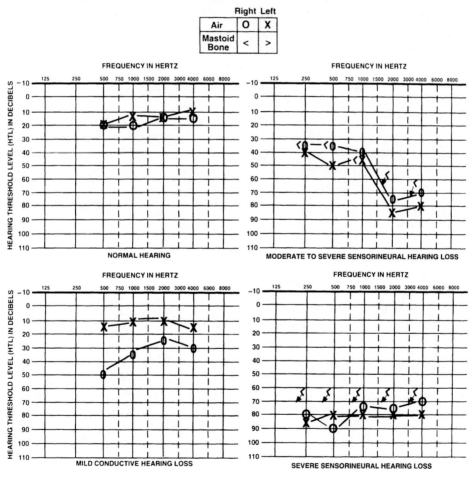

Figure 4.6. Sample audiograms from VRA assessment.

provide the precision necessary to quantify the degree, type, and configuration of any existing hearing impairment. This places limitations on the use of behavioral observation audiometry for determining sensitivity. However, another important goal of the audiologic evaluation is to examine auditory *function*. Although electrophysiologic procedures can quantify auditory sensitivity in infants with compromised neuromotor function, BOA can provide very useful insight into the quality of the child's auditory responsiveness.

BOA is no longer recommended for assessing frequency-specific threshold sensitivity in newborns, young infants (<5 months), or those children whose developmental disabilities preclude them learning the operant VRA procedure. However, BOA can provide an estimate of functional capabilities useful in planning intervention. Secondly, behavioral observation of orienting responses may be useful for examining neuromotor development in high-risk newborns. There is some evidence that very low birthweight infants demonstrate poorer auditory orienting abilities than full-term babies even when ages for both groups are corrected for prematurity (Kurtzburg et al. 1979). They also demonstrate later impaired cognitive and linguistic function (Wallace et al. 1982).

Limitations of Behavioral Observation Audiometry

A major, probably uncontrollable, limitation of BOA is that it is a test of responsiveness and not absolute sensitivity. Infants under five months of age developmentally generally display reflexive and orienting responses to external stimuli. Reflexive responses in BOA include head or limb reflex, whole body startle, nonnutritive sucking, and eye-blink or flutter. Orienting or attentive-type behaviors include increased and decreased motion, eye widening, searching, and localization. Test parameters of BOA are generally discussed in terms of the factors that influence response behavior. For example, the probability of a response occurring is dependent on the state of the infant, the nature of the auditory stimulus, the ambient noise levels, and agreement among observers that a response occurred. Together, these factors lead to high false-positive and false-negative rates when BOA is utilized as a screening test of sensitivity in conventional audiologic applications. As a result, there are serious concerns about the effectiveness of BOA for newborn hearing screening.

For example, using BOA in a screening application, Plotnick and Leppler (1986) identified only two severely hearing-impaired infants among 356 newborns in the neonatal intensive care unit (NICU). Assuming a very conservative 2-percent prevalence of significant sensorineural hearing loss in an NICU, at least three times as many hearing-impaired infants should have been identified in the group tested. Because of the high stimulus intensity required to elicit reflexive response behaviors, BOA is likely to miss an infant with a mild-to-moderate bilateral hearing loss as well as one with unilateral impairment. False negative rates of 40 to 86% have been reported for BOA (Alberti et al. 1983; Durieux-Smith et al. 1985; Jacobson and Morehouse 1984), meaning that many infants with significant hearing impairments pass behavioral screening and are thus lost to immediate follow-up.

Babies cared for in an NICU may show generally decreased responsiveness to external stimuli due to immature or compromised neurodevelopmental processes or poor health. Thus, they may demonstrate absent or unorganized responses to sensory stimuli. Reflexive responses or auditory orienting may be absent in infants with normal hearing sensitivity. Thus, behavioral observations of responses to auditory stimuli have been of limited value in screening for neonatal hearing loss in neurodevelopmentally at-risk infants.

Although BOA is no longer viewed as an effective screening procedure, there are still some proponents of the technique as evidenced by a small handheld screener now being marketed as a convenient and inexpensive alternative to more elaborate and costly instrumentation. Because of its poor sensitivity and specificity, BOA cannot be recommended for neonatal hearing screening.

Application to Special Populations

Audiologists are challenged to interpret the auditory behavior of children with special needs: those who have severely compromised cognitive function and those who are challenged with multiple neuromotor disabilities. Electrophysiologic techniques (e.g., frequency-specific air- and bone-conducted ABR, EOAEs, acoustic immittance) are critical for delineating hearing sensitivity in this population. Once hearing sensitivity has been established, an examination of the auditory responsiveness or function of these youngsters is important for maximizing individual developmental potential through habilitational strategies, for determining realistic goals for educational intervention, for providing assistance for family dynamics, and in helping to predict areas of potential difficulty with various forms of auditory input. In this regard, audiologists should always include behavioral observation audiometry in their assessment of these populations.

With respect to children who are low functioning, retarded, or multiply-impaired, Gans and Flexer (1983) found that level of responsiveness is closely related to the general developmental level of a child. As expected, responsiveness to low-intensity sounds is less for children at lower developmental ages. These investigators showed that, with a systematic approach to testing, BOA could separate normal hearing and mild hearing loss from moderate, severe, and profound hearing loss in this population. However, concerning past criticisms of BOA, test methodology must be approached with a clear understanding of the limitations of BOA.

BOA Test Methodology

The restrictions imposed by stimulus factors, the state of the child, and examiner bias on the outcome of BOA procedures with youngsters must be considered in developing BOA protocols. Moreover, judgments should not be elevated to a level of precision beyond that defined by the resolving power of the instrument. Because BOA does not involve conditioning, it is inherently a test of responsiveness and not of sensitivity.

Stimulus Factors

Bandwidth appears to be a factor that affects responsivity for both normal infants (Gerber and Dobkin 1984) and for children with multiple disabilities (Flexer and Gans 1985). Figure 4.7 (Thompson and Thompson 1972) shows the percentage of responses to five different stimuli across four different intensity levels in normally developing infants seven to twelve months of age. These data show clearly the interaction of stimuli with different bandwidths at different presentation levels on responses observed from a BOA procedure. Flexer and Gans (1985) investigated four stimuli (broadband noise, 2000-Hz narrowband noise, speech, and bandpass filtered speech centered at 2000 Hz) with young infants and children with multiple and severe developmental disabilities. Their results agreed with Thompson and Thompson (1972), showing that narrow bandwidth

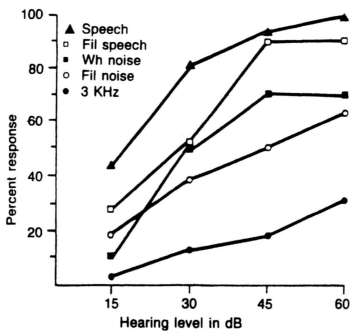

Figure 4.7. Percent response to five stimuli as a function of hearing level. Infants 7 to 12 months of age (from Thompson and Thompson 1972).

stimuli, regardless of meaningfulness, are simply not as effective as broader bandwidth stimuli in eliciting responses from infants and youngsters who are developmentally compromised. The same is true for normal, well newborns (Gerber and Mencher 1979). Moreover, Gerber and Dobkin (1984) showed that elimination of low frequencies diminishes responsiveness of full-term well newborns. The results from Flexer and Gans also revealed that there were no group differences for responsivity. That is, auditory responsiveness of normal infants can be extrapolated to youngsters who are multiply-handicapped and of similar developmental ages.

Test Considerations

Behavioral observation audiometry procedures usually require several examiners. The use of multiple examiners allows one examiner to present auditory stimuli, one examiner to monitor state changes and to cue signal presentations when the child's state is appropriate, and an optional additional examiner to be responsible for videorecording responses. Besides specific responsibilities for testing, multiple examiners are necessary to judge response behavior. Multiple judges are designed to reduce two forms of error associated with observational judgments: (1) judging that a response occurred when in reality there was no response and (2) judging that no response occurred when in reality a response did occur.

Because a variety of response behaviors is monitored (e.g., head or limb reflex, increased motion, decreased motion, whole body startle, eye widening, nonnutritive sucking, searching, eyeblink or flutter, localization, smiling, laughing, pointing), another source of concern that must be minimized in judging responses is preinformation bias—that is, the examiner's expectations of the outcome of the test. The expectation of the examiner is different if prior knowledge exists regarding developmental status, previous test results, or medical status. Therefore, examiners should have minimal information about each patient before testing.

Another form of bias may occur in the test situation. When the examiner is aware of the sound stimuli presentations (test trials), he or she adopts a different criterion in defining responses than in test protocols in which the examiner is naive as to trial type and in which control trials (no sound) are included. Children who are developmentally disabled often are active during testing and frequently change attentional states. The purpose of the control trial is to identify this random behavior. Response behavior during control trials is documented and serves as the basis for scoring response behavior. The occurrence of test trials and control trials initiates an observation interval during which responses are judged. If a response occurs during a test trial (signal present), it is considered a correct detection. If, however, a response occurs during a control trial (that is, when no acoustic stimulus is presented), it is considered a false-positive response. Control trials are interspersed among test trials on a random schedule.

The presence or absence of false-positive responses during control trials allows the examiner to calculate the percentage of false-positive responses.

It should be stressed that the presence of multiple examiners does not overcome the problem of observer bias. A single examiner, if naive to trial type, is a more reliable observer than two or more observers who are aware of the presence of test signals.

Scoring

Gans (1987) recommends the use of a six-point certainty scale for judging response behavior. In addition, it is important to list the elicited response behaviors. The scale recommended is as follows: 1 = real sure, no; 2 = pretty sure, no; 3 = not sure, no; 4 = not sure, yes; 5 = pretty sure, yes; 6 = real sure, yes. Following a 4, 5, or 6 rating, judges should list the specific response behavior. Judging responses can be done "live" or from subsequent review of a videorecording. The relationship between responsiveness during a test trial and a control trial is examined in each judge's scoring by subtracting the nearest adjacent control trial rating from that for the test trial. The resultant value is called a difference score. The difference score can range from −5 (1 = test trial; 6 = control trial) to +5 (6 = test trial; 1 = control trial). A positive difference score is an indication that a youngster exhibited a greater change in background behavior during a test trial (signal presented) than during a control trial interval. A zero or negative difference score is interpreted as indicating that no differential change of behavior occurred for the "test" versus "catch" trial condition.

Test State

The state of an infant or youngster under test affects responsiveness and thus the ability to judge responses accurately. For example, in rating sleep in stages from deep sleep to fully awake, it has been shown that the middle states allow the highest response ratios (Downs and Sterritt 1964; Eisenberg et al. 1964). It has become clear that the quiet awake condition is best for eliciting robust organized orienting responses from newborns. Thus, for the qualitative clinical application of BOA, the youngster under test should be encouraged to observe passively or play quietly with colorful, non-noisy toys. The auditory stimulus should not be presented if the youngster is vocalizing, sleeping, fretting, crying, or moving excessively.

Assessment Outcomes

Results from BOA do not indicate a true auditory threshold but instead reflect a level of responsiveness. Yet, under ideal test conditions, responses from youngsters may reflect a minimum response level. Developmental age level can have a strong effect on response level. Gans (1987) suggests that, for children (normally developing or disabled) with developmental ages above five months, minimum response levels equal to or better than 50 dB HL can be achieved with BOA. For children with developmental ages of less than two months, however, minimum response levels from BOA are usually greater than 80 dB HL. It is important to consider the data of Thompson and Weber (1974), who showed the wide ranges of intra- and intersubject variability in infants and young children up to six years of age. Nevertheless, Gans (1987) provides detailed information showing that a 50 dB cut-off can be applied with confidence in BOA applications to children who have severe developmental disabilities. That is, when minimum response levels of 50 dB or better are obtained, moderate, severe, and profound hearing losses can be ruled out.

Response behaviors seen during BOA can be separated into those that are attentive-type (increased and decreased motion, eye widening, searching, localization, smiling, laughing, pointing) and those considered reflexive (head or limb reflex, whole body startle, sucking, eye-blink or flutter). Analyzing response behaviors may provide useful information in determining how youngsters attach meaning to sound. If response behavior is reflexive from a child known to have near normal hearing, it may indicate a child unlikely to use auditory input as a primary input mechanism or one who does not attach much meaning to sound. On the other hand, children who show orienting responses to sound are perhaps demonstrating a higher level of cortical functioning.

Application of BOA in Neurobehavioral Assessment

The cognitive difficulties encountered by children born at very low birthweight (VLBW <1500 grams) have been well documented (DeHirsch, Jansky, and Langford 1966; Drillien, Thompson, and Burgoyne 1980; Wallace et al. 1982). For example, children born at VLBW have a greater prevalence of impaired intellectual functioning. Moreover, when compared to their full-term counterparts, children born at VLBW frequently display perceptual-motor, language, and cognitive disabilities. Frequently, these deficits are recognized only when the child enters school and is faced with the challenge of learning to read, write, and manipulate numbers. Since early therapeutic intervention appears beneficial in minimizing later disabilities, neonatal identification of infants who manifest compromised neuromotor function would foster timely intervention.

There has been evidence that some aspects of neonatal neurobehavioral performance are predictive of later cognitive abilities. For example, Scarr and Williams (1971), using Brazelton's Neonatal Behavioral Assessment Scale, and Grellong et al. (1981), using the Einstein Neonatal Neurobehavioral Assessment Scale (ENNBAS), have found that assessments that include basic orienting (visual following, auditory orienting) with assessments of motoric functions were related to later cognitive status.

Wallace et al. (1982) investigated the relationship between results of the ENNBAS and six-year cognitive outcome (i.e., verbal IQ, performance IQ, visual-motor integration, reading, and sentence repetition). The results of this study provide evidence that some aspects of neonatal neurobehavioral performance predicted cognitive abilities at six years of age. A high correlation was found between the three summary scores of the ENNBAS (auditory orienting, visual following, and motility) and five cognitive outcome measures. Yet, among the ENNBAS components, only the items testing orientation to acoustic stimuli accounted for the predictive power of the neonatal instrument. Moreover, among the highly intercorrelated outcome measures, the measures that involved verbal and language processes were most highly related to the neonatal neurobehavioral performance. These findings are significant regarding an application of BOA to newborns. That is, these results suggest that even simple indices of acoustic processing in the newborn can index later language-related abilities. Furthermore, it is possible that since language acquisition, which underlies verbal intelligence, depends on auditory processes, audition may play a key role in cognitive development.

TEST CONSIDERATIONS: Three factors must be considered in the application of BOA as a neurobehavioral assessment tool. The behavior, the method to monitor the behavior, and the eliciting stimulus must be chosen to yield a sensitive and specific indicator of auditory orienting behavior.

The behavior to be monitored is an orienting behavior. Orienting behavior is shown by quieting, eyes widening with searching behavior, and finally, head turning to the side of sound (Gerber 1969). Concerning the issue of development of localization, Muir and Field and associates (Field et al. 1979, 1980; Muir et al. 1979; Muir and Field 1979) have presented a series of studies showing that neonates will consistently turn their heads toward a sound source. Their experimental procedure involved the use of videoscoring and other controls for potential observer bias. In most cases, the latency of the neonates' responses was long: 2.5 seconds to the beginning of the head-turn response and 5.5 seconds to the end of the response. Comparing these collective findings of Muir and Field and associates to the literature in pediatric audiology, it becomes clear that our ideas about the development of localization responses may have seriously underestimated the actual abilities of infants.

Testing must be performed in a well-controlled environment. One such environment, dubbed the NEST (an acronym for Neonatal Environment for Sensitivity Testing), has been proposed (Bernstein and Gravel 1992). The NEST is an enclosure designed to provide a controlled auditory and visual environment. In addition, the NEST is lined with three inches of acoustic foam to minimize echoes. Loudspeakers are mounted on two walls of the NEST at the level of the baby. Provisions have been made to support the infant on a slightly inclined mattress and to image the infant's head with a closed-circuit television.

When monitoring orienting behavior in newborns, it is absolutely necessary to incorporate signal and control trials. Although the response is defined, the actual determination of response behavior is made when signal trials are compared with control intervals. Newborn infants tend to perform certain behaviors because of sound being presented (orienting) and have less of a tendency to perform the same behaviors in the absence of an eliciting stimulus. Based on the baby's behaviors, the examiner decides whether a response occurred. The examiner receives immediate feedback regardless of whether a signal was presented. Subsequently, comparisons between response behavior and trial type lead to the performance characteristics of the test (i.e., response present or absent during signal trials; response present or absent during control trials). The outcome of these comparisons indicates the robustness of response behavior.

When a trial is initiated, one of three events occurs: (1) the stimulus is presented from the right; (2) the stimulus is presented from the left; and (3) no stimulus is presented. Observers are required to decide, on each trial, whether the eliciting stimulus was presented. The examiner is blind to trial type; and, therefore, decisions on response behavior are based solely on the observation of infants' behaviors.

For years, clinicians agonized over selecting a signal for BOA that achieved an appropriate compromise between the frequency-restricted stimulus we would like to use to determine configuration of a hearing loss and a signal that was sufficiently complex to maximize auditory responses in infants. When the focus changes from sensitivity to responsivity in BOA, stimulus characteristics are not a limiting factor. That is, wideband stimuli as well as band-limited stimuli can be used. Yet, clinicians should define signal characteristics in terms of intensity, bandwidth, rise time, and duration. Signal characteristics may be relevant in the analysis of response behavior with different population groups. Speech, filtered speech, white and complex noise, as well as band-limited noise can be used in this application because the acoustic characteristics can be specified. Noisemakers have also been used in this application of BOA; however, it may be impossible to attribute precise intensity and frequency measurements to most noisemakers (Gerber 1982).

Clinical Application

A principal objective of neonatal neurobehavioral assessment is the identification of deviant infants and the characterization of their aberrant performance. Perhaps more so with this type of assessment than with others, a detailed battery of measures must be evaluated to obtain a relevant picture of an infant's neurobehavioral status. Information on both the neurologic integrity of the newborn and the behavioral characteristics that influence the newborn's interaction with the environment are necessary in evaluating the infant's developmental potential and possible problem areas. It is clear from early evidence that auditory orienting behavior is an excellent tool for separating full term from low birthweight infants and that auditory orienting may play a key role in cognitive development. To the extent that impairment of specific sensory and motor systems can be detected, it may be possible to make some prediction about areas of potential handicap. Perhaps more importantly, the identification of deviant neurobehavioral performance, employing a sensitive and comprehensive assessment battery, pinpoints a given infant as a candidate for more detailed neurological evaluation and close developmental observation. Moreover, establishing goals for intervention emphasizes auditory activities that are developmentally based.

SUMMARY

CLEARLY, conditioned behavioral procedures can be valid and reliable for both assessment and screening purposes. Observational techniques, on the other hand, are useful in examining global auditory function. Current behavioral and electrophysiologic procedures have provided the pediatric audiologist with a powerful test armamentarium. The clinician is cautioned, however, that, although auditory evoked potentials and EOAE procedures can make substantial contributions to our knowledge of a child's auditory sensitivity, only behavioral procedures offer the unique ability to examine functional use of hearing. Behavioral methods offer insight into audition that is beyond the level of the cochlea and brainstem; higher-order abilities that are essential for informed and productive habilitation, parent counseling, and follow-up.

REFERENCES

Alberti, P.W., M.L. Hyde, K. Riko, H. Corgin, and S. Ambramovich. 1983. An equivalent of BERA for hearing screening in high-risk neonates. *Laryngoscope* 93:1115–1121.

Bergstrom, L. 1984. Congenital hearing loss. In *Hearing disorders*, 2d ed., ed. by J.L. Northern. Boston: Little, Brown and Co.

Bernstein, R.S., and J.S. Gravel. 1992. Orienting as a means of assessing hearing in newly born infants. In *Screening children for auditory function*, ed. F.H. Bess and J.W. Hall III. Nashville: Bill Wilkerson Center Press.

Bond, E.K. 1972. Perception of form by the human infant. *Psychological Bulletin* 77: 225–245.

Bradford, L.J. 1975. Respiration audiometry. In *Physiological measures of the audiovestibular system*, ed. L.J. Bradford. New York: Academic Press.

Caron, R.F., and A.J. Caron. 1968. The effects of repeated exposure and stimulus complexity on visual fixation in infants. *Psychonomic Science* 10:207–208.

———. 1969. Degree of stimulus complexity on visual fixation in infants. *Psychonomic Science* 14:78–79.

Davis, H., and S. Onishi. 1969. Maturation of auditory evoked potentials. *International Audiology* 8:24–33.

Davis, H., and S. Zerlin. 1966. Acoustic relations of the human vertex potential. *Journal of the Acoustical Society of America* 39:109–116.

DeHirsch K., J. Jansky, and W.S. Langford. 1966. Comparisons between prematurely and maturely born children at three age levels. *American Journal of Orthopsychiatry* 36: 610–628.

Downs, M.P. 1976. Early identification of hearing loss: Where are we? Where do we go from here? In *Early identification of hearing loss*, ed. G.T. Mencher. Basel: S. Karger.

Downs, M.P., and G.M. Sterritt. 1964. Identification audiometry for neonates: A preliminary report. *Journal of Auditory Research* 4:69–80.

———. 1967. A guide to newborn and infant hearing screening. *Archives of Otolaryngology* 85:15–22.

Drillien, C.M., A.M. Thompson, and K. Burgoyne. 1980. Low birthweight children at early school age: A longitudinal study. *Developmental Medicine and Child Neurology* 22: 26–47.

Durieux-Smith, A., T. Picton, C. Edwards, J.T. Goodman, and B. MacMurray. 1985. The crib-o-gram in the NICU: An evaluation based on brain stem electric response audiometry. *Ear and Hearing* 6:20–24.

Eilers, R.E., E. Miskiel, O. Ozdamar, R. Urbano, and J.E. Widen. 1991a. Optimization of automated hearing test algorithms: Simulations using an infant response model. *Ear and Hearing* 12:191–198.

Eilers, R.E., O. Ozdamar, and M.L. Steffens. 1993. Classification of audiograms by sequential testing: Reliability and validity of an automated behavioral hearing screening algorithm. *Journal of the American Academy of Audiology* 4:172–181.

Eilers, R.E., J.E. Widen, R. Urbano, T.M. Hudson, and L. Gonzales. 1991b. Optimization of automated hearing test algorithms: A comparison of data from simulations and young children. *Ear and Hearing* 12:199–214.

Eisenberg, R.B. 1969. Auditory behavior in the human neonate: Functional properties of sound and their ontogenetic implications. *International Audiology* 8:34–45.

Eisenberg, R.B., E.J. Griffen, D.B. Coursin, and M.A. Hunter. 1964. Auditory behavior in the human neonate: A preliminary report. *Journal of Speech and Hearing Research* 7: 245–269.

Field, J., D. DiFranco, P. Dodwell, and D. Muir. 1979. Auditory-visual coordination in two and one-half-month-old infants. *Infant Behavior and Development* 2:113–122.

Field, J., D. Muir, R. Pilon, M. Sinclair, and P. Dodwell. 1980. Infants' orientation to lateral sounds from birth to three months. *Child Development* 51:295–298.

Flexer, C., and D.P. Gans. 1985. Comparative evaluation of the auditory responsiveness of normal infants and profoundly multihandicapped children. *Journal of Speech and Hearing Research* 28:163–168.

Gans, D.P. 1987. Improving behavior observation audiometry testing and scoring procedures. *Ear and Hearing* 8:92–100.

Gans, D.P., and C. Flexer. 1983. Auditory response behavior of severely handicapped children. *Journal of Auditory Research* 23:137–148.

Gerber, S.E. 1969. Auditory behavioral responses of some hearing infants. *Volta Review* 71:340–346.

———. 1982. The use of noise-making toys as audiometric devices. *International Journal of Pediatric Otorhinolaryngology* 4:309–315.

Gerber, S.E., and M.S. Dobkin. 1984. The effect of noise bandwidth on the auditory arousal response of neonates. *Ear and Hearing* 5:195–198.

Gerber, S.E., and G.T. Mencher. 1979. Arousal responses of neonates to wide band and narrow band noise. Paper presented at the annual convention of the American Speech-Language-Hearing Association.

Gravel, J.S., and D.N. Traquina. 1992. Experience with the audiologic assessment of infants and toddlers. *International Journal of Pediatric Otorhinolaryngology* 23:59–71.

Greenberg, D.B., W.R. Wilson, J.M. Moore, and G. Thompson. 1978. Visual reinforcement audiometry VRA with young Down's syndrome children. *Journal of Speech and Hearing Disorders* 43:8–458.

Grellong, B., H.G. Vaughan, Jr., L. Rotkin, et al. 1981. Neonatal performance, cognitive and neurologic outcome to 40 months among low birthweight infants. Presented at Biennial Meeting, Society for Research in Child Development, Boston.

Hecox, K., and R. Galambos. 1974. Brainstem auditory evoked responses in human infants and adults. *Archives of Otolaryngology* 99:30–33.

Jacobson, J.T., and C.R. Morehouse. 1984. A comparison of auditory brainstem response and behavioral screening in high risk and normal newborn infants. *Ear and Hearing* 5: 247–253.

Joint Committee on Infant Hearing. 1972. Supplementary statement on infant hearing screening. *Asha* 16:160.

Kurtzberg, D., H.G. Vaughan, Jr., C.M. McCarton-Daum, B.A. Grellong, S. Albin, and L. Rotkin. 1979. Neurobehavioral performance of low birth weight infants at 40 weeks conceptional age: Comparison with normal full-term infants. *Developmental Medicine and Child Neurology* 21:590–607.

Lewis, M., and S. Goldberg. 1969. The acquisition and violation of expectancy: An experimental paradigm. *Journal of Experimental Psychology* 1:75–86.

Lidén, G., and A. Kankkunen. 1969. Visual reinforcement audiometry. *Acta Oto-Laryngologica* 67:281–292.

Lipsitt, L.P., and J.S. Werner. 1981. The infancy of human learning processes. In *Developmental plasticity: Behavioral and biological aspects of variations in development*, ed. E.S. Gollin. New York: Academic Press.

Mencher, G.T., B. McCullouch, A.J. Derbyshire, and R. Dethlefs. 1977. Observer bias as a factor in neonatal hearing screening. *Journal of Speech and Hearing Research* 20:27–34.

Moore, J.M., G. Thompson, and M. Thompson. 1975. Auditory localization of infants as a function of reinforcement conditions. *Journal of Speech and Hearing Disorders* 40: 29–34.

Moore, J.M., W.R. Wilson, and G. Thompson. 1977. Visual reinforcement of head-turn responses in infants under 12 months of age. *Journal of Speech and Hearing Disorders* 42:328–334.

Muir, D., W. Abraham, B. Forbes, and L. Harris. 1979. The ontogenesis of an auditory localization response from birth to four months of age. *Canadian Journal of Psychology* 33:320–333.

Muir, D., and J. Field. 1979. Newborn infants orient to sounds. *Child Development* 50:431–436.

Plotnick, C.H., and J.G. Leppler. 1986. Infant hearing assessment: A program for identification and habilitation within four months of age. *The Hearing Journal* 39:23–25.

Primus, M.A., and G. Thompson. 1985. Response strength of young children in operant audiometry. *Journal of Speech and Hearing Research* 28:539–547.

Scarr, S., and M.L.Williams. 1971. The assessment of neonatal and later status of low birthweight infants. Presented at meeting of the Society for Research in Child Development, Minneapolis.

Schulman, C.A. 1973. Heart rate audiometry. Part I. An evaluation of heart rate response to auditory stimuli in newborn hearing screening. *Neuropaediatrie* 4:362–374.

Stein, L., S. Clark, and N. Kraus. 1983. The hearing-impaired infant: Patterns of identification and habilitation. *Ear and Hearing* 4:232–236.

Stein, L., T. Jabaley, R. Spitz, D. Stoakley, and T. McGee. 1990. The hearing-impaired infant: Patterns of identification and habilitation revisited. *Ear and Hearing* 11:128–133.

Suzuki, T., and Y. Ogiba. 1960. A technique of pure-tone audiometry for children under three years of age: Conditioned orientation reflex (COR) audiometry. *Revue de Laryngologie, Otologie, Rhinologie* 81:33–45.

Tharpe, A.M., and D.H. Ashmeade. 1993. Computer simulation technique for assessing pediatric auditory test protocols. *Journal of the American Academy of Audiology* 4:80–90.

Thompson, G., and R.C. Folsom. 1984. A comparison of two conditioning procedures in the use of visual reinforcement audiometry (VRA). *Journal of Speech and Hearing Disorders* 49:241–245.

Thompson, G., and B.A. Weber. 1974. Responses of infants and young children to behavior observation audiometry (BOA). *Journal of Speech and Hearing Disorders* 39:140–147.

Thompson, G., W.R. Wilson, and J.M. Moore. 1979. Application of visual reinforcement audiometry (VRA) to low-functioning children. *Journal of Speech and Hearing Disorders* 44:80–90.

Thompson, M., and G. Thompson. 1972. Response of infants and young children as a function of auditory stimuli and test method. *Journal of Speech and Hearing Research* 15:699–707.

U.S. Department of Health and Human Services, Public Health Service. 1990. *Healthy People 2000: National Health Promotion and Disease Prevention Objectives*. Washington, D.C.: U.S. Government Printing Office.

Wallace, I.F., S.K. Escalona, C.M. McCarton-Daum, and H.G. Vaughan. 1982. Neonatal precursors of cognitive development in low birth weight children. *Seminars in Perinatology* 6:327–333.

Weber, B.A. 1969. Validation of observer judgements in behavioral observation audiometry. *Journal of Speech and Hearing Disorders* 34:350–355.

Widen, J.E. 1990. Behavioral screening of high-risk infants using visual reinforcement audiometry. *Seminars in Hearing* 11:342–356.

———. 1993. Adding objectivity to infant behavioral audiometry. *Ear and Hearing* 14:49–57.

Wilson, W.R. 1978. Behavioral assessment of auditory function in infants. In *Communicative and cognitive abilities: Early behavioral assessment*, ed. F.D. Minifie and L.L. Lloyd. Baltimore: University Park Press.

Wilson, W.R., and G. Thompson. 1984. Behavioral audiometry. In *Pediatric audiology: Current trends*, ed. J. Jerger. San Diego: College-Hill Press.

5

Speech Audiometry for Children

Jane R. Madell

PURPOSES OF SPEECH AUDIOMETRY

SPEECH audiometry, appropriately used, can be an exceptionally valuable part of the clinical audiologic test battery, particularly in evaluating and monitoring auditory function in children. Pure tone testing provides information about degree and type of hearing loss but tells us nothing about function: how a person uses hearing for perception of speech. Speech perception is critical for the development of spoken language and for accurate speech production. Speech perception testing is the only method available at present for assessing how a child hears speech. Unfortunately, it is frequently overlooked or used only in a limited fashion, thereby failing to maximize its potential usefulness.

Assessing speech perception can be very helpful in determining what difficulties a child may be having, if any, and in planning remediation. Word recognition scores that are poorer than expected when compared to pure tone thresholds at normal and soft conversational levels can be strong indicators for aggressive treatment: medical, audiological, or a combination of the two. Testing at soft conversational levels and in the presence of competing noise can effectively demonstrate the need for hearing aids, an FM system in the classroom, or auditory training.

Information from evaluation of large numbers of adults indicates that word recognition ability decreases as the degree of hearing loss increases. This is also true for children (Boothroyd 1984). However, the effect of hearing loss on children is much more significant than on adults because of the negative impact that even a mild hearing loss can have on the development of speech and language (Friel-Patti et al. 1982; Ross and Giolas 1978; Wallace et al. 1988). Word recognition testing is an important technique for evaluating the extent to which a child's hearing loss has adversely affected speech perception, putting development of speech and language at risk.

For children with identified hearing losses or auditory processing disorders, word recognition testing can monitor progress during treatment. Almost everyone agrees that, despite the mode of communication that families choose in educating their hearing-impaired children, all children should be given the opportunity to maximize their auditory skills. Providing appropriate amplification is a necessary but incomplete step toward this goal. Even young children with profound hearing loss can be taught to use audition for the reception of language. The use of audition will positively affect language growth and accurate speech production. The audiologist who evaluates a child annually, semiannually, or quarterly may be in a better position to evaluate auditory progress than the therapist who sees the child several times a week. If a therapy program is successful, the child's word recognition should continue to improve, and, over time, the child should be able to perform more difficult auditory tasks. The audiologist can monitor the child's progress and assist the therapist in modifying treatment goals to improve the child's auditory functioning. This, to my mind, is a most exciting aspect of pediatric audiology.

EVALUATING AUDITORY PERCEPTION

THE goal of speech audiometry is to obtain as much information as possible about a child's speech perception abilities. There are several ways to evaluate speech perception, and each procedure provides different information. Erber and Alencewicz (1976) and Erber (1979) described an auditory skills matrix that is useful when thinking about the different components of speech perception testing and auditory training.

There are four different response tasks that can be used to assess perception. *Detection* is the ability to tell when a stimulus is present. *Discrimination* is the ability to determine whether two stimuli are the same or different. *Identification* is the ability to recognize the stimulus being presented and to identify it by repeating, pointing, or writing. *Comprehension* is the ability to understand what the stimulus means.

Each response task can be assessed using several different stimuli, from phonemes, syllables, words, phrases, and sentences to connected discourse. Phoneme testing is the most difficult task in the stimulus hierarchy because it is the least redundant and provides the fewest cues. However, it yields valuable information. It can be presented in either a closed or open set format, produces specific information about which sounds are not correctly perceived, and can test many stimuli in a short period. Connected discourse, on the other hand, is easier to understand but will afford very little information about which specific phonemes are causing perceptual difficulties because the listener may correctly extrapolate words not correctly perceived from contextual cues.

Erber (1979) suggests that, to assess fully a person's speech perception abilities, it is necessary to utilize all the different stimuli using each response task. The resultant complex evaluation will supply the kind of comprehensive information that is necessary to understand fully each child's auditory functioning. It is invaluable for planning an auditory training program for a hearing-impaired child or for a child with an auditory processing disorder. Fortunately, because of the time it requires, it is not a necessary part of every audiological evaluation. It is useful, however, for the audiologist to keep the auditory skills matrix in mind when selecting tests for evaluating a particular child and for determining which tests and how many are needed to measure fully that child's auditory functioning.

FACTORS TO CONSIDER IN SELECTING SPEECH PERCEPTION TESTS

Closed Set vs. Open Set Testing

WORD recognition tests may be divided into two categories: closed set tests and open set tests. In closed set testing, the number of possible items is restricted. The child being tested understands what all the possible test stimuli are and will select a response from that limited number of potential items. Items might be numbers, body parts, alphabet letters, or pictures placed in front of the child. Open set testing provides no clues. The child may know that the stimulus will be a one- or two-syllable word but will know nothing else about it. Any word in the vocabulary is a possibility. Sometimes children may be asked to repeat what they hear even if it isn't a word so that the audiologist can determine exactly what perceptual errors the child is making. Open set testing is much more difficult than closed set testing and will frequently result in lower scores, but it may furnish a more realistic picture of speech perception abilities in conversation than closed set testing does.

Vocabulary Level

It is essential that the tester know the child's vocabulary level in order to select the appropriate test. If possible, determine the child's vocabulary age by using a standardized vocabulary test, by obtaining information from tests done at another evaluation, or from reporting by parents or teachers. When these alternatives are not available, use information obtained from observation and conversation with the child. Test materials that contain vocabulary not in the child's lexicon will result in a score that is not a true reflection of speech perception abilities.

Degree of Hearing Loss

Degree of hearing loss should not be a factor in selecting tests of speech perception. Tests should be selected based on the individual child's abilities. It is unfair to the child to make assumptions about performance based on the pure tone audiogram alone. Many children with profound hearing losses are capable of using residual hearing for reception of auditory information. However, it is undoubtedly true that profound hearing loss makes it more difficult to receive information using the auditory channel. For children who have not had the opportunity for early intervention, who have not been trained in a program that emphasizes the use of audition, or who do not have the ability to use audition, special tests have been developed that make word recognition testing possible. (See Tests for Severe and Profound Hearing Loss in this chapter and Cochlear Implants, chapter 11).

Phoneme Scoring vs. Whole Word Scoring

Most of the tests we use to evaluate speech perception are scored according to whether the person correctly identifies the whole word. If the person makes an error on one phoneme, the entire word is scored as wrong. This method of scoring may be depriving us of useful information. Arthur Boothroyd has written extensively about phoneme scoring and its advantages and has developed a test that uses phoneme scoring (1968, 1984, 1988). But phoneme scoring can be used with any test. By recording the phoneme errors that a child makes during any speech perception test, we can learn what parts of the spectrum are not being appropriately perceived. Vowel errors indicate insufficient low frequency information; inability to perceive sibilants correctly indicates insufficient high frequency information or possible upward spread of masking caused by too much low frequency amplification. Knowing the specific frequencies of the misperceived sibilants will yield even more specific information. Such knowledge may permit us to make changes in the frequency response of the child's amplification system and to make suggestions about auditory training goals.

Half List vs. Full List

The issue of half list vs. full list has been debated in the field of audiology for some time. Obviously, using a full fifty-word list reduces the chance of error in scoring. However, when working with young children, many factors need to be considered. With young children, time is essential. It is necessary to obtain a great deal of information in a short period of time, and it may not be possible to obtain all the necessary test results if too much time is spent on any one test. However, the necessity for speed does not permit using fewer than the required number of stimuli. Short lists should be used only when that protocol has been validated. The number of words used must be sufficient to acquire all the data necessary to assess the child's speech perception abilities. This evaluation can usually be done with twenty-five words on most tests but not with ten. Except in rare cases—such as the Isophonemic Word Lists (Boothroyd 1968) that have been standardized on ten-word lists—ten words will not provide a sufficient number and variety of stimuli to obtain an accurate score.

Use of a Carrier Phrase

Most word recognition tasks were designed for use with a carrier phrase, which alerts the child to attend and places the word in a sentence context that more accurately represents its use in normal conversation. The carrier phrase should end with a vowel so that the phrase does not influence the word. Common carrier phrases are "show me the . . ." or "tell me. . . ."

Recorded vs. Monitored Live Voice

Recorded testing has the advantage of being easier to compare from test session to test session. It also avoids the possibility of the tester's voice being modified either intentionally or unintentionally to assist the child in obtaining a higher score. On the other hand, recorded testing is more time consuming and prevents the audiologist from making adaptations that are sometimes needed when testing children. Children may need more off time between stimuli to be able to attend than the recording permits. If they get distracted and begin to talk to the tester, they may need to have an item repeated; they may also require time out for encouragement. It is certainly possible to stop the tape or CD player and rewind, but this is often difficult to do efficiently. My experience has indicated that, if the tester is aware of the pitfalls of monitored live voice testing, then it is possible to obtain accurate results using live voice.

Is One Test Enough?

With both children and adults, optimal information will be acquired by using more than one test during an evaluation. Figure 5.1 presents test results of a child with a profound hearing loss. Word recognition testing with a four-item forced-choice closed set test (NU-CHIPS) indicated that he had excellent word recognition skills. Because this was a closed set test, the results may not be a realistic assessment of how he will do in conversation. A repetition of the test in an open set format (no pictures) indicated that he had much poorer skills than the closed set test had indicated. Both tests provided important information and, taken together, give an accurate picture of this child's auditory skills.

Figure 5.2 contains the test results for a child who appeared to have very poor word recognition abilities when using open set testing. When closed set testing was performed, it became clear that he indeed had some word recognition abilities. The additional use of phoneme scoring can also tell us which sounds the child can perceive correctly and which he cannot. Armed with this information, we can provide more amplification in the frequency areas where perception is poor, and we can stress these phonemes in auditory training.

Using Visual Clues

Most speech perception testing is performed using audition alone. However, when children have very poor word recognition skills or very little confidence in their auditory abilities, it may be useful to test using vision alone, audition alone, and both vision and audition together. When the examiner uses vision and audition together, the child is permitted to watch the face of the examiner and listen at the same time. This permits a combined approach to listening that is more similar to what is actually experienced in daily activities. At the same time, it is critical to obtain information using only audition, since that alone will provide the necessary data for setting amplification and planning auditory training. By testing using vision alone, audition alone, and comparing these scores to the combined vision-audition test, we can ascertain how much each sense contributes to reception.

THRESHOLD SPEECH TESTS

AUDIOLOGISTS frequently begin evaluations with adults using pure tone stimuli, but many pediatric audiologists begin with speech stimuli. Any audiologist who works with children is aware that speech, probably because of

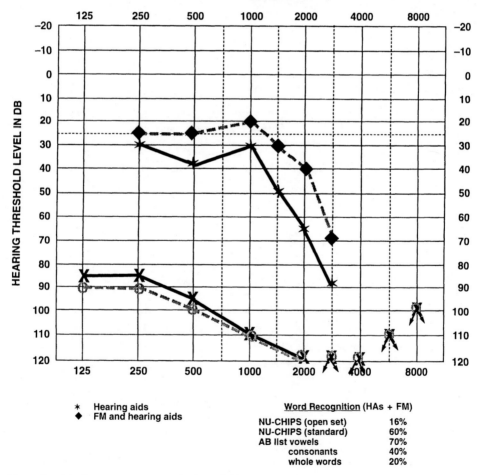

Figure 5.1. Word recognition test results for a child with a profound hearing loss, comparing an open set test, a closed set test, and phoneme scoring (from Madell 1992 with permission).

its familiarity and interest, can more easily attract the attention of a young child than pure tone or noise band stimuli. The choice of stimulus will be determined by the child's speech and language skills. Speech awareness or reception thresholds furnish some basic auditory data that can help determine the level at which to begin when presenting pure tone or noise band stimuli for threshold testing and to confirm the pure tone thresholds.

Speech Awareness or Speech Detection Thresholds

The speech awareness (SAT) or speech detection (SDT) threshold is a test that uses speech stimuli to determine threshold: the lowest intensity level at which a

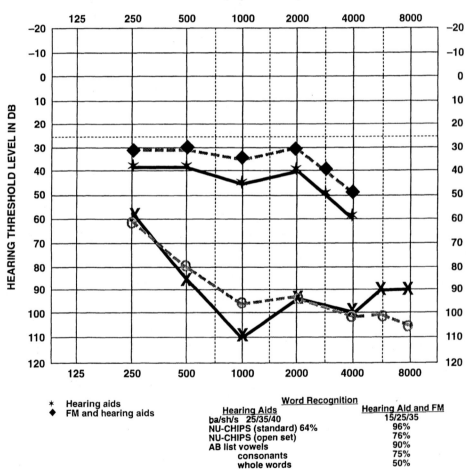

PURE TONE AUDIOMETRY (RE ANSI 1969) - FREQUENCY IN Hz
DAVID (4 years old)

	Word Recognition	
Hearing aids *	**Hearing Aids**	**Hearing Aid and FM**
FM and hearing aids ◆	ba/sh/s 25/35/40	15/25/35
	NU-CHIPS (standard) 64%	96%
	NU-CHIPS (open set)	76%
	AB list vowels	90%
	consonants	75%
	whole words	50%

Figure 5.2. Word recognition test results for another child with a profound hearing loss, comparing an open set test, a closed set test, and phoneme scoring (from Madell 1992 with permission).

person can detect the presence of the stimulus 50% of the time. Speech awareness thresholds are generally used only when more complex speech stimuli cannot be used. Such situations might occur when testing a very young child without the vocabulary for other speech testing or when testing a person with extremely poor or no word recognition ability.

A variety of different stimuli can be used. The most common stimulus is conversational voice. The audiologist may call the child's name or use music either by singing or playing recorded children's songs. However, the information obtained will be limited, since both music and conversation are broadband stimuli, and the threshold obtained will be close to that obtained at the frequency the child hears at the lowest levels.

More worthwhile information is derived by employing the Ling Five Sound Test (Ling 1978). The test items—/a/, /i/, /u/, /sh/, and /s/—are selected to provide frequency-specific information. The vowels assess perception of low-frequency stimuli, /sh/ measures perception of mid-high-frequency stimuli, and /s/ gauges perception of high-frequency stimuli. An adapted version (Madell 1990) uses /ba/ or /bu/ for assessing low-frequency stimuli, /sh/ for measuring mid-high frequency stimuli, and /s/ for gauging high-frequency stimuli. Although it takes slightly longer to obtain three thresholds than it does to obtain one, the information elicited is much more valuable than that obtained using a single broad-frequency stimulus. It is frequency specific and tells us how a person can be expected to perceive speech stimuli across the frequency range needed for speech. In addition, since the test is frequency specific, it can be compared more directly to pure tone thresholds.

Speech Reception Thresholds

The speech reception threshold (SRT) determines the lowest level at which a person can identify speech stimuli 50% of the time. It differs from detection tasks that require only that the person be aware of the presence of speech, not identify it. The test materials selected will depend on the individual being tested. When possible, it is desirable to use test materials and procedures that are standardized on adults so that results are comparable. This will obviously not be possible with all children, but that does not mean you cannot obtain useful information. Older children with good language skills will be able to perform well on standard tests that were developed for adults. Young children may not have the vocabulary or may be too shy to repeat what the tester has said. For these children, a picture-pointing task or a task requiring pointing to body parts will be easier and will tender useful results.

The test procedure for SRTs requires that the examiner be familiar with the material being presented. Familiarity makes testing easier and results in a threshold at a lower level than that obtained with open set testing, in which any vocabulary word might be used. Standard testing uses spondee words (two-syllable words with equal stress on both syllables.) With children who can perform this task, the audiologist reads the list of words at a comfortably loud level, permitting speechreading if necessary, with the child repeating the word to verify that it is understood. Once the child is familiar with the words, the audiologist begins testing using audition alone and reduces the intensity until the child begins making errors. The audiologist then increases and decreases intensity establishing the level at which the child can correctly repeat the words 50% of the time. American Speech-Language-Hearing Association guidelines for speech reception threshold testing (1988) describe a complex procedure that, while resulting in an accurate threshold, may be time consuming. Cramer and Erber (1974) found that best results were obtained by asking the child to say the word and point at the same time. This combined task may increase the child's attention to the task and, therefore, result in improved scores.

For children who cannot perform using standard techniques, the audiologist can use pictures or objects representing the spondee words. The presence of the items will make the task easier. If the child's vocabulary is not sufficient for the use of standard spondees, similar information can be obtained using familiar objects, pictures, or body parts. Even very young children (younger than two years of age) are likely to be able to point to eyes, nose, mouth, ears, hair, shoes, and so on. For children whose speech perception is very poor, it may be possible to obtain an SRT using numbers from one to ten, since number recognition requires only vowel perception.

Siegenthaler and Haspiel (1966) developed a threshold test called Threshold by the Identification of Pictures (TIP). This is a picture identification test that uses monosyllabic words rather than the standard bisyllabic words. Monosyllabic words are less redundant than bisyllabic words—making the task more difficult—and may affect test results adversely.

WORD RECOGNITION TESTING

WORD recognition tests evaluate a child's ability to understand speech under different listening conditions. Unlike threshold testing, word recognition testing is performed at suprathreshold levels. Testing may be conducted at different intensities and under various conditions of competing noise. The selection of test materials and conditions will depend on the child's vocabulary level and ability to cooperate. Scoring requires accurate perception of all the phonemes in any word to obtain a correct score. By modifying the response task and types of reinforcement, it is possible to learn a great deal about a child's speech perception skills, without which information an audiological evaluation is incomplete.

Word Recognition Tests

Closed Set Tests

NUMBERS: Identification of numbers may be the easiest word recognition task since the vocabulary is familiar to most children and requires only vowel recognition. Erber (1980) developed a test called the Auditory Numbers Test (ANT), which used pictures of one, two, three, four or five ants on cards that also had the numbers from one to five. This is simply a more formalized way of testing number recognition, but the pictures may hold more interest for young children than simply repeating numbers.

BODY PARTS OR OTHER FAMILIAR OBJECTS: Pointing to body parts is an easy task even for very young children. This can usually be made into an interesting game. This same task can also be done using pictures or objects with which the child is familiar. Because only a limited number of stimuli is being used, the results must be interpreted with care.

ALPHABET TEST (APAL): The APAL test was designed to overcome the difficulties caused by reduced vocabulary in many children with impaired hearing and to evaluate the type of errors they make (Ross and Randolph 1990). The test requires that the child be able to identify spoken letters of the alphabet. Responses may be made orally, using finger spelling, or by pointing to a response board. A recorded version of the test is available. The tester uses the carrier phrase "the letters are . . ." and then says two letters, which the child must identify in sequence.

The scoring sheet provides three weighted categories developed to analyze errors based on their perceptual distance from the stimulus. For example, if the stimulus is /p/ and the child identifies /b/, the response is off by only one distinctive feature (voicing); this is a Category I error. If the response is off by two features, it is a Category II error, and all other errors are Category III errors. The test form permits easy scoring.

NORTHWESTERN UNIVERSITY CHILDREN'S PERCEPTION OF SPEECH (NU-CHIPS): The NU-CHIPS, created by Elliott and Katz (1980), is a four-item, forced-choice picture identification test. It has fifty stimulus pages and can be used in whole- or half-list format. Two versions are available, providing a total of four fifty-word lists or eight twenty-five word lists. The vocabulary is at the three-year level and can frequently be used with two-year-olds. A recorded version is available with a choice of either male or female speakers.

WORD INTELLIGIBILITY BY PICTURE IDENTIFICATION (WIPI): The WIPI, developed by Ross and Lerman (1970), is a six-item, forced-choice picture identification test with twenty-five items and four test forms. This test requires the vocabulary of a three-and-a-half-year-old and is available in recorded format. A good alternative for slightly older children, the test is somewhat more difficult than the NU-CHIPS because it is a six-item test and because the vocabulary is more difficult.

DISCRIMINATION IN PICTURES (DIP): Siegenthaler and Haspiel (1966) devised the DIP, a two-item, forced-choice picture identification test. It contains forty-eight pairs of monosyllabic words. Because there are only two choices for each item, there is a 50% chance of getting the item correct randomly, which makes interpreting the test results difficult.

PEDIATRIC SPEECH INTELLIGIBILITY TEST (PSI): The Pediatric Speech Intelligibility Test (Jerger and Jerger 1982) is a picture-pointing test designed to provide both central and peripheral auditory processing information. It is intended to assist in locating the site of a lesion. The test uses both monosyllabic words and sentence materials and tests performance-intensity functions and message-to-competition functions. Sentences form the competing message. The test comes in a five- and a three-tape screening version and is intended for use in a recorded format only. The focus group of the test is children three years of age and up.

SPEECH PATTERNS CONTRAST TEST (SPAC): The SPAC (Boothroyd 1984, 1987) is a four-alternative, forced choice test of speech perception. It was originally designed as a research tool to measure the perception of speech contrasts by hearing-impaired children with different degrees of hearing loss. The test measures four suprasegmental and eight segmental contrasts. These include location of stress, sex of speaker, presence or absence of pitch variation, direction of pitch change, vowel height and place, presence or absence of voicing of initial and final consonants, continuance vs. stop plosion of initial and final consonants, and place of articulation of initial and final consonants. It requires that the child be able to read the response alternatives, so it is useful only for older children.

Boothroyd concluded that, as a group, children with less hearing loss had better speech perception skills than children with greater hearing loss. However, it was not possible to predict an individual child's speech perception based on the pure tone audiogram alone. Many different factors influence speech perception abilities, and each child must be evaluated individually. Tests such as the SPAC can provide much more specific data than the more global tests commonly used. The SPAC thus enables us to determine the specific auditory skills an individual possesses and to design a therapy program that will promote them.

Open Set Tests

NU-CHIPS OR WIPI WORDS WITHOUT PICTURES: The vocabulary used in the NU-CHIPS is at the three-year level, while that in the WIPI is at the three-and-one-half-year level. Both of these word lists are excellent for testing young children who can perform using an open set format. The vocabulary level makes the words good choices for open set testing of very young children. Recorded versions of these tests are available.

PHONETICALLY BALANCED KINDERGARTEN LIST (PBK): The PBKs (Haskins 1949) are fifty-item, phonemically balanced, monosyllabic word lists selected from the spoken vocabulary of normal-hearing kindergarten children. Research by Sanderson-Leepa and Rintelman (1976) has demonstrated that the test should not be used for children younger than kindergarten age because the vocabulary will be too difficult, resulting in depressed scores. There is no recorded version of this test.

ISOPHONEMIC WORD LISTS (AB LISTS): The Isophonemic Word lists (Booth-royd 1968, 1984) consist of fifteen word lists, each containing ten CVC words. Each list uses the same thirty phonemes, of which ten are vowels and twenty are consonants. The test, which does not use a carrier phrase, may be presented in a recorded or monitored live voice format. Subjects are asked to repeat what they hear and are scored on the number of phonemes repeated correctly. As previously discussed, phoneme scoring is an excellent way to determine exactly what perception errors the child is making. Because only ten words are used, the test can be administered quickly, and the thirty items provide sufficient information to make comparisons between different amplification or competing message conditions.

CONNECTED DISCOURSE OR SENTENCE TESTING: Using a nonstandardized procedure, we are able to formulate some impression of a child's ability to understand conversational speech using connected discourse. We must interpret these results with caution, however, since context will provide a great deal of information to the child. Connected discourse tracking, developed by De Filippo and Scott (1978), scores the child's ability to repeat correctly phrases and sentences read by the examiner in a five-minute period. A standardized open set sentence test is included as part of the Minimal Auditory Capabilities Battery (MAC) (Owens et al. 1985).

Tests for Severe and Profound Hearing Loss

Auditory Numbers Test (ANT)

This test (Erber 1980) was discussed previously as both an SRT and a word recognition test. It is a closed set test that assesses vowel perception (see Word Recognition: Numbers.)

Monosyllable, Trochee, Spondee Test (MTS)

The MTS (Erber and Alencewicz 1976) consists of twelve words: four monosyllables, four trochees (two-syllable words with stress on the first syllable), and four spondees. All twelve pictures are placed in front of the child, who is asked to point to the picture identified by the examiner. The test is scored in two ways: percentage of words correct and percentage of words categorized correctly by stress pattern. For example, if the word presented is a trochee, and the child chooses the wrong trochee, it will be scored wrong for the word but correct for stress pattern. The test was designed for children over the age of five years but can be used for younger children who have the necessary vocabulary.

Glendonald Auditory Screening Procedure (GASP)

The GASP (Erber 1982) was designed as a closed set test, one portion of which uses the concept of the MTS. It contains twelve words: three monosyllables, three trochees, three spondees, and three polysyllables. In addition, it contains ten everyday sentences and a phoneme detection task. Berliner and Eisenberg (1985) report using it in an open set format for evaluating children with cochlear implants.

Discrimination after Training Test (DAT)

The DAT (Thielemeir 1982) is intended for use with children and adults who are prelingually deaf. The stimulus items are taken from the MTS and proceed through twelve levels of difficulty, beginning with speechreading, to determine whether the child understands the stimulus. Testing evaluates speech detection, gross duration and timing cues, and discrimination of speech pattern perception. The test is administered live voice.

Early Speech Perception Test (ESP)

The ESP (Geers and Moog 1989; Moog and Geers 1990) was originated to meet the needs of very young profoundly hearing-impaired children with limited vocabulary and language skills. The vocabulary is familiar to hearing-impaired children by the age of six years, the words used are easily depicted with pictures, and the test takes less than an hour to complete. It is administered using monitored live voice, first using a combination of vision and audition to be certain that the child has the vocabulary, and then using audition alone.

The test contains a pattern perception subtest and two word identification subtests. The pattern perception subtest is adapted from the GASP and presents the same twelve pictures and four stress categories. Part two is a twelve-item spondee identification test with each item having a different vowel. Part three is a twelve-item monosyllabic word identification test containing similar words. All words begin with /b/, and most end with a plosive. Children who do very well are then tested with the WIPI or the PBK. There is a "low-verbal" version for children who do not have sufficient vocabulary for the standard version. It uses real objects instead of pictures and small sets consisting of two or three objects.

Minimal Auditory Capabilities Battery (MAC)

The MAC (Owens et al. 1985) is a recorded test battery that comprises thirteen auditory tests and one speechreading test. These tests examine phonemic discrimination, sentence identification, suprasegmental features, identification of environmental sounds, and visual enhancement with and without amplification. Because the test is complex, it yields a great deal of information, although it is not applicable for young children.

Test of Auditory Comprehension (TAC)

The TAC (Los Angeles County 1980) is a closed set recorded test that evaluates perception of both environmental sounds and speech. It has ten subtests, beginning with the ability to perceive the difference between linguistic and nonlinguistic sounds (speech vs. cough), and proceeds to the comprehension of speech in the presence of competing messages. The child responds by pointing to pictures.

Speech Patterns Contrast Test (SPAC)

The SPAC, previously discussed, is a suitable test for assessing a variety of speech contrasts in children. (See Closed Set Tests.)

Evaluation of Speech Perception in Infants

Several researchers have demonstrated that infants can discriminate among different sounds very early in life (Eilers 1977; Eimas 1974; Kuhl and Miller 1975; Morse 1972). Eilers, Wilson, and Moore (1977) developed the Visually Reinforced Infant Speech Discrimination paradigm (VRISD). This recorded test requires presentation of two phonemes during a four-second interval; the child is reinforced using a three-dimensional toy for a head turn when the sound is changed. Initially, the second stimulus is presented at a higher intensity than the first. Once the child has learned the task, the intensities are equated. Although this has been used primarily as a research tool, the potential for clinical use is genuinely exciting. It would be especially effective in assessing amplification benefits for infants who cannot yet perform other speech perception tasks.

Test Conditions for Assessing Speech Perception

Evaluating Monaural Functioning

To assess fully a child's speech perception abilities, an audiologist must perform several tests under different conditions. Earphone testing—usually performed at 40 dB SL or at MCL—will provide information about the child's speech perception abilities in each ear separately. If retrocochlear pathology is a concern, PB-PI functions (Bess, Josey, and Humes 1979) can be determined with any of the word recognition tests discussed previously. Since most speech perception testing is conducted at what should be comfortably loud levels, we may not derive information about everyday functioning. To acquire this knowledge, the audiologist should test the child at normal and soft conversational levels, preferably in soundfield.

Soundfield Evaluation

Every child should have auditory functioning evaluated regardless of the basic reason for the evaluation (NIH 1993). Even a child with a mild conductive hearing loss who performs well under earphones at 40 dB SL may have difficulty with word recognition at soft conversational levels or in the presence of competing noise. Figure 5.3 shows test results for just such a child. The information obtained by testing at soft conversational levels and with competing noise will be valuable in helping physicians, parents, classroom teachers, and the children themselves recognize the effect of a mild hearing loss on classroom functioning.

Testing should be conducted routinely at normal (50 dB HL) and soft (35 dB HL) conversational levels (Madell 1990). If test results are extremely poor at normal levels, they need not be obtained at soft levels. After testing in quiet, testing should be repeated at normal and soft conversational levels in the presence of competing noise. The most useful competing message is recorded four- or twelve-talker babble. Because the stimulus is speech, it will be more distracting than speech noise or white noise and more like the message competition that the child faces every day.

Testing is usually conducted at +5 or +6 dB S/N. If good results are obtained at that level, testing can be repeated at 0 dB S/N. For soundfield testing, the child should be seated facing the loudspeaker at 0 degrees azimuth with the speech stimulus coming from the front speaker. The competing message can be presented from the same loudspeaker, from 180 degrees (directly behind the child), or from 90 degrees on both sides of the child. The level (in dBA) at which the child achieves 80% may be an acceptable norm (McCormick 1993). When a child has a unilateral hearing loss, it is useful to test with the loudspeakers at 45 or 90 degrees on each side of the child, with speech directed to the side of the poorer ear and the competing message directed to the better ear. This will tax the child's auditory capability maximally.

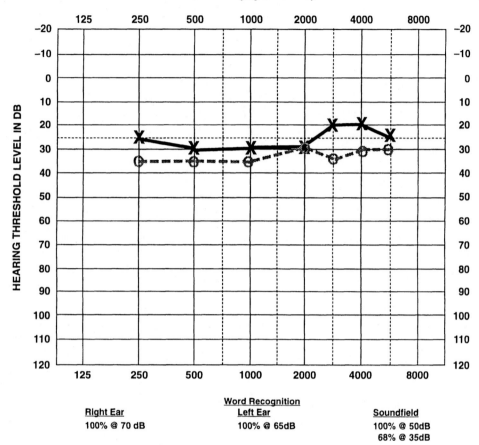

PURE TONE AUDIOMETRY (RE ANSI 1969) - FREQUENCY IN Hz
RACHAEL (5 years old)

	Word Recognition	
Right Ear	Left Ear	Soundfield
100% @ 70 dB	100% @ 65dB	100% @ 50dB
		68% @ 35dB

Figure 5.3. Word recognition testing for a child with a mild hearing loss at normal and soft conversation levels

A child whose word recognition drops significantly in the presence of competing noise may be demonstrating auditory processing difficulties. Figure 5.4 demonstrates test results of a child with normal hearing and good word recognition at normal conversational levels but with poor word recognition at soft levels and in the presence of competing noise. Identification of the problem helps the parent, teacher, and child understand some aberrant academic and behavior patterns that do not stem from inattention, but from a very real perceptual problem.

Testing with Amplification

The assessment of amplification follows unaided testing, so soundfield test results at normal and soft conversational levels in quiet and in the presence of a competing message will already be available. The same tests should be repeated

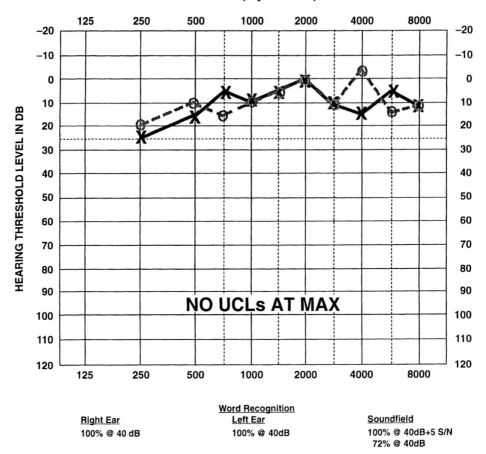

Figure 5.4. Word recognition testing in quiet and in the presence of a competing message for a child with normal hearing and a presumed auditory processing disorder

with amplification. If there is any doubt, this type of testing should verify the benefit obtained from amplification. If aided test results indicate reduced functioning in quiet or in the presence of a competing message, a good case can be made for the use of FM systems in the classroom and in other situations in which distance from the talker or competing noise is a factor.

Describing Auditory Functioning

A part of each audiologic report should include a description of the child's auditory functioning. This will help the reader to understand what to expect from the child in a variety of situations and will assist the teacher and therapist in planning remediation if needed. What can you expect from the child when speech is presented at normal and soft conversational levels? What happens in the presence of noise? Can the child perform in an unclued (open set) situation, or is it necessary for the child to be clued (closed set or topic information) in order to understand? Does the child require paragraph or sentence material to follow conversation, or can she follow single words? Does the child require repetition in order to understand? If the child wears hearing aids, functioning should be compared unaided, aided, and with an FM system to develop a complete picture of the child's auditory strengths and weaknesses.

SUMMARY

SPEECH perception testing is an exciting and challenging part of the audiologic test battery. By fully assessing speech perception, we are able to obtain valuable information about a child's use of audition that cannot be obtained in any other way. A large variety of speech perception tests is available. Combining them appropriately, under different test conditions, allows us to evaluate children of all ages, with all levels of vocabulary, and with all degrees and types of hearing loss. These tests afford us an opportunity to assist in maximizing every child's communication abilities. Speech perception testing is an essential part of our test battery, and in-depth testing should be routinely included in every child's audiological evaluation. By doing so, we fulfill our responsibility to do more than simply identify the presence or absence of hearing loss and do what audiology was intended to do: assess and improve communication function.

REFERENCES

American Speech-Language-Hearing Association. 1988. Guidelines for determining threshold level for speech. *Asha* 30:85–89.

Berliner, K.I., and L.S. Eisenberg. 1985. Methods and issues in the cochlear implantation of children: An overview. The cochlear implant: An auditory prosthesis for the profoundly deaf child. *Ear and Hearing* (Suppl. 6) 3:6S–13S.

Bess, F.H., A.F. Josey, and L.E. Humes. 1979. Performance intensity functions in cochlear and eighth nerve disorders. *American Journal of Otolaryngology* 1:27–31.

Boothroyd, A. 1968. Developments in speech audiometry. *Sound* 2:3–10.

———. 1984. Auditory perception of speech contrasts by subjects with sensorineural hearing loss. *Journal of Speech and Hearing Research* 27:134–144.

———. 1987. Perception of speech pattern contrasts via cochlear implants and limited hearing. *Annals of Otology, Rhinology, and Laryngology* (Suppl. 128) 96:58–62.

———. 1988. Amplitude compression and profound hearing loss. *Journal of Speech and Hearing Research* 31:362–376.

Cramer, K.D., and N.P. Erber. 1974. A spondee recognition test for young hearing-impaired children. *Journal of Speech and Hearing Disorders* 39:304–311.

De Filippo, C.L., and B.L. Scott. 1978. A method for training and evaluating the reception of ongoing speech. *Journal of the Acoustical Society of America* 63:1186–1192.

Eilers, R.E. 1977. Context-sensitive perception of naturally produced stop and fricative consonants by infants. *Journal of the Acoustical Society of America* 61:1321–1336.

Eilers, R.E., W.R. Wilson, and J.M. Moore. 1977. Developmental changes in speech discrimination in infants. *Journal of Speech and Hearing Research* 20:766–780.

Eimas, P.D. 1974. Auditory and linguistic processing of cues for place of articulation by infants. *Perception and Psychophysics* 16:513–521.

Elliott, L.L., and D. Katz. 1980. *Northwestern University children's perception of speech (NU-CHIPS)*. St. Louis: Auditec.

Erber, N.P. 1979. An approach to evaluating auditory speech perception ability. *The Volta Review* 81:16–24.

———. 1980. Use of the auditory numbers test to evaluate speech perception abilities of hearing impaired children. *Journal of Speech and Hearing Disorders* 45:527–532.

———. 1982. *Auditory training.* Washington, D.C.: A.G. Bell Association

Erber, N.P., and C.M. Alencewicz. 1976. Audiologic evaluation of deaf children. *Journal of Speech and Hearing Disorders* 41:256–267.

Friel-Patti, S., T. Finitzo-Hieber, G. Conti, and K. Brown. 1982. Language delay in infants associated with middle ear disease and mild fluctuating hearing impairment. *Pediatric Infectious Disease* 1:104–109.

Geers, A., and J. Moog. 1989. Evaluating speech perception skills: Tools for measuring benefits of cochlear implants, tactile aids, and hearing aids. In *Cochlear implants in young deaf children*, ed. E. Owens and D. Kessler. Boston: College-Hill Press.

Haskins, H. 1949. A phonetically balanced test of speech discrimination for children. Master's thesis, Northwestern University.

Jerger, S., and J. Jerger. 1982. Pediatric speech intelligibility test: Performance-intensity characteristics. *Ear and Hearing* 3:325–333.

Kuhl, P.K., and J.D. Miller. 1975. Speech perception in early infancy: Discrimination of speech-sound changes. *Journal of the Acoustical Society of America* (Suppl. 1) 58:566.

Ling, D. 1978. Auditory coding and recoding: An analysis of auditory training procedures for hearing impaired children. In *Auditory management of hearing impaired children*, ed. M. Ross and T. Giolas. Baltimore: University Park Press.

Los Angeles County, Office of the Los Angeles County Superintendent of Schools, Audiology Services, and Southwest School for the Hearing Impaired. 1980. *Test of auditory comprehension*. North Hollywood: Forworks.

McCormick, B. 1993. Behavioural hearing tests 6 months to 3; 6 years. In *Paediatric audiology, 0–5 years*, 2d ed., ed. B. McCormick. London: Whurr Publishers.

Madell, J.R. 1990. Audiological evaluation. In *Hearing-impaired children in the mainstream*, ed. M.Ross. Parkton, MD: York Press.

———. 1992. FM systems as primary amplification for children with profound hearing loss. *Ear and Hearing* 13: 102–107.

Moog, J., and A. Geers. 1990. *Early speech perception test for profoundly hearing-impaired children*. St. Louis: Central Institute for the Deaf.

Morse, P.A. 1972. The discrimination of speech and non-speech stimuli in early infancy. *Journal of Experimental Child Psychology* 14:477–492.

National Institutes of Health (NIH). 1993. Early identification of hearing impairment in infants and young children. *NIH Consensus Statement* 11:1–24.

Owens, E., D.K. Kessler, M.W. Raggio, and E.D. Schubert. 1985. Analysis and revision of the minimal auditory capabilities (MAC) battery. *Ear and Hearing* 6:280–290.

Ross, M., and T.G. Giolas. 1978. *Auditory management of hearing-impaired children: Principles and prerequisites for intervention.* Baltimore: University Park Press.

Ross, M., and J. Lerman. 1970. A picture identification test for hearing-impaired children. *Journal of Speech and Hearing Research* 13:44–53.

Ross, M., and K. Randolph. 1990. A test of the auditory perception of alphabet letters for hearing impaired children: The APAL test. *The Volta Review* 92:237–244.

Sanderson-Leepa, M.E., and W.F. Rintelmann. 1976. Articulation function and test-retest performance of normal-hearing children on three speech discrimination tests: WIPI, PBK 50, and NU auditory test no. 6. *Journal of Speech and Hearing Disorders* 41:503–519.

Siegenthaler, B., and G. Haspiel. 1966. *Development of two standardized measures of hearing for speech by children.* Cooperative research program project #2372. Washington, D.C.: United States Office of Education.

Thielemeir, M.A. 1982. *Discrimination after training test.* Los Angeles: House Ear Institute.

Wallace, I.F., J.S. Gravel, C.M. McCarton, and R.J. Ruben. 1988. Otitis media and language development at 1 year of age. *Journal of Speech and Hearing Disorders* 54:245–251.

6

Acoustic Immittance

Shlomo Silman and Carol A. Silverman

Basic Concepts of Acoustic Immittance

Components

ACOUSTIC immittance can be defined in terms of acoustic impedance or admittance. Acoustic impedance is defined as the rejection offered by an acoustico-mechanical system to the flow of energy. The unit of acoustic impedance is the acoustic ohm. Acoustic admittance is the reciprocal of acoustic impedance. The unit of acoustic admittance is the acoustic mho.

Acoustic impedance consists of three components: acoustic mass reactance, acoustic stiffness reactance, and acoustic resistance. Acoustic mass reactance is the rejection offered by the mass of a system to a flow of energy. Acoustic stiffness reactance is the rejection offered by the stiffness of a system to a flow of energy. The acoustic mass reactance and acoustic stiffness reactance components function in opposition to each other.

An acoustic system can be described as mass-dominated or stiffness-dominated, depending on which component—acoustic mass reactance or acoustic stiffness reactance—is larger. In the early literature, the normal human middle ear was erroneously described as a stiffness-dominated system. The normal human middle ear is indeed a stiffness-dominated system for low-frequency probe tones. At frequencies below 900 Hz, the normal middle ear is stiffness dominated, and at probe-tone frequencies above 1200 Hz, it is mass dominated. The acoustic resistance is largely unaffected by probe-tone frequency.

Acoustic admittance is defined as the ease with which acoustic energy passes through a system. The admittance components include acoustic stiffness susceptance, acoustic mass susceptance, and acoustic conductance. Acoustic stiffness susceptance is the ease with which energy flows into a stiff system. Acoustic mass susceptance is the ease with which energy flows into a mass system. Acoustic conductance is the ease with which energy flows into friction.

Acoustic Reflex

When the acoustic reflex is activated at low probe-tone frequencies, the acoustic middle-ear impedance, which is measured at the tympanic membrane, changes. Acoustic-reflex activation consists primarily of contraction of the stapedius muscle. With acoustic-reflex activation, the ossicular chain is stiffened, causing increased acoustic middle-ear reactance and, therefore, increased middle-ear impedance.

Acoustic-reflex activation is bilateral, even when stimulation is unilateral. Therefore, the acoustic reflex can be monitored in the stimulated ear (ipsilateral acoustic-reflex assessment) or in the ear contralateral to the stimulated ear (contralateral acoustic-reflex assessment). In ipsilateral acoustic-reflex measurement, both the probe-tone signal (used to measure the acoustic-immittance change) and the acoustic-reflex activating signal are presented to the same ear through the probe tube. On the other hand, in contralateral acoustic-reflex measurement, the activating signal is presented to one ear through an earphone or ear insert, and the probe tone is presented to the opposite ear through a probe tube. The acoustic-reflex threshold (ART) is the lowest intensity for the activating signal resulting in a measurable change in acoustic immittance at the tympanic membrane, which is monitored in the probe ear.

Advantages of ipsilateral over contralateral acoustic-reflex assessment include independent ear evaluation and elimination of collapsed ear-canal effects. Ipsilateral acoustic-reflex assessment has certain disadvantages that, for the most part, are not shared by contralateral acoustic-reflex assessment. One disadvantage of ipsilateral acoustic-reflex measurement results from the presentation of both the acoustic-reflex activating and probe-tone signals into the same tube, yielding artifact problems. Presentation of both into the same tube frequently results in acoustic interaction between these signals. Consequently, the sound-pressure level of the probe tone is altered, falsely signaling acoustic-impedance change associated with acoustic-reflex contraction.

The occurrence of additive and subtractive artifacts can be prevented through the use of a multiplexing circuit (incorporated in some commercially available electroacoustic-immittance devices) in which the tones are rapidly pulsed in an alternating fashion. The admittance measures are determined from probe-tone measurements while the activator is off between pulses.

Another disadvantage of ipsilateral acoustic-reflex measurement (and of contralateral acoustic-reflex measurement that presents stimulation through an ear insert instead of an earphone) is the calibration of the intensity level in a 2-cm^3 rather than the 6-cm^3 coupler employed for calibration of intensities in clinical audiometers. Therefore, ipsilateral ARTs cannot be compared directly with contralateral ARTs, even when the thresholds are reported in dB HL.

As probe-tone frequency increases, the magnitude of the change in acoustic middle-ear impedance with acoustic-reflex activation decreases (Bennett 1984;

Bennett and Weatherby 1982). Beginning at the probe-tone frequency of approximately 600–700 Hz, the acoustic middle-ear impedance decreases rather than increases with acoustic-reflex activation. (The reversing probe-tone frequency is approximately 665 Hz.) That is, at higher probe-tone frequencies, the magnitude of the acoustic resistance decreases and exceeds the magnitude of any change in acoustic reactance.

Acoustic-reflex adaptation (ARA) (or decay) is the decrease in magnitude of the change in acoustic-immittance during sustained acoustic stimulation. With ARA or decay, the decrease in magnitude of the change in acoustic-immittance reflects the increase in middle-ear admittance during sustained acoustic stimulation.

ARTs in Normal Persons

As shown in Table 6.1, the 90% range between the 5th and 95th percentiles for the ipsilateral acoustic-reflex thresholds for the 226-Hz probe tone in normal-hearing adults is 72–90 dB HL for the 500-Hz tonal activator, 75–90 dB HL for the 1000-Hz tonal activator, 77–95 dB HL for the 2000-Hz tonal activator, and 55–75 dB HL for the broadband noise (BBN) activator (Wiley, Oviatt, and Block 1987).

Table 6.1 also shows that the contralateral acoustic-reflex thresholds for the 220-Hz probe tone range (2 SD above and below the mean) are between 75 and 95 dB HL for the 500-Hz tonal activator, between 75 and 100 dB HL for the 1000-Hz tonal activator, and between 80 and 100 dB HL for the 2000-Hz tonal activator in normal-hearing adults (Silman and Gelfand 1981). The mean contralateral ART for normal-hearing adults is approximately 85–90 dB HL for the 500- 1000-, and 2000-Hz tonal-activating signals and approximately 70–75 dB HL for the BBN noise activating signal obtained with the 220-Hz probe tone (Silman and Gelfand 1981; Silman, Gelfand, Howard, and Showers 1982; Silverman, Silman, and Miller 1983). The difference between the contralateral ART for tonal activating signals and the contralateral ART for broadband noise activators is approximately 10–20 dB.

Tympanometry

With tympanometry, the acoustic-immittance of the middle or total (outer and middle) ear is measured as air pressure in the ear canal is varied. The results of

Table 6.1. 90% Range for the Ipsilateral[a] ARTs and 2 SD Range for the Contralateral[b] ARTs

Mode	500 Hz	1000 Hz	2000 Hz	BBN
Ipsilateral	72–90 dB HL	75–90 dB HL	77–95 dB HL	55–75 dB HL
Contralateral	75–95 dB HL	75–100 dB HL	80–100 dB HL	—

[a] For the 226-Hz probe tone, based on the data of Wiley et al. (1987).

[b] For the 220-Hz probe tone, based on the data of Silman and Gelfand (1981).

tympanometry yield (a) the tympanometric peak pressure at which maximum middle-ear (or total-ear) admittance is obtained and (b) the amplitude and shape of the function relating air pressure in the ear canal to the magnitude of the acoustic immittance of the middle ear or total ear.

Static-Acoustic Middle-Ear Admittance

The static-acoustic middle-ear admittance is derived by subtracting the static ear-canal admittance obtained at an extreme air pressure in the ear canal (e.g., +200 daPa or −400 daPa) from the static total-ear admittance obtained at the tympanometric peak pressure. The static-acoustic middle-ear admittance is reported in acoustic millimhos (mmhos), and the static-acoustic middle-ear impedance is reported in acoustic ohms.

The normal range for static-acoustic middle-ear admittance depends on (a) whether a relative or absolute acoustic-admittance device was employed, (b) whether +200 or −400 was used to determine the outer-ear admittance, and (c) the pump speed for the air-pressure variation in the ear canal. (A pump speed not exceeding 50 daPa/s is generally used in diagnostic evaluations, whereas a pump speed of 200 daPa/s is generally used for screening.) The data by Jerger, Jerger, and Mauldin (1972), based on older children and adults, indicate that the range of normal static-acoustic middle-ear admittance between the 10th and 90th percentiles is 0.39–1.30 mmhos (or cc), using a pump speed of 50 daPa/s and the +200 daPa pressure point to determine the ear-canal volume.

With an absolute acoustic-admittance device, the data of Van Camp, Margolis, Wilson, Creten, and Shanks (1986) suggest that the range of normal static-acoustic middle-ear admittance between the 5th and 95th percentiles (using −400 daPa as the pressure point to determine the ear-canal volume) is 0.50–1.75 mmhos for a pump speed not exceeding 50 daPa/s; the range is 0.57–2.00 for the 200 daPa/s pump speed (going from a positive to a negative direction). The ASHA (1990) guidelines for screening for hearing impairment and middle-ear disorders based on Margolis and Heller's (1987) data defined the 90% range of normal static-acoustic middle-ear admittance between the 5th and 95th percentiles (using +200 as the pressure point to determine the ear-canal volume) as 0.3–1.4 mmhos for a pump speed of 200 daPa/s (going from a positive to a negative direction).

Based on the normative ranges, ears with stiffening pathology—such as otosclerosis, congenital ossicular fixation, otitis media, and cholesteatoma—would be expected to have acoustic-admittance values of less than approximately 0.50–0.57 mmhos. Similarly, ears with loosening pathology—such as partial erosion of the ossicular chain and complete ossicular disarticulation—would have admittance values greater than approximately 1.75–2.00 mmhos. These expectations are not completely fulfilled since many pathologic ears have admittance and impedance values within the normal range. Therefore, the static-acoustic middle-ear admittance cannot be used as the only audiologic tool for

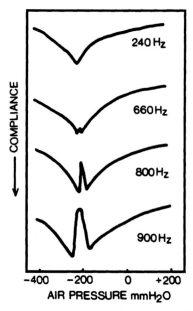

Figure 6.1. Effect of probe frequency on tympanogram in a patient with grossly abnormal tympanic membrane. Note that the "W" shape is obvious at 800 and 900 Hz, but only barely discernible at 660 Hz. (Reprinted by permission of Alberti and Jerger.)

diagnosis of middle-ear disorders; it must be used in conjunction with the audiometric and other acoustic-immittance findings.

Tympanometric Peak Pressure

It cannot be assumed that the tympanometric peak pressure represents the middle-ear pressure for the following reasons: Variation in ear-canal pressure during tympanometry is associated with variation in middle-ear volume with movement of the tympanic membrane, leading to changes in tympanometric peak pressure. This effect is exacerbated in persons with flaccid tympanic membranes. Also, some acoustic-immittance devices have electronic circuits that do not rapidly track large acoustic-immittance changes, such as those that occur with a flaccid tympanic membrane.

The tympanometric peak pressure in adults with normal middle ears generally ranges between $+50$ and -50 daPa (Brooks 1980; Holmquist and Miller 1972; Peterson and Lidén 1972; Porter 1974).

Amplitude and Shape

With an absolute acoustic-immittance device, the amplitude of the tympanogram (from peak to tail) directly yields the static-acoustic middle-ear immittance. With a relative acoustic-immittance device, the amplitude of the tympanogram does not directly yield the static-acoustic middle- or outer-ear immittance. Therefore, amplitude and shape are discussed for the relative acoustic-immittance device, whereas shape is discussed for the absolute acoustic-immittance device; amplitude is addressed in the section on static-acoustic middle-ear admittance.

Figure 6.1 shows the effect of probe-tone frequency on tympanograms obtained with relative acoustic-impedance meters in normal middle ears (with normal or abnormal tympanic membranes). This figure illustrates that there is no notching of the tympanogram for the 240-Hz probe tone although there is a slight w-shaped notching of the tympanogram for the 660-Hz probe tone and more pronounced notching at higher probe-tone frequencies.

The lower limit of the normal range of peak amplitude for relative acoustic-impedance meters varies from one manufacturer to another. The shaded areas in Figures 6.2 and 6.3 show the normal range of peak amplitude for an American Electromedics 83 acoustic-impedance meter and Madsen ZO–73 acoustic-impedance meter, respectively. The normal range of peak amplitude is 5–10 arbitrary acoustic-immittance units for the former vs. 3–10 units for the latter device.

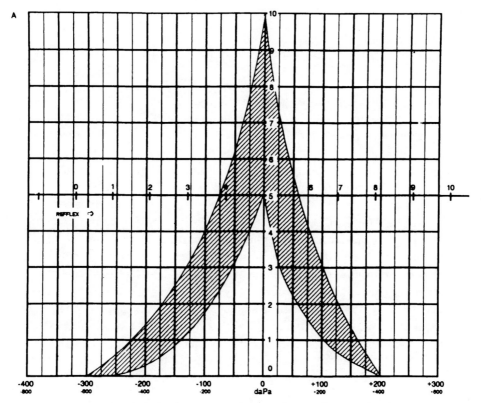

Figure 6.2. Tympanogram form for the American Electromedics impedance meter (relative acoustic-impedance device) (Reprinted with permission of American Electromedics Corp.)

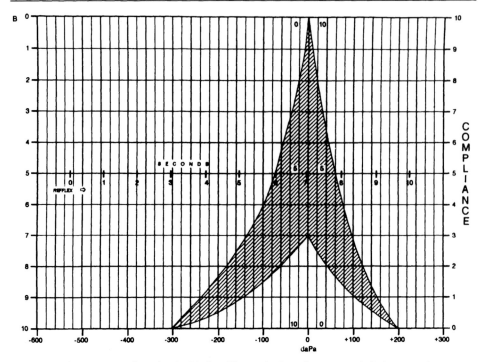

Figure 6.3. Tympanogram form for the Madsen Electronics impedance meter (relative acoustic-impedance device). (Reprinted with permission of Madsen North America, Inc.)

Figure 6.4 shows the susceptance, conductance, and admittance tympanograms obtained with an absolute acoustic-admittance meter for the 226- and 678-Hz probe-tone frequencies in a normal middle ear. This figure reveals that, for the 226-Hz probe tone, the admittance tympanogram has one peak and is relatively shallow; the susceptance tympanogram is similar in shape, and the conductance tympanogram is very shallow. For the 678-Hz probe tone, the admittance, susceptance, and conductance tympanograms are multipeaked.

For the 660-Hz probe tone, there are four normal susceptance and conductance tympanometric patterns (Vanhuyse, Creten, and Van Camp 1975). Figure 6.5 reveals that the 1B1G tympanometric pattern is defined by single-peaked susceptance and conductance tympanograms. This figure also reveals that the 3B1G tympanometric pattern is defined by three peaks (i.e., three extrema) for the susceptance tympanogram and a single-peaked conductance tympanogram. The 3B3G tympanometric pattern is defined by triple-peaked (three extrema) susceptance and conductance tympanograms. The 5B3G tympanometric pattern is defined by a susceptance tympanogram with five peaks (five extrema) and a triple-peaked (three extrema) conductance tympanogram.

In the Vanhuyse et al. (1975) classification system, a normally notched tympanogram must meet the following criteria: (1) The number of extrema must not exceed five for the susceptance (B) and three for the conductance

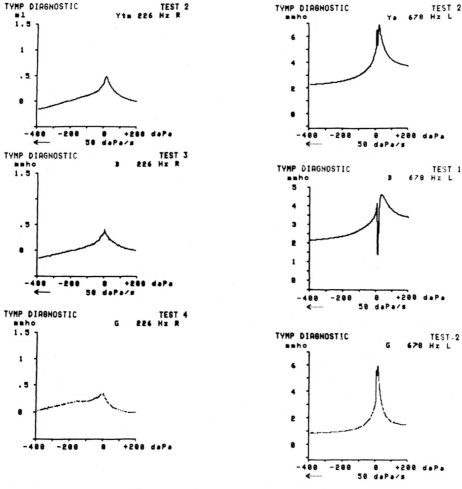

Figure 6.4a. Susceptance, conductance, and admittance tympanograms for the 226-Hz probe tone from the normal middle ear, obtained using an absolute acoustic-immittance device.

Figure 6.4b. Susceptance, conductance, and admittance tympanograms for the 678-Hz probe tone from a normal middle ear, obtained using an absolute acoustic-immittance device.

(G) tympanograms; (2) the distance (in decapascal) between the outermost conductance maxima must be smaller than the distance between the susceptance maxima; and (3) the distance between the outermost maxima must not exceed 75 daPa for tympanograms with three extrema (e.g., 3B3G) and must not exceed 100 daPa for tympanograms with five extrema (e.g., 5B3G). (Shanks 1984, p. 274)

Gradient and Tympanometric Width

The tympanometric gradient or width is a measure of the sharpness of the tympanometric peak. Figure 6.6 illustrates one of the European definitions of tympanometric gradient. According to Brooks (1969), the tympanometric gradient is the ratio hp/ht.

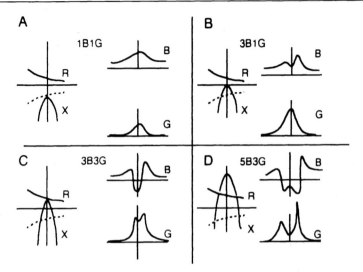

Figure 6.5. Four normal high-frequency tympanometric patterns modeled in acoustic impedance [resistance (R) and reactance (X)] and acoustic admittance [conductance (G) and susceptance (B)]. (Vanhuyse et al. 1975. Reprinted with permission from Shanks 1984.)

Figure 6.7 illustrates the American procedure for determining the tympanometric gradient. According to ASHA (1990), the tympanometric width is the pressure interval corresponding to 50% reduction in static-acoustic middle-ear admittance during tympanometric measurement. In order to determine this pressure interval, the ear-canal volume (admittance) at +200 daPa is subtracted from the tympanometric peak amplitude. A horizontal line is drawn through the tympanogram at the point representing half of this amplitude difference; in

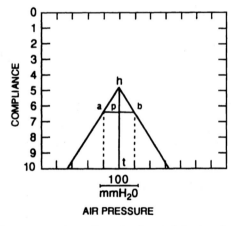

Figure 6.6. Definition of tympanometric gradient. Gradient is defined as the ratio *hp/ht*, where *ht* equals the overall height of the tympanogram, and *hp* equals the vertical distance from the peak of the tympanogram to a horizontal line intersecting the tympanogram; its width between the points of intersection (a,b) is 100 mm H₂0. The higher the ratio hp/ht, the steeper the gradient. (Adapted from Brooks 1969. Reprinted with permission from Paradise, Smith, and Bluestone 1976.)

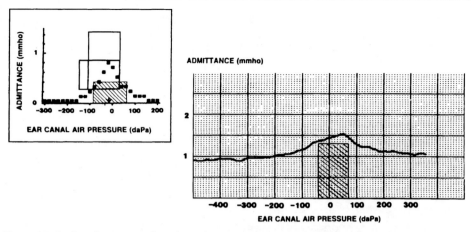

Figure 6.7. In these figures, templates for evaluating tympanometric width are shown for two tympanograms, one recorded from a preschool-aged child (top) and one recorded from an adult (bottom). The shaded regions in each figure represent templates with widths of 150 daPa (bottom), the upper limits of the 90-percent ranges for children and adults, respectively. The template is placed at the ordinate value corresponding to one half of the distance from the peak to the tail value. If the template can be placed at the appropriate admittance value without intersecting the tympanogram, the tympanometric width is outside the normal range. The tympanogram in the upper panel has a tympanometric width of 90 daPa, within the normal range for a preschool-aged child. The tympanogram in the lower panel has a tympanometric width of 165 daPa, an abnormally wide tympanometric width for an adult.

For typanograms that are automatically corrected for ear-canal volume, the tail value is always zero and the template is placed at the admittance value corresponding to one half of the peak. This is the case for the example in the upper panel. When the tympanogram is not corrected for ear-canal volume (lower panel), the template is placed at the value that lies midway between the peak and the positive tail [if the norms in Appendix A of the ASHA (1990) guidelines are used]. If the negative tail value is used, normative data obtained in that manner must be employed (such as those provided by Shanks and Wilson 1986). [Reprinted with permission from ASHA (1990).]

addition, vertical lines from the intersection of the horizontal line and the tympanogram to the abscissa are drawn. The pressure interval is defined by the intersection of the vertical lines with the abscissa.

According to ASHA, the 95th percentile for tympanometric width in normal adults is 110 daPa for a pump speed of 200 daPa/s (going from a positive to a negative direction) and the 226-Hz probe tone. ASHA recommended that, if measurement parameters other than those they recommended in 1990 are used, then normative data should be obtained for those measurement parameters.

The smaller the tympanometric gradient or the larger the tympanometric width, the less sharp or more broad is the tympanometric peak.

MATURATIONAL EFFECTS

Acoustic Reflex

Neonates and Infants

THE acoustic reflex is difficult to measure in neonates at low probe-tone frequencies, for there is essentially no observable acoustic-impedance change at probe-tone frequencies up to approximately 500 Hz (Bennett 1984; Weatherby and Bennett 1980). At the low probe-tone frequencies, there is mismatch between the low acoustic impedance of the eardrum, where the acoustic-impedance change is measured, and the high acoustic-impedance of the middle ear (associated with high acoustic resistance). Therefore, the low acoustic impedance of the eardrum diverts the high impedance of the middle ear, making it difficult to "read" the change in middle-ear impedance associated with acoustic-reflex activation in neonates. At probe-tone frequencies between approximately 500 and 1200 Hz, the mechanism of acoustic-impedance change in neonates is essentially similar to that in adults between 220 and 665 Hz. The reversing probe-tone frequency at which the magnitude of the acoustic impedance begins to decrease (rather than increase) with acoustic-reflex activation is approximately 1200 Hz in neonates (as compared with 665 Hz in adults). The mechanism of acoustic-impedance change at probe-tone frequencies above 1200 Hz in neonates is essentially similar to that in adults above the probe-tone frequency of 665 Hz (Bennett 1984; Weatherby and Bennett 1980).

Most investigations showed a high percentage of absent contralateral acoustic reflexes for the low-frequency probe tone (e.g., 220 or 226 Hz) in neonates and infants (McMillan, Bennett, Marchant, and Shurin 1985; S. Jerger, J. Jerger, Mauldin, and Segal 1974). It is difficult to compare the contralateral ARTs between neonates or infants and adults because of the confounding effects of ear-canal volume in which the sound pressure develops for neonates or infants vs. adults and the coupler volume size. No normative studies on the contralateral ARTs of neonates and infants have been done that have controlled for these procedural problems. Investigators have also reported a high percentage of absent ipsilateral acoustic reflexes for the 220-Hz probe tone (McMillan et al. 1985). As for the contralateral acoustic reflexes, a lower percentage of ipsilateral acoustic reflexes was absent in neonates for the 660-Hz than for the 220-Hz probe tone.

The clinical techniques employed for ipsilateral and contralateral acoustic-reflex threshold measurement do not control for variation in sound-pressure level developed in the ear canal because of large intersubject variability in ear-canal volume in neonates and infants. Therefore, we recommend that absence vs. presence of the acoustic reflexes rather than the ART levels in neonates and infants be evaluated for the purpose of determination of middle-ear effusion or prediction of hearing impairment.

Weatherby and Bennett (1980) reported that the percentage of reflexes present in newborns increases with probe-tone frequency, becoming similar to that in adults by 800 Hz, at least for the broadband noise activator. It is suggested that the presence vs. absence of the acoustic reflex be established for the 800-Hz or higher frequency probe tone. If the acoustic reflex is absent for the tonal activators, then the broadband noise activator should be employed.

The findings of Hirsch, Margolis, and Rykken (1992) illustrate some of the problems of acoustic-reflex assessment in newborns. They found that infant movement prevented the obtaining of acoustic-reflex data in approximately 15% of their high-risk newborns.

Children

Several investigators have shown that the mean contralateral ART for tonal and broadband noise activators decreases as age increases to approximately twelve years (Himmelfarb, Shanon, Popelka, and Margolis 1978; S. Jerger et al. 1974; Osterhammel and Osterhammel 1979; Robertson, Peterson, and Lamb 1968). The data of S. Jerger et al. (1974) suggest that the contralateral tonal ARTs for the 220-Hz probe tone exceeded 110 dB HL in approximately 20% of normal children from birth to three years of age, approximately 15% of normal children between three and four years of age, approximately 12% of normal children between four and five years of age, and approximately 6% of normal children between five and six years of age. The data of J. Jerger (1970), based on 49 normal children between six and thirteen years of age, suggest that approximately 4% of these children have contralateral tonal ARTs for the 220-Hz probe tone exceeding 110 dB HL. These data show that the percentage of contralateral ARTs for the 220-Hz probe tone exceeding 110 dB HL falls below 10% in children five or more years of age and approaches adult values at approximately thirteen years of age.

Hall and Weaver's (1979) data suggest that the 95th percentiles for the contralateral acoustic reflexes for the 220-Hz probe tone in 539 normal-hearing children between one and twenty years of age who had "minor tympanogram abnormalities" (deep tympanogram and/or negative tympanometric peak pressure between −50 and −100 daPa) are approximately 10 dB higher than those in normal-hearing adults.

The possibility of a maturation effect for the ipsilateral as well as contralateral acoustic reflex for tonal and broadband noise activators cannot be ruled out.

Static-Acoustic Immittance

Neonates and Infants

There are maturational effects on static-acoustic reactance and resistance. For the 220-Hz probe tone in neonates, the magnitude of the static-acoustic resistance component greatly exceeds that of the static-acoustic reactance component of middle-ear acoustic impedance. This relation is the reverse of that in adults. In two- to four-month-old infants, the magnitude of the static-acoustic reactance is smaller than in neonates but is still larger than that of acoustic resistance. By approximately four months of age, the relation between reactance and resistance is similar to that in adults.

The magnitude of the static-acoustic middle-ear impedance is greater in neonates than adults at probe tone frequencies above approximately 350 Hz. Below 350 Hz, the magnitude of the static-acoustic middle-ear impedance appears to be greatly decreased and is similar to that in adults (Weatherby and Bennett 1980). This reduced static-acoustic impedance at the low (as compared with the high) frequency probe tone in neonates reflects resonance related to the characteristics of the tympanic membrane in this population. In neonates, the acoustic impedance of the tympanic membrane is much lower that that of the middle ear, so the higher impedance of the middle ear is shunted, making static-acoustic middle-ear impedance measurement inaccurate at low probe-tone frequences such as 226 Hz (Weatherby and Bennett 1980).

In neonates, measurement of the static-acoustic middle ear impedance is also inaccurate at higher probe-tone frequencies such as 678 Hz. This inaccuracy results from the contaminating effect of increased volume of the ear canal because of distention of the soft tissue of the ear canal (in neonates) with the introduction of positive air pressure in tympanometry. The acoustic reactance is inversely related to the product of probe-tone frequency and volume. Therefore, the increased ear-canal volume from positive air pressure introduced into the ear canal during tympanometry will result in decreased reactance and, in turn, decreased impedance, particularly at higher probe-tone frequencies.

Because of the problems associated with high resistance for the low probe-tone frequencies and increased ear-canal volume with air-pressure variation, no normative static-acoustic immittance data are presently available for neonates and infants.

Children

In general, the static-acoustic middle-ear admittance is lower in children than in adults (Jerger et al. 1972; Van Camp et al. 1986). Brooks (1971) obtained normative data on the static-acoustic middle-ear admittance on children using a relative acoustic-admittance device with calculation of the ear-canal static-acoustic admittance at +200 daPa and a probe-tone frequency of 220 Hz. The range between the 10th and 90th percentiles was 0.35 to 1.05 mmhos.

Van Camp et al. (1986) obtained normative data on the static-acoustic middle-ear admittance on children between three and five years using an absolute acoustic-immittance device with calculation of the ear-canal static-acoustic admittance at −400 daPa and a probe-tone frequency of 226 Hz. For low pump speeds (≤50 daPa/s), the range between the 5th and 95th percentiles was 0.35 to 0.90 mmhos. For a high pump speed (200 daPa/s), the range between the 5th and 95th percentiles was 0.40 to 1.03 mmhos.

Silman, Silverman, and Arick (1992) obtained normative data on the static-acoustic middle-ear admittance of children between three and ten years using an absolute acoustic-immittance device with calculation of the ear-canal static-acoustic admittance at +200 daPa, probe-tone frequency of 226 Hz, and pump speed of 50 daPa/s. The range between the 5th and 95th percentiles was 0.35 to 1.25 mmhos.

Tympanometric Peak Pressure

The Eustachian tube is usually collapsed in infants and young children because it has less cartilage; furthermore, that cartilage is more compliant in this population than in adults, and the tensor veli palatini functions less effectively in this population than in adults. As a result, negative tympanometric peak pressures occur more frequently in normal infants and young children than in adults. The tympanometric peak pressure approaches adult values between approximately seven and thirteen years of age.

There are discrepant findings regarding the normal range for tympanometric peak pressure in neonates, infants, and children. A methodologic shortcoming of many of the normative investigations on tympanometric peak pressure is the use of criteria other than otoscopic findings for the establishment of middle-ear normalcy. Until normative data are obtained using otoscopic findings for the establishment of middle-ear pressure, we suggest that the lower limit of normal tympanometric peak pressure be −100 daPa in neonates, infants, and children up to thirteen years of age.

Tympanometric Amplitude and Shape

The characteristics of the outer and middle ears in neonates differ from those in adults. In neonates, the osseous portion of the external ear canal is not developed, rendering the infant ear highly compliant in comparison with the adult ear. Further, the tympanic ring is not fully developed until the end of the first year. Finally, the outer- and middle-ear volumes in infants are smaller than those in adults. Consequently, the tympanometric patterns seen in infants are different from those seen in adults.

Margolis and Shanks (1985) stated that the introduction of positive ear-canal air pressure during tympanometry is associated with a distention of the ear-canal walls, producing an increase in the outer-ear volume, susceptance, and admittance at the 220-Hz probe-tone frequency. Therefore, tympanometry with the 220-Hz probe tone is a less accurate clinical audiologic tool in neonates than adults. The increase in outer-ear volume during tympanometry in neonates is tripled in value for the 660-Hz probe tone since the acoustic susceptance is directly related to the product of probe-tone frequency and volume. As a result, the 660-Hz tympanogram is even less accurate than the 220-Hz tympanogram in neonates. The problems that confound tympanometric assessment in neonates also confound static-acoustic middle-ear admittance assessment in neonates. By four months of age, the amplitude and shape of the tympanogram approach those of adults.

Tympanometric Gradient or Width

The gradient is considered to be normal in children if it is greater than 0.15, according to some investigators (Brooks 1969; Paradise, Smith, and Bluestone 1976) or if it is greater than 0.1, according to other investigators (e.g., Fiellau-Nikolajsen 1983). The 95th percentile for the tympanometric width in children, according to ASHA (1990), is 150 daPa for the 200 daPa/s (positive-to-negative direction) pump speed. Silman et al. (1992), using a pump speed of 50 daPa/s (positive-to-negative direction), reported that the 95th percentile for the tympanometric width is 180 daPa for their sample of normal children.

ACOUSTIC-IMMITTANCE TEST BATTERY: PROCEDURE

Acoustic-Reflex Threshold

FOR measurement of the ART, the starting intensity should be well below the expected threshold. For clinical purposes, intensity is increased in 5-dB steps until a just noticeable change in acoustic immittance occurs, as evidenced by needle deflection on the meter of the acoustic-immittance device or analysis (which may be retrospective) of the acoustic-immittance change displayed on a monitor or oscilloscope. The ART is the lowest intensity associated with a measurable change in acoustic immittance. To verify the intensity yielding the ART, present a stimulus that is 5-dB greater; this stimulus also should be associated with an acoustic-immittance change that is not necessarily larger than the change at threshold levels. Figure 6.8 illustrates the acoustic-immittance changes at several intensities and the level associated with the ART.

Some manufacturers of absolute acoustic-immittance devices recommend that the ART be based on a predetermined amount of acoustic-immittance change, such as 0.02 mmho; some computer-generated ARTs are indeed based on this definition of the ART. We recommend that the ART be based on the smallest detectable acoustic-immittance change rather than a predetermined magnitude of acoustic-immittance change for these reasons: (a) the latter is not necessarily the smallest detectable acoustic-immittance change, and (b) many of the normative data on the ART, including the Silman and Gelfand (1981) 90th percentiles for differential diagnosis, are based on the smallest detectable acoustic-immittance change. The ARTs are commonly obtained for the 500-Hz, 1000-Hz, 2000-Hz, and broadband noise (BBN) activators.

Acoustic-Reflex Adaptation (Reflex Decay)

For ARA testing, the activating signal intensity should be 10 dB SL for the acoustic-reflex threshold. The activating signal is presented for ten seconds, and the change in acoustic immittance at the tympanic membrane is monitored in the probe ear.

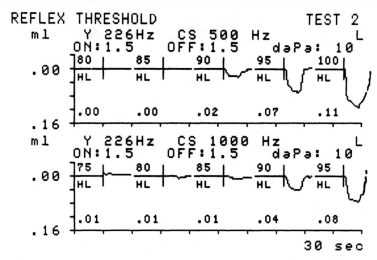

Figure 6.8. The acoustic-immittance change at successive 5-dB levels for the 500-Hz (top row) and 1000-Hz (bottom row) tonal activators. Note that the smallest, visible acoustic-immittance change occurs at 90 dB HL for the 500-Hz tonal activator. A visible acoustic-immittance change is also observable at 95 dB HL, confirming selection of 90 dB HL as the ART at 500 Hz. At 1000 Hz, note that the smallest, visible acoustic-immittance change occurs at 85 dB HL. A visible acoustic-immittance change is also observable at 90 dB HL confirming selection of 85 dB HL as the ART at 1000 Hz.

To determine whether abnormal ARA is present, the height between the baseline (postactivating stimulus) and the acoustic middle-ear admittance at five (or ten) seconds and the height between the baseline (postactivating stimulus) and onset of the acoustic middle-ear admittance change are measured. If the former is 50% or less of the latter, abnormal ARA is present. Figure 6.9 illustrates the procedure for determining whether abnormal ARA is present.

Anderson, Barr, and Wedenberg (1969) considered abnormal ARA to be present if the acoustic-reflex magnitude decayed by at least 50% within the first five seconds. Several investigators use the criterion of 50% or greater ARA within the first ten rather than five seconds (J. Jerger, Harford, Clemis, and Alford 1974; Olsen, Noffsinger, and Kurdziel 1975). ARA is evaluated for the 500-Hz and 1000-Hz tonal activators.

Static-Acoustic Admittance

With a relative acoustic-impedance meter, the clinician must make two measurements to derive the static-acoustic middle-ear impedance or acoustic-admittance equivalent air volume. The static-acoustic middle-ear admittance is actually obtained during tympanometry. For the first measurement, the ear canal is subjected to an extreme pressure of +200 or −400 daPa. The potentiometer is then adjusted (balanced) to bring the needle deflection in the balance meter to 0. The outer-ear admittance is usually read from the device in acoustic-admittance equivalent air volume. The air pressure in the ear canal is then reduced until it reaches the tympanometric peak pressure, the point of maximum

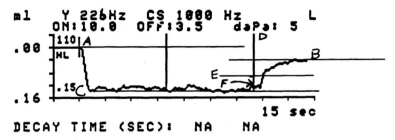

Figure 6.9. Results of the acoustic-reflex adaptation test on a normal-hearing person. The magnitude of the acoustic-immittance change is shown as a function of time. Because of baseline shift, the poststimulus tail (B) is lower than the prestimulus tail (A). Therefore, a horizontal line should be drawn from the poststimulus tail. A horizontal line should also be drawn from the peak magnitude at the onset of the activator stimulation (C). The vertical line (D) is a marker set at 10 seconds from the signal onset. The half-amplitude point between the two horizontal lines (50 percent decay point) should be determined (B to E distance along the D vertical line) and compared with the amplitude associated with the magnitude of the acoustic-immittance change at 10 seconds poststimulus activation (B to F distance along the vertical line). If the amplitude of B–F is greater than that of B–E, abnormal acoustic-reflex adaptation is not present. (If the 5-second rather than the 10-second marker is employed as the criterion for adaptation, the procedure is modified accordingly, with amplitudes determined based on the 5-second marker.)

deflection of the needle in the balance meter to the left (if +200 daPa was used for the first measurement) before reversing direction. (If −400 daPa was used for the first measurement, the tympanometric peak pressure is reached at the point of maximum deflection of the needle in the balance meter to the right before reversing direction.) At the tympanometric peak pressure, the potentiometer is again adjusted (balanced) to bring the needle deflection in the balance meter to 0 to yield the second measurement. The total-ear admittance is then read from the device in acoustic-admittance equivalent air volume. The first result (the outer-ear static-acoustic admittance in equivalent air volume) is subtracted from the second result (the total-ear static-acoustic admittance in equivalent air volume) to yield the middle-ear static-acoustic admittance in equivalent air volume.

With an absolute acoustic-admittance meter, the two measurements are automatically made by the acoustic-immittance device during tympanometry and read directly from the graph of the acoustic-admittance-pressure function. Figure 6.10 shows the acoustic-admittance pressure function (tympanogram) obtained with an absolute acoustic-impedance meter. Figure 6.10 reveals that the static-acoustic admittance in mmhos is shown on the ordinate and the ear-canal air pressure in daPa is shown on the abscissa. The static-acoustic middle-ear admittance is the static-acoustic admittance from the tympanometric peak pressure (highest point on the tympanogram) to the baseline on the negative or positive side of the tympanogram (see B in Figure 6.10). If the baseline feature of the device is employed, the static-acoustic ear-canal admittance will not be shown in the tympanogram, and the static-acoustic middle-ear admittance is the difference between the static-acoustic admittance at the peak pressure and that at the

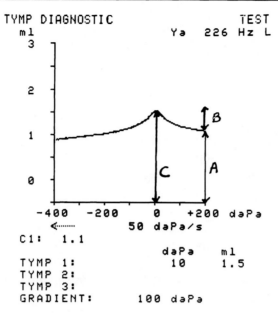

Figure 6.10. Admittance tympanogram obtained with the 226-Hz probe tone and recorded on the GS 1733 otoadmittance meter (absolute acoustic-admittance device) from a normal middle ear. (A) Outer ear static-acoustic admittance; (B) Middle-ear static-acoustic admittance; (C) Total (combined outer and middle) ear static-acoustic admittance.

abscissa. If the baseline feature of the device is not employed, the static-acoustic ear-canal admittance will be shown on the tympanogram as the difference between the static-acoustic admittance at the baseline of the tympanogram and that at the abscissa (see A in Figure 6.10).

The static-acoustic ear-canal admittance will be smaller if it is based on −400 rather than +200 daPa. If the static-acoustic ear-canal admittance is based on −400, the static-acoustic middle-ear admittance may be spuriously large and may result in lack of detection of some stiffening middle-ear lesions. Therefore, we recommend basing the static-acoustic ear-canal admittance on +200 rather than −400 daPa.

Tympanometric Peak Pressure

In Figure 6.10, the tympanometric peak pressure is 0 daPa as it is the pressure associated with the greatest tympanometric amplitude. In order to obtain a tympanometric peak pressure that is less affected by the direction of the air-pressure change (positive to negative vs. negative to positive), it is recommended that the tympanometric peak pressure be obtained twice, once while varying the air pressure from positive to negative and once while varying the air pressure from negative to positive. The average of the two tympanometric peak pressures will yield a more accurate tympanometric peak pressure. This procedure is recommended when a borderline normal tympanometric peak pressure is obtained.

Tympanometric Gradient and Width

The procedure for the tympanometric gradient or width follows that for obtaining the tympanogram. With a relative acoustic-immittance device, +200 daPa is introduced into the ear canal, and the potentiometer is adjusted until the deflection needle points to the extreme right of the range, indicating the highest impedance or lowest admittance (relative units). Then the air pressure is decreased gradually to −200 or −400 daPa, and the sound-pressure change with air pressure is recorded automatically or manually plotted at 50-daPa intervals. The procedure is similar for an absolute acoustic-immittance device except there is no adjustment of the potentiometer and the middle ear or combined outer- and middle-ear admittance at various ear canal pressures is recorded. Then, one of the methods mentioned earlier for calculation of the tympanometric gradient or width is applied to the tympanogram.

ACOUSTIC-IMMITTANCE FINDINGS FOR VARIOUS PATHOLOGIES

THE acoustic-immittance findings are presented for the more commonly occurring outer ear, middle ear, cochlear, eighth nerve, and brainstem disorders in neonates, infants, and children, which can affect aural acoustic immittance. Acoustic immittance findings are generally diagnostic of auditory site rather than disorder. Nevertheless, acoustic immittance findings in conjunction with other audiologic findings and case history may be suggestive of a particular auditory disorder.

Outer Ear Disorders

External Otitis

In cases of severe external otitis, one finds a mild hearing impairment and elevated or absent contralateral acoustic reflexes (when the stimulus ear is the affected ear). The elevated or absent contralateral acoustic reflexes result from the presence of significant air-bone gaps. If the external otitis results in a mass growth on the floor of the external ear canal, the tympanometric amplitude and shape will reflect mass effects (Shanks 1984), which lower the resonant frequency of the middle ear. These mass effects can be detected at high probe-tone frequencies. Therefore, the tympanometric amplitude and shape will be normal for the 226-Hz probe tone but will be abnormal for the 678-Hz probe tone, showing an abnormally wide separation between the outermost extrema, according to the Vanhuyse et al. (1975) criteria. Other acoustic-immittance findings are normal for external otitis.

Figure 6.11 illustrates the admittance tympanogram for the 220-Hz probe tone and the susceptance and conductance tympanograms for the 660-Hz probe tone for a five-year-old child with external otitis. Note the 5B tympanometric pattern that became a 1B pattern after the otitis externa resolved.

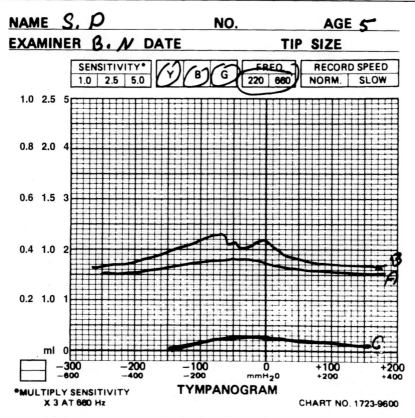

Figure 6.11. Admittance tympanogram (A) for the 220-Hz probe tone and the susceptance (B) and conductance (C) tympanograms for the 660-Hz probe tone for a five-year-old child with otitis externa.

Collapsed Ear Canal

The acoustic-immittance findings are unaffected by collapsed canals when the activating transducer and the probe-tone transducer are inserts that alleviate the collapsed ear canal. Some acoustic-immittance devices employ earphones rather than inserts for the activating signal transducer. In such cases, the contralateral acoustic reflexes will be elevated or absent when the stimulated ear is the affected ear as the collapsed canal will result in a blockage in the ear canal that reduces the intensity of the activating signal. If the collapse is unilateral, the contralateral acoustic reflexes are affected unilaterally. If the collapse is bilateral, the contralateral acoustic reflexes are affected bilaterally. Other acoustic-immittance findings will be normal for collapsed ear canals.

Cerumen Impaction

With cerumen impaction, the probe tone energy is directed against the hard wall of the cerumen rather than against the tympanic membrane. Resultantly, air-pressure variation in the ear canal will produce no acoustic immittance changes in the ear as the probe tone will essentially be totally reflected off the hard wall of the cerumen at all air pressures. Therefore, the static-acoustic outer-ear admittance and total-ear admittance will be below normal limits and essentially equivalent, yielding a static-acoustic middle-ear admittance near zero. Also, a tympanometric peak pressure will be absent. The acoustic reflexes will be absent for all activating frequencies for ipsilateral and contralateral stimulation when the probe ear is the affected ear. When the stimulus ear is the affected ear, the contralateral acoustic reflex will be elevated or absent, depending upon the air-bone gap at the activating frequency. Similar findings are also obtained for a probe assembly that is incorrectly inserted, with the result that the probe tone is reflected off the ear-canal wall.

Middle-Ear Disorders

Tympanic Membrane Disorders

PERFORATION: With a perforated tympanic membrane, the probe tone is always directed against the promontory of the cochlea. Therefore, air-pressure variation in the ear canal will produce no acoustic-immittance changes in the ear as the probe tone will essentially be totally reflected off the bony promontory of the cochlea at all air pressures. Therefore, as in the case of impacted cerumen, the static-acoustic outer-ear admittance and total-ear admittance will be equivalent, yielding a static-acoustic middle-ear admittance near zero. Unlike the case of impacted cerumen, however, the ear-canal static-acoustic admittance with a perforated tympanic membrane will be abnormally increased, exceeding 2.0 mmho, as the perforation causes inclusion of the middle-ear volume when the ear-canal volume is being measured. As in the case of impacted cerumen, a tympanometric peak pressure will be absent in ears with a perforated tympanic membrane. Also, the acoustic reflexes will be absent for ipsilateral and contralateral stimulation when the probe ear is the affected ear. When the stimulus ear is the affected ear, the contralateral acoustic reflex could occur at normal levels if no significant air-bone gaps are present; or it may be elevated or absent, depending upon the magnitude of the air-bone gaps at the activating test frequency, if a significant air-bone gap is present at that frequency.

FLACCID: Some persons are born with a flaccid tympanic membrane. A flaccid tympanic membrane (one with decreased stiffness) can also result from a healed perforation. The effect of decreased stiffness is to lower the resonant frequency of the middle ear to approximately 600–800 Hz. Therefore, at the low probe-tone frequency (e.g., 226 Hz), a flaccid tympanic membrane will behave like a compliant system, and a large amount of probe-tone energy will be admitted into the middle ear. The static-acoustic middle-ear admittance will be abnormally increased, with tympanometric amplitude therefore increased, but other acoustic admittance findings will be normal for the low-frequency probe tone.

At the high probe-tone frequency (e.g., 678 Hz), the tympanometric amplitude and shape will tend to reflect resonance effects as evidenced by multiple peaks in the susceptance and conductance tympanograms, although the tympanograms will still be normal, according to the Vanhuyse et al. (1975) criteria. The tympanometric findings for the high-frequency probe tone are similar for external otitis and a flaccid tympanic membrane. The findings for the former, however, are related to an increase in the mass component of the ear; the latter are related to a decrease in stiffness of the middle ear, lowering the resonant frequency of the system. A flaccid tympanic membrane does not result in significant air-bone gaps.

TYMPANOSCLEROSIS: In children, tympanosclerosis is the condition of scar tissue on the tympanic membrane, usually as a result of chronic middle-ear effusion. The scar tissue can slightly increase the mass component of the middle ear. The static-acoustic middle-ear admittance is generally normal or slightly increased. The other acoustic-immittance findings are generally normal for the low-frequency probe tone. At the high probe-tone frequency (e.g., 678 Hz), the tympanometric amplitude and shape will tend to reflect increased mass effects (which lower the resonant frequency of the middle ear), yielding multiple peaks in the susceptance and conductance tympanograms; the tympanograms, however, will still be normal, according to the Vanhuyse et al. (1975) criteria.

The tympanometric findings for the high-frequency probe tone are similar to those for external otitis and a flaccid tympanic membrane. The findings for tympanosclerosis and external otitis, however, are related to an increase in the mass component of the ear, whereas the findings for a flaccid tympanic membrane are related to a decrease in stiffness of the middle ear. Tympanosclerosis is not associated with significant air-bone gaps.

Eustachian Tube Dysfunction

Normative pediatric data are lacking on Eustachian tube testing for the Valsalva, Toynbee, inflation, and deflation maneuvers to identify abnormal Eustachian tube function, differentiate between functional and mechanical obstruction, and differentiate between obstruction and abnormal patency. Therefore, tympanometric Eustachian tube tests for the Valsalva, Toynbee, inflation, and deflation maneuvers in children are not recommended at this time.

A tympanometric peak pressure more negative than −100 daPa is consistent with Eustachian tube dysfunction in children up to thirteen years of age. Tympanometric peak pressures less than −100 daPa are present in 10% of newborns, 18% of three-month-old infants, and 39% of six-month-old infants (Gersdorff 1992). In children older than thirteen years of age, a negative tympanometric peak pressure less than −50 daPa is consistent with Eustachian tube dysfunction (as it is for adults). The static-acoustic middle-ear admittance may be slightly reduced or within normal limits.

Significant air-bone gaps are occasionally present. As the ear-canal pressure is routinely adjusted to equal the tympanometric peak pressure in acoustic-reflex assessment, the contralateral and ipsilateral acoustic reflexes obtained when the probe ear is the affected ear are usually within the normal range or are slightly elevated. The contralateral and ipsilateral acoustic reflexes obtained when the stimulus ear is the affected ear are within normal limits or are slightly elevated according to the magnitude of the air-bone gap at the activating signal frequency.

Middle-Ear Effusion

The acoustic immittance results for middle-ear effusion (MEE) are generally consistent with those for a stiffening middle-ear pathology. Therefore, when the static-acoustic middle-ear admittance is affected, it is reduced (J. Jerger et al. 1974). The tympanometric peak pressure usually is significantly negative (i.e., more negative than the lower limit of the normal range) or absent (J. Jerger 1970). Reduced gradients (e.g., less than or equal to 0.1) and large tympano-metric widths (e.g., greater than 150 daPa in children) are associated with the presence of MEE. The contralateral and ipsilateral acoustic reflexes generally are absent for all stimulus activators when the affected ear is the probe ear; they are elevated or absent, depending upon the magnitude of the air-bone gap when the affected ear is the stimulus ear. Significant (15 dB or more) air-bone gaps are generally present. Silman, Silverman, and Arick (1994) reported that 100% of their sample of children with MEE who failed the ASHA (1990) pure-tone screening and 92% of their sample of children with MEE who passed the ASHA (1990) pure-tone screening had significant air-bone gaps at one or more frequencies.

Children

Silman (1990) and Silman et al. (1992) investigated the sensitivity and specificity of the acoustic-immittance measures in detection of MEE. Table 6.2 shows the results of their investigation for the total sample of 82 middle ears with effusion, the subgroup of middle ears with effusion and hearing loss greater than 20 dB HL at 1000, 2000, and/or 4000 Hz, the subgroup of middle ears with effusion and normal hearing threshold levels at 1000–4000 Hz, and a group of 53 middle ears without effusion. This table reveals fair to poor sensitivity for the ASHA (1990) tympanometric width and static-acoustic middle-ear admittance, respectively, and excellent sensitivity for the tympanometric peak pressure and ipsilateral acoustic reflex measures for the total MEE sample. In the MEE subgroup with normal-hearing threshold levels, only the ipsilateral acoustic reflex measure had excellent sensitivity, approximating 90%. The value of the acoustic reflex was substantiated by Cavaliere, Masieri, Liberini, Proietti, and Magalini (1992),

Table 6.2. Results for ASHA (1990) TW, Static-Acoustic ME Admittance,
IAR, and TPP in MEE and in Control Ears

Group	ASHA (1990) TW		Static-Acoustic ME Admittance		IAR		TPP	
	P	F[a]	P	F[b]	P	F[c]	P	F[d]
MEE (N=82)								
	23	77	39	61	7	93	11	89
MEE having 1kHz, 2kHz, and/or 4kHz > 20 dB HL (N=44)								
	7	93	14	86	9	91	2	98
MEE having 1kHz, 2kHz, and 4kHz ≤ 20 dB HL (N=38)								
	42	58	68	32	5	95	21	79
ME without effusion having normal-hearing thresholds (N=53)								
	81	19	77	23	84	16	83	17

P = pass rate (%); F = failure rate (%)

[a] > 180 daPa (pump speed 50 daPa/s); [b] < 0.35 mmho (pump speed 50 daPa/s); [c] absent at 110 dB HL at 1000 Hz; [d] ≤ −100 daPa. Reprinted with permission from Silman et al. (1992).

who reported that abnormal or absent acoustic reflexes in a sample of unconscious patients in the intensive care unit usually were associated with MEE or Eustachian tube dysfunction. Silman (1990) and Silman et al. (1992) also reported that the specificity ranged between approximately 81 and 84% for the ASHA (1990) tympanometric width, ipsilateral acoustic reflex, and tympanometric peak pressure and was below 80% for the static-acoustic middle-ear admittance.

Ovesen, Passke, and Elbrond's (1993) findings are in accord with those of Silman et al. (1992). They reported that the specificity of an acoustic-immittance protocol (based on absent or negative tympanometric peak pressure) that does not include the acoustic reflex is low (52.9%). The presence vs. absence of MEE was established upon myringotomy following otomicroscopy.

Nozza et al. (1992) investigated the acoustic-immittance findings in children between one and eight years of age who were brought to the operating room for myringotomy and tube surgery. Their sample consisted of 81 middle ears with effusion and 30 middle ears without effusion. When the criterion for MEE based on the static-acoustic middle-ear admittance was less than or equal to 0.3 mmho, the sensitivity and specificity were only 73% and 80%, respectively. Although the sensitivity of the tympanometric gradient (Paradise et al. 1976, based on Brooks 1969) was high at 91%, the specificity was low at 70% when the criterion was less than or equal to 0.2. The ipsilateral acoustic reflex measure (110 dB HL at 1000 Hz) was the only acoustic-immittance measure characterized by high rates for both sensitivity (88%) and specificity (85%).

Smith, Wiley, and Pyle (1993) also evaluated the efficacy of the individual acoustic-immittance measures in detection of MEE. Data were obtained from subjects with surgically-confirmed MEE. The sensitivity and specificity of the static-acoustic middle-ear admittance were 60% and 80%, respectively. The sensitivity and specificity of the tympanometric width were only 74% and 48%, respectively. The sensitivity and specificity of an absent (at 90 dB HL) contralateral acoustic reflex for pulsed broadband noise (which was absent for at least two of three activator presentations) were 84% and 63%, respectively.

The ASHA (1990) protocol for detection of MEE was based on the static-acoustic middle-ear admittance and tympanometric width. Silman (1990) and Silman et al. (1992) proposed a protocol for detection of MEE, based on the ASHA (1990) tympanometric width, ipsilateral acoustic reflex, and tympanometric peak pressure. That is, either (a) increased tympanometric width, reduced static-acoustic middle-ear admittance, and absent ipsilateral acoustic reflex (at 110 dB HL at 1000 Hz), or (b) significantly negative tympanometric peak pressure (less than or equal to −100 daPa) and absent ipsilateral acoustic reflex are consistent with middle-ear effusion. They compared the sensitivity and specificity of their proposed protocol with those for the ASHA protocol, as shown in Table 6.3.

Table 6.3 reveals that the sensitivity is poor for the ASHA protocol but excellent for the Silman et al. proposed protocol for the MEE group with normal-hearing threshold levels. Similarly, the specificity of the Silman et al. proposed protocol is markedly higher than that for the ASHA protocol. Smith et al. (1993) reported that the sensitivity and specificity of the ASHA protocol were only 74% and 69%, respectively, based on data from subjects with surgically-confirmed MEE. Smith et al. reported that the sensitivity and specificity of an acoustic-immittance protocol increased to 83% and 82%, respectively, when the contralateral BBN acoustic reflex was combined with the static middle-ear admittance.

For detection of MEE in children, we recommend the use of the Silman

Table 6.3. Results for the Silman et al. (1992) Proposed Protocol and ASHA (1990) Protocol in MEE and in Control Ears

Group	ASHA (1990) Protocol		[(Static + TW + IAR) or (TPP + IAR)] *	
	P	F	P	F
MEE (N=82)	19.5	81.5	10.0	90.0
MEE having 1kHz, 2kHz, and/or 4kHz > 20 dB HL (N=44)	7.0	93.0	9.0	91.0
MEE having 1kHz, 2kHz, and 4kHz ≤ 20 dB HL (N=38)	37.0	63.0	10.5	89.5
ME without effusion having normal-hearing thresholds (N=53)	79.0	21.0	92.5	7.5

P = pass rate (%); F = failure rate (%)

* Proposed Silman et al. (1992) protocol based on (a) reduced static-acoustic middle-ear admittance, increased tympanometric width, and absent ipsilateral acoustic reflex, or (b) significantly negative tympanometric peak pressure and absent ipsilateral acoustic reflex. Adapted from Silman et al. (1992).

et al. protocol, if the acoustic-immittance device permits ipsilateral acoustic-reflex testing at 110 dB HL at 1000 Hz with a multiplexing circuit to control for artifacts. Otherwise, the Smith et al. protocol is recommended. For diagnostic purposes, the acoustic-reflex threshold should be established as acoustic reflexes frequently are obtained below the criterion level of 110 dB HL for the ipsilateral tonal acoustic reflex and 90 dB HL for the contralateral BBN acoustic reflex.

Neonates and Infants up to Four Months of Age

As mentioned earlier, the static-acoustic middle-ear admittance and tympano-metric amplitude and shape measures are insensitive to middle-ear pathology in neonates and infants up to four months of age.

We suggest that the following be considered as consistent with the presence of MEE in neonates and infants up to four months of age: (a) absence of the con-tralateral and ipsilateral acoustic reflexes for the 1000-Hz tonal and BBN activa-tors for the 226-, 678-, and 1000-Hz (if available) probe-tone frequencies together with a significantly negative tympanometric peak pressure (less than or equal to −100 daPa); or (b) absent tympanometric peak pressure. Neonates and infants with absent acoustic reflexes but a tympanometric peak pressure less than −100 daPa should be followed up as MEE cannot be ruled out in such cases.

Congenital Ossicular Fixation

Congenital ossicular fixation, a stiffening middle-ear pathology, is frequently ac-companied by significant air-bone gaps. The static-acoustic middle-ear admit-tance and, consequently, tympanometric amplitude for the 226-Hz probe tone can be reduced or normal. Tympanometric shape is unaffected for the low- and high-frequency probe tones. When the affected ear is the probe ear, the ipsilat-eral and contralateral acoustic reflexes will be absent for all activators. When the affected ear is the stimulus ear, the contralateral and ipsilateral acoustic reflexes will be elevated or absent, depending on the magnitude of the air-bone gap at the activating frequency.

Some children present with both a flaccid tympanic membrane and ossicular fixation. In such cases, the static-acoustic middle-ear admittance reflects the most lateral pathology (i.e., the flaccid tympanic membrane) and is abnormally increased.

Cholesteatoma

In cases exhibiting cholesteatoma, significant air-bone gaps are usually present. With advanced cholesteatoma, tympanic membrane perforation and ossicular necrosis can occur. The tympanometric peak pressure frequently is negative. This stiffening pathology results in an abnormally reduced static-acoustic middle-ear admittance (J. Jerger et al. 1974). Compared with congenital ossicular fixation, middle-ear effusion, and tympanosclerosis, this is the only stiffening middle-ear pathology characterized by static-acoustic middle-ear admittance values that do not overlap with those for normal middle ears. The tympanometric amplitude or shape can be reduced or flat for the low-frequency probe tone. The tympanometric pattern resembles that for ossicular discontinuity if ossicular necrosis occurs. When the affected ear is the probe ear, the pathology results in absence of the contralateral and ipsilateral acoustic reflexes for all activators. When the affected ear is the stimulus ear, the contralateral and ipsilateral acoustic reflexes are absent or elevated, depending upon the magnitude of the air-bone gap at the activating frequency. These findings also are generally characteristic of other tumors of the middle ear.

Ossicular Discontinuity

Ossicular discontinuity is associated with large air-bone gaps throughout the frequency range, which are often larger at the high frequencies. Ossicular discontinuity substantially increases the mass component of the middle ear. The static-acoustic middle-ear admittance is increased or normal; consequently, the tympanometric amplitude for the low-frequency probe tone can be increased or normal. The tympanometric shape for the low-frequency probe tone is normal. Because of the increase in the mass component of the middle ear, the tympanometric shape and amplitude are abnormal for the high-frequency probe tone (e.g., 678 Hz). That is, for the high-frequency probe tone, more than five extrema in the susceptance tympanogram, or more than three extrema in the conductance tympanogram, or greater than 75 daPa distance between the outermost extrema in a tympanogram with three extrema, and/or greater than 100 daPa distance between the outermost extrema in a tympanogram with five extrema exist. Congenital ossicular fixation with a flaccid tympanic membrane as well as ossicular discontinuity may present with significant air-bone gaps and abnormally increased static-acoustic middle-ear admittance. The tympanometric pattern for the high-frequency probe tone (e.g., 678 Hz) will differentiate between these pathologies as the former condition will be associated with normal, high-frequency tympanometric shape whereas the latter will be associated with an abnormal, high-frequency tympanometric shape. Figure 6.12 contrasts the susceptance and conductance tympanograms for a child with congenital ossicular fixation and a flaccid tympanic membrane with those for a child with ossicular discontinuity.

With ossicular discontinuity, the acoustic-reflex pattern is dependent on the location of the break. A break lateral to the insertion of the stapedius on the stapes will interrupt the connection between the insertion point of the stapedius on the stapes and the eardrum. In this case, the contralateral and ipsilateral acoustic reflexes will be absent for all activators when the affected ear is the probe ear. When the affected ear is the stimulus ear, the contralateral and ipsilateral acoustic reflexes are generally absent because of the large air-bone gaps.

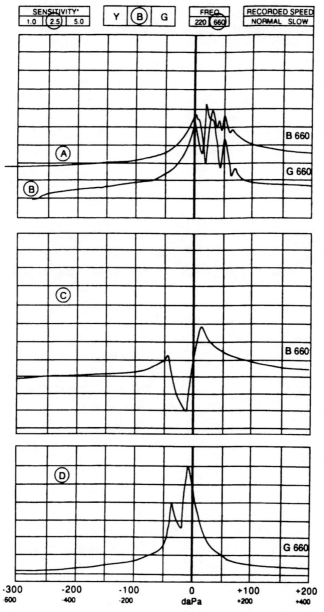

Figure 6.12. Tympanograms obtained using an absolute acoustic-immittance device using the 660-Hz probe tone. (A) Susceptance tympanogram from the ear with ossicular discontinuity. (B) Conductance tympanogram from the ear with ossicular discontinuity. (C) Susceptance tympanogram from the ear with otosclerosis and a flaccid tympanic membrane or healed perforation of the tympanic membrane. (D) Conductance tympanogram from the ear with otosclerosis and flaccid tympanic membrane. (Reprinted with permission from Silman and Silverman 1991.)

A break medial to the insertion of the stapedius on the stapes will not interrupt the connection between the insertion point of the stapedius on the stapes and the eardrum. In this case, the contralateral and ipsilateral acoustic reflexes will be present at normal or near normal levels when the affected ear is the probe ear. Nevertheless, the contralateral and ipsilateral acoustic reflexes will generally be absent because of the large air-bone gaps when the affected ear is the stimulus ear.

Cochlear Disorders

In persons with hearing impairment not exceeding approximately 50 to 55 dB HL, the contralateral tonal ARTs for the low-frequency probe tone (e.g., 220 Hz) are similar to those for normal-hearing persons. Therefore, the tonal ARTs in such cases are generally unaffected by hearing impairment of cochlear etiology (Alberti and Kristensen 1970; Beedle and Harford 1973; Jepsen 1963; J. Jerger 1970; J. Jerger et al. 1972; Metz 1946; Peterson and Lidén 1972). Hearing impairment of cochlear etiology exceeding approximately 50 to 55 dB HL affects the afferent acoustic reflex arc. When the magnitude of the hearing impairment exceeds approximately 50 dB HL, the contralateral tonal ART for the low-frequency probe tone increases directly with the degree of hearing impairment (Gelfand, Piper, and Silman 1983; Holmes and Woodford 1977; Keith 1979; Martin and Brunette 1980; Norris, Stelmachowicz, and Taylor 1974; Popelka 1981; Silman and Gelfand 1979, 1981; Silman, Popelka, and Gelfand 1978; Silman et al. 1982).

The 90th percentiles for the contralateral tonal ARTs as a function of magnitude of hearing impairment at 500, 1000, and 2000 Hz for the 220-Hz tonal activator in adults (Silman and Gelfand 1981) are shown in Table 6.4. These data show that the 90th percentiles increase with increasing magnitude of cochlear hearing impairment beyond approximately 50 dB HL. Silman and Gelfand also reported that the frequency of absent contralateral acoustic reflexes for the 220-Hz probe tone is 30% or less for the 500-, 1000-, and 2000-Hz tonal activators when the magnitude of hearing impairment does not exceed 85 dB HL; however, it increases to 56% for the 500-Hz tonal activator, 40% for the 1000-Hz tonal activator, and 58% for the 2000-Hz tonal activator when the magnitude of the hearing impairment is 90 dB HL or greater. Thus, the Silman and Gelfand 90th percentiles are feasible for clinical application when the magnitude of the hearing impairment is less than 90 dB HL at 500, 1000, and 2000 Hz.

Neonates and Infants

The contralateral acoustic reflexes for the 220-Hz probe tone are absent in a majority of neonates and infants. Therefore, the Silman and Gelfand (1981) ninetieth contralateral tonal ART percentiles for normal-hearing thresholds and cochlear hearing impairment cannot be applied to neonates and infants.

Table 6.4. 90th Percentiles (dB HL) for the Contralateral Tonal ARTs

Hearing loss (dB HL)	S&G[a] (1981) 13+ years (dB HL)			S&G (1981) + 5 dB 9–13 years (dB HL)			S&G (1981) + 10 dB 5–9 years (dB HL)		
	500	1000	2000	500	1000	2000	500	1000	2000
0–5	95	100	95	100	105	100	105	110	105
10–15	95	100	100	100	105	105	105	110	110
20–25	95	100	100	100	105	105	105	110	110
30–35	100	100	105	105	105	110	110	110	115
40–45	100	105	105	105	110	110	110	115	115
50–55	105	105	110	110	110	115	115	115	120
60–65	105	110	115	110	115	120	115	120	125
70–75	115	115	125	120	120		125	125	
80–85	125	125	125						

[a] Silman and Gelfand.

Children

The percentage of contralateral tonal ARTs exceeding 110 dB HL falls below 10% in children who are five or more years of age and approaches adult values by thirteen years of age (S. Jerger et al. 1974). Also, the 95th percentiles for the contralateral tonal ARTs for the 220-Hz probe tone are approximately 10 dB higher in normal-hearing children with minor tympanic membrane abnormalities than normal-hearing adults.

Based on these data, we suggest that 10 dB be added to the Silman and Gelfand (1981) 90th percentile levels for the contralateral ARTs for the low-frequency probe tone to derive the interim 90th percentile levels for children between five and nine years of age. We also suggest that 5 dB be added to the Silman and Gelfand 90th percentile levels for the contralateral ARTs for the low-frequency probe tone to derive the interim 90th percentile levels for children between nine and thirteen years of age. The Silman and Gelfand 90th percentile levels can be applied without correction to children who are thirteen or more years of age. The results of the application of the 10-dB and 5-dB correction factors to the Silman and Gelfand 90th percentile levels for the contralateral tonal ARTs are shown in Table 6.4. The application of the 5- or 10-dB correction to the 90th percentiles limits their clinical utility to children with magnitudes of hearing impairment of less than 80 dB HL at 500 and 1000 Hz and less than 70 dB HL at 2000 Hz. It is recommended that these derived, interim 90th percentile levels be employed until normative 90th percentile, large-sample data are obtained.

It is recommended that, for children between four months and five years of age, the contralateral tonal ARTs for the low-frequency probe tone be compared with the adult or proposed interim norms for children. If the ARTs do not exceed the proposed pediatric or adult norms, the results can be considered as consistent with normal-hearing thresholds or hearing impairment of cochlear etiology. If the ARTs exceed both the adult and proposed pediatric norms, then the 90th percentiles (either corrected or uncorrected) are not applicable.

Eighth Nerve and Low Brainstem Disorders

Eighth nerve and low brainstem disorders affecting the afferent acoustic-reflex arc (e.g., at the level of the superior olivary complex, trapezoid body, ventral cochlear nuclei, facial-nerve nuclei) are generally associated with elevated or absent ARTs and abnormal acoustic-reflex adaptation when the stimulus ear is the affected side (Anderson et al. 1970; Silman, Gelfand, and Chun 1978). Other acoustic-immittance findings are unaffected by eighth nerve and low brainstem disorders. The acoustic reflexes are generally unaffected by higher level central auditory disorders.

Eighth Nerve Disorders

Eighth nerve disorders in children, such as those that can result from bacterial meningitis and neurosyphilis (congenital or acquired), are frequently bilateral. Eighth nerve tumors in children, except for those associated with Von Reckling-hausen neurofibromatosis, are rare. With unilateral eighth nerve pathology, the contralateral acoustic reflexes (when the stimulus ear is the affected side) are elevated or absent beyond the 90th percentile levels, and the ipsilateral acoustic reflexes also are elevated or absent. Contralateral and ipsilateral acoustic-reflex adaptation frequently is abnormal when the stimulus ear is the affected side. With bilateral eighth nerve pathology, the contralateral and ipsilateral acoustic reflexes are usually bilaterally elevated or absent; contralateral and ipsilateral acoustic-reflex adaptation is usually abnormal bilaterally.

Low Brainstem Lesions

In children, unlike adults, the majority (65%) of brain tumors develop in the posterior fossa (Green, Waggener, and Kriegsfeld 1976). The most common pattern of acoustic reflex abnormality is bilaterally elevated or absent contralateral acoustic reflexes and bilaterally normal ipsilateral acoustic reflexes. Frequently, contralateral acoustic-reflex adaptation is abnormal bilaterally with bilaterally normal ipsilateral acoustic-reflex adaptation. When the lesion is extensive, affecting the ventral cochlear nuclei or facial nerve nuclei unilaterally or bilaterally, then the ipsilateral acoustic-reflex threshold and adaptation also can be abnormal for the affected side(s).

Facial Nerve or Stapedial Muscle Pathology

The distinguishing acoustic-immittance feature in cases of facial nerve pathology medial to the insertion on the stapedius muscle or stapedius muscle disorders is abnormality of the acoustic-reflex threshold (Alford, Jerger, Coats, Peterson, and Weber 1973) or adaptation (Silman et al. 1988; Wilson, Shanks, and Lilly 1984), when the affected side is the probe ear. Disorders of the medial part of the facial nerve or of the stapedius represent a lesion of the efferent part of the acoustic-reflex arc. Lesions of the efferent acoustic-reflex arc are manifested when the affected side is the probe ear. Facial nerve pathology lateral to the insertion on the stapedius muscle does not affect the acoustic reflex.

ACOUSTIC-IMMITTANCE SCREENING FOR DETECTION OF MIDDLE EAR WITH EFFUSION

THE ASHA (1990) guidelines for screening to detect MEE were based on the history, visual inspection, identification audiometry, and tympanometry. The history was done at the time of screening or in advance (especially from parents) to establish whether there was recent occurrence of otalgia (ear pain) or otorrhea (ear discharge). ASHA recommended immediate medical referral if the history of ear pain or otorrhea was positive. ASHA also recommended visual inspection by the unaided eye or otoscopy. If visual inspection reveals (a) structural defects of the ear, head, or neck; (b) ear-canal abnormalities (blood or effusion, occlusion, inflammation, excessive cerumen, tumor, foreign material); or (c) apparent eardrum abnormalities (abnormal color, bulging eardrum, fluid line or bubbles, perforation, or tympanic-membrane retraction), the ASHA guidelines also recommend immediate medical referral.

The ASHA guidelines included identification audiometry for the purposes of (a) detection of a significant communication problem in conjunction with abnormal acoustic-immittance findings and (b) detection of sensorineural hearing impairment. The procedure for identification (pure-tone screening) audiometry recommended by the ASHA guidelines was in conjunction with the ASHA (1985) identification audiometry guidelines. Therefore, pure-tone (air-conduction) screening was based on 1000, 2000, and 4000 Hz at 20 dB HL if the screening program included acoustic-immittance assessment; it was based on 500 Hz as well as 1000, 2000, and 4000 Hz at 20 dB HL if the screening program did not include acoustic-immittance assessment. Referral for a complete audiologic evaluation was based on failure to respond to the recommended screening levels at any frequency in either ear. Pure-tone rescreening, preferably within the same test session, was mandatory to reduce the failure rate.

The ASHA (1990) acoustic-immittance measures were based on a 226-Hz probe tone, +200 daPa ear canal volume correction, and a pump speed of −200 daPa/s (going from a positive to a negative direction). Interim normative data for children who are three or more years of age and adults were provided by ASHA for use until more complete normative data become available. ASHA recommended that normative data should be collected if acoustic-immittance screening is based on other combinations of ear canal correction and pump speed. ASHA stated that the test procedures could be performed by audiologists or personnel other than audiologists, provided they were sufficiently trained and supervised by a clinical audiologist with appropriate training and experience related to the test protocol.

The acoustic-immittance measures included equivalent ear canal volume, static-acoustic middle-ear admittance, and tympanometric width. Equivalent ear canal assessment was recommended for detection of many tympanic membrane perforations. The presence of an equivalent ear canal volume exceeding the 90% range at 1.0 cm³ (based on +200 daPa and a −200 daPa/s pump speed) together with an absent tympanometric peak pressure constituted the basis for immediate medical referral. Detection of other middle-ear disorders, such as chronic or recurrent MEE as opposed to transient, spontaneously recovering serous otitis media, was based on static-acoustic middle-ear admittance and tympanometric width.

Based on ASHA's (1990) normative data for children and acoustic-immittance screening parameters, reduced static-acoustic middle-ear admittance below 0.9 mmho (the lower limit of the 90% range) or increased tympanometric width exceeding 150 daPa (the upper limit of the 90% range), which is determined using the ASHA method, constitutes a basis for retesting. That is, reduced static-acoustic middle-ear admittance and/or increased tympanometric width warrants medical referral only if also present upon a retest after four to six weeks.

Limitations

Research has shown that a protocol for detection of MEE based on reduced static-acoustic middle-ear admittance or increased tympanometric width, such as the ASHA (1990) protocol, is characterized by low sensitivity, especially in children with normal-hearing thresholds, and low specificity. In fact, Roush, Drake, and Sexton (1992) reported that the sensitivity of the revised ASHA acoustic-immittance test/retest protocol (84%) was lower than that for the ASHA (1979) acoustic-immittance test-retest protocol (95%). Roush et al. reported a low specificity for the 1979 protocol as compared with the revised protocol, probably because of the low screening level for the ipsilateral acoustic reflex, which did not account for maturational effects as mentioned earlier. The high specificity reported by Roush et al. for the revised protocol contradicts the low specificity for the revised protocol reported by Smith et al. (1993). The Silman et al. (1992) proposed acoustic-immittance protocol (based on tympanometric width and peak pressure, static-acoustic middle-ear admittance, and ipsilateral acoustic reflex) has sensitivity and specificity that are high and greater than those for the ASHA (1990) protocol.

ASHA (1990) recognized that a one-shot screening could not detect recurrent or chronic MEE. Therefore, they recommend retesting failures at four to six weeks post-initial test. The findings of Silman et al. (1994) illustrated the fact that MEE can resolve spontaneously or persist beyond six to eight weeks. Conversely, MEE that is absent on an initial test may be present on a retest. Therefore, screening protocols that refer based only on failure upon initial test and retest, such as the ASHA (1990) protocol, will fail to detect children with MEE who pass the initial test and fail a retest.

It is recommended that screening for detection of OME (i.e., MEE) be based on the ASHA (1990) pure-tone and acoustic-immittance guidelines, modified to incorporate the Silman et al. (1992) proposed acoustic-immittance battery (based on the four acoustic-immittance measures) in place of the ASHA (1990) acoustic-immittance battery (essentially based on tympanometric width and static-acoustic middle-ear admittance). The acoustic-immittance battery based on the static-acoustic middle-ear admittance and contralateral pulsed BBN activator (Smith et al. 1993) is recommended in place of the Silman et al. (1992) battery if the acoustic-immittance screening device does not permit ipsilateral acoustic-reflex assessment at 110 dB HL at 1000 Hz while controlling for artifacts.

PREDICTION OF HEARING IMPAIRMENT FROM THE ACOUSTIC-REFLEX THRESHOLD

THE ART has been used to predict the presence vs. absence of sensorineural hearing impairment. The basic principle underlying prediction of the presence vs. absence of sensorineural hearing impairment from the ART is the relation between the tonal ARTs and BBN ART for the low-frequency probe tone. As the magnitude of the hearing impairment increases, the tonal ARTs remain essentially unchanged until approximately 50 dB HL, and then increase directly with the degree of hearing impairment. On the other hand, the BBN ART increases directly with the magnitude of hearing impairment until approximately 50 dB HL and then remains essentially unchanged (Popelka 1981; Silman 1976; Silman, Popelka, and Gelfand 1978). Resultantly, the noise-tone difference (tonal ARTs minus BBN ART) is small for persons with mild-moderate hearing impairment but large and essentially equivalent for persons with normal hearing as for persons with severe hearing impairment. These principles underlie the bivariate-plot procedure for prediction of the presence vs. absence of sensorineural hearing impairment from the ART.

With the traditional bivariate-plot procedure (Popelka, Margolis, and Wiley 1976; Popelka 1981), two acoustic reflex quantities that increase directly with the magnitude of hearing impairment are plotted as coordinates on a bivariate graph. The ART for a single tonal activator or the average of the ARTs for three tonal activators is represented on the ordinate (in dB SPL). The ratio of the ART for a noise activator (usually BBN) to the ART (in dB SPL) for a tonal activator (or the average of the ARTs for several tonal activators, usually 500, 1000, and 2000 Hz), times 100, is represented on the abscissa.

To construct a traditional bivariate-plot template, the ART data are plotted for a group of young, normal-hearing subjects. Two line segments (one vertical and one diagonal) with a slope of -1.0 are drawn, such that at least 90% of the data from the subjects are located within the delineated (left) region of the graph as shown in Figure 6.13. The normal-hearing region should not be drawn to include any obvious "outliers" since their inclusion will decrease the sensitivity (hit) rate for the bivariate-plot procedure. The bivariate-plot template then should be drawn showing the ordinate, abscissa, horizontal, and diagonal lines without the individual data points for future clinical use. We recommend that the miss and false alarm rates of the bivariate plot be determined by plotting the ART data from a group of hearing-impaired subjects who have known mild, high-frequency impairment (PTA between 20 and 29 dB HL or hearing threshold >20 dB HL at 2000 or 4000 Hz) as well as significant hearing impairment (PTA ≥30 dB HL) along with the ART data from a group of normal-hearing subjects. The miss rate for the significantly hearing-impaired ears is the percentage of significantly hearing-impaired ears that fall into the normal-hearing (left) region of the graph. The miss rate for the mild, high-frequency hearing-impaired ears is the percentage of mild, high-frequency hearing-impaired ears that fall into the normal-hearing region of the graph. The false-positive data are the percentage of normal-hearing ears that fall into the hearing-impaired (right) region of the graph.

Silman et al. (1984b) reported that the traditional bivariate-plot procedure was characterized by hit rates of 86% for ears with significant hearing impairment (PTA ≥30 dB HL) and 66% for ears with mild or high-frequency hearing impairment. Questionable findings associated with data points on the slope segment of the bivariate plot were obtained for 3% of the persons with significant or mild, high-frequency hearing impairment. The false alarm rate was 3%.

Silman et al.'s (1984b) modified bivariate-plot procedure improved predictive accuracy in comparison with that for the classical bivariate-plot procedure. The modified bivariate-plot procedure differed from the classical bivariate-plot procedure as follows:

1. The bivariate-plot was applied to persons younger than forty-five years of age.
2. The ART data from hearing-impaired as well as normal-hearing persons were plotted before drawing the line segments.
3. The line segments were drawn to obtain a sensitivity of at least 90% (for mild, high-frequency as well as significantly hearing-impaired ears) without incurring a large false alarm rate (the diagonal line segment is drawn with any slope, in contrast with the -1.0 slope employed in the classical bivariate-plot procedure). An example of the modified bivariate plot is shown in Figure 6.14.

According to Silman et al. (1984b), the sensitivity of the modified bivariate-plot procedure was 96% for significantly hearing-impaired ears as well as for the mild, high-frequency hearing-impaired ears; the false positive rate was 14%.

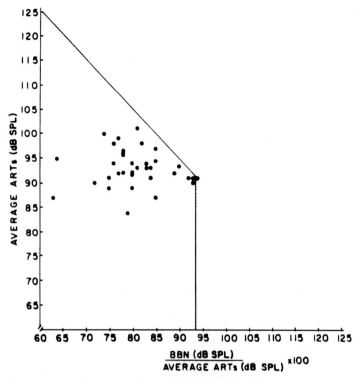

Figure 6.13. Illustration of the traditional bivariate plot as described by Popelka (1981). The ordinate represents the average of the ARTs for the 500-, 1000-, and 2000-Hz tonal activators, and the abcissa represents the ratio of the ART for the BBN activator to the average of the ARTs for the 500-, 1000-, and 2000-Hz tonal activators multiplied by 100. The line segments were drawn after plotting the data points for the normal-hearing ears. The line segments consist of the vertical segment and a diagonal segment with a slope of −1.0. The line segments were drawn so that at least 90% (here, 97%) of the data points for the normal-hearing ears were located to the left of them. (Reprinted by permission of Silman, Gelfand, Piper, Silverman, and Van Frank 1984a.)

Because of the higher sensitivity and specificity, the modified procedure is preferred in children as well as adults, despite the lower occurrence of mild, high-frequency hearing impairment in children.

The use of the bivariate-plot procedure can easily be employed in children thirteen years of age or older, whose contralateral ARTs are similar to those for adults. As mentioned previously, a maturation effect exists for the contralateral ART up to approximately thirteen years of age, and the ARTs for children who are five to nine years of age are higher than those for children who are nine to thirteen years of age. Therefore, the bivariate-plot procedure can be adapted for use with children between five and thirteen years of age by constructing two bivariate-plot templates: one based on ART data from children who are five to nine years of age and one based on ART data from children who are nine to thirteen years of age.

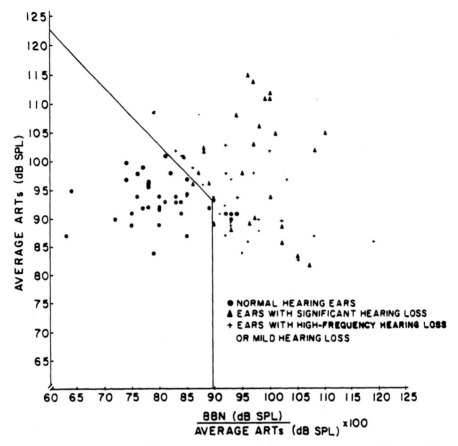

Figure 6.14. The modification of the bivariate-plot procedure involves adjustment of the vertical line segment to the left (with the diagonal line segment adjusted for the best separation between the normal-hearing and hearing-impaired ears) until at least 90 percent of the mild and high-frequency and significantly hearing-impaired ears lay in the hearing-impaired region. (Reprinted by permission of Silman, Silverman, Showers, and Gelfand 1984)

In neonates and infants, the standard deviations for the contralateral ARTs at low and high probe-tone frequencies are considerable, especially for the BBN activator, for both low- and high-frequency probe tones (McMillan et al. 1985; Sprague et al. 1985). These large standard deviations primarily reflect variability in sound-pressure levels associated with variability in ear-canal volume as well as maturational effects. Therefore, the bivariate-plot procedure has limited potential clinical utility in neonates and infants, regardless of probe-tone frequency. The data of S. Jerger et al. (1974) suggest that the standard deviations of the contralateral tonal ARTs for the low-frequency probe-tone and percentage of occurrence of the acoustic reflexes do not approach adult values until approximately five years of age.

Functional Hearing Impairment

The presence of acoustic reflex thresholds at or below the pure-tone thresholds is consistent with the presence of functional (nonorganic) hearing impairment (Terkildsen 1964).

Silman (1988) investigated the applicability of the modified bivariate-plot procedure for the low-frequency probe tone in young adults with functional hearing impairment. The sensitivity of the modified bivariate-plot procedure was 100%; the false-positive rate was 17%. The use of the modified bivariate-plot procedure for the low-frequency probe tone is applicable for detection of functional hearing impairment in persons older than thirteen years of age, nine to thirteen years of age, and five to nine years of age, providing the bivariate-plot template is appropriately developed.

REFERENCES

Alberti, P.W.R., and J.F. Jerger. 1974. Probe-tone frequency and the diagnostic value of tympanometry. *Archives of Otolaryngology* 99:206–210.

Alberti, P.W.R., and R. Kristensen. 1970. The clinical application of impedance audiometry. *Laryngoscope* 80:735–746.

Alford, B., J.F. Jerger, A. Coats, C. Peterson, and S. Weber. 1973. Neurophysiology of facial nerve testing. *Archives of Otolaryngology* 97:214–217.

American Speech-Language-Hearing Association. 1979. Guidelines for acoustic immittance screening of middle ear function. *Asha* 27:49–52.

———. 1985. Guidelines for identification audiometry. *Asha* 40:49–52.

———. 1990. Guidelines for screening for hearing impairments and middle ear disorders. *ASHA* (Suppl. 2) 32:17–30.

Anderson, H., B. Barr, and E. Wedenberg. 1969. Intra-aural reflexes in retrocochlear lesions. In *Nobel symposium 10: Disorders of the skull base region*, ed. C.A. Hamberger and J. Wersall. Stockholm: Almqvist and Wiksell.

———. 1970. Early diagnosis of VIIIth-nerve tumours by acoustic reflex tests. *Acta Oto-Laryngologica* 262, 232–237.

Beedle, R.K., and E.R. Harford. 1973. A comparison of acoustic reflex and loudness growth in normal and pathological ears. *Journal of Speech and Hearing Research* 16:271–281.

Bennett, M. 1984. Impedance concepts relating to the acoustic reflex. In *The acoustic reflex: Basic principles and clinical applications*, ed. S. Silman. New York: Academic Press.

Bennett, M.J., and L.A. Weatherby. 1982. Multiple probe frequency acoustic reflex measurements. *Scandinavian Audiology* 12:3–9.

Brooks, D.N. 1969. The use of the electroacoustic impedance bridge in the assessment of the middle ear function. *International Audiology* 8:563–569.

———. 1971. A new approach to identification audiometry. *Audiology* 10:334–339.

———. 1980. Impedance in screening. In *Clinical impedance audiometry*, 2d ed., ed. by J. Jerger and J.L. Northern. Acton, MA: American Electromedics Corporation.

Cavaliere, R., S. Masieri, L. Liberini, R. Proietti, and S.I. Magalini. 1992. Tympanometry for middle-ear effusion in unconscious ICU patients. *European Journal of Anaesthesiology* 9:71–75.

Fiellau-Nikolajsen, M. 1983. Tympanometry and secretory otitis media. *Acta Oto-Laryngologica* (Suppl. 394):1–73.

Gelfand, S.A., N. Piper, and S. Silman. 1983. Effects of hearing levels at the activator and other frequencies upon the expected levels of the acoustic reflex threshold. *Journal of Speech and Hearing Disorders* 48:11–17.

Gersdorff, M.C.H. 1992. Diagnostic value of tympanometry in otitis media with effusion. *Acta Oto-Rhino-Laryngolgica Belgica* 46:361–368.

Green, J., J. Waggener, and B. Kriegsfeld. 1976. Classification and incidence of neoplasms of the central nervous system. In *Advances in neurology*, ed. R. Thompson and J. Green. New York: Raven Press.

Hall, J.W., and T. Weaver. 1979. Impedance audiometry in a young population: The effect of age, sex, and tympanogram abnormalities. *Journal of Otolaryngology* 3: 210–221.

Himeelfarb, M.Z., E. Shanon, G.R. Popelka, and R.H. Margolis. 1978. Acoustic reflex evaluation in neonates. In *Early diagnosis of hearing loss*, ed. S.E. Gerber and G.T. Mencher. New York: Grune and Stratton.

Hirsch, J.E., R.H. Margolis, and J.R. Rykken. 1992. A comparison of acoustic reflex and auditory brain stem response screening of high-risk infants. *Ear and Hearing* 13:181–186.

Holmes, D.E., and C.M. Woodford. 1977. Acoustic reflex threshold and loudness discomfort level: Relationships in children with profound hearing losses. *Journal of the American Auditory Society* 2:193–196.

Holmquist, J., and J. Miller. 1972. Eustachian tube evaluation using the impedance bridge. In *Mayo Foundation impedance symposium*, ed. D. Rose and L. Keating. Rochester, MN: Mayo Foundation.

Jepsen, O. 1963. Middle ear muscle reflexes in man. In *Modern developments in audiology*, ed. J.F. Jerger. New York: Academic Press.

Jerger, J. 1970. Clinical experience with impedance audiometry. *Archives of Otolaryngology* 92:311–324.

Jerger, J., L. Anthony, S. Jerger, and L. Mauldin. 1974. Studies in impedance audiometry: Middle ear disorders. *Archives of Otolaryngology* 99:165–171.

Jerger, J., E. Harford, J. Clemis, and B. Alford. 1974. The acoustic reflex in eighth nerve disorders. *Archives of Otolaryngology* 99:409–413.

Jerger, J., S. Jerger, and L. Mauldin. 1972. Studies in impedance audiometry: I. Normal and sensorineural ears. *Archives of Otolaryngology* 96:513–523.

Jerger, S., J. Jerger, L. Mauldin, and P. Segal. 1974. Studies in impedance audiometry: II. Children less than 6 years old. *Archives of Otolaryngology* 99:1–9.

Keith, R.W. 1979. Loudness and the acoustic reflex: Cochlear-impaired listeners. *Journal of the American Auditory Society* 5:65–70.

Margolis, R.H., and J.W. Heller. 1987. Screening tympanometry: Criteria for medical referral. *Audiology* 26:197–208.

Margolis, R.H., and J.E. Shanks. 1985. Tympanometry. In *Handbook of clinical audiology*, 2d ed., ed. by J. Katz. Baltimore: Williams and Wilkins.

Martin, F.N., and G.W. Brunette. 1980. Loudness and the acoustic reflex. *Ear and Hearing* 1:106–108.

McMillan, P.M., M.J. Bennett, C.D. Marchant, and P. Shurin. 1985. Ipsilateral and contralateral acoustic reflexes in neonates. *Ear and Hearing* 6:320–324.

Metz, O. 1946. The acoustic impedance measured on normal and pathologic ears. *Acta Oto-Laryngologica* (Suppl. 63):1–254.

Norris, T.W., P.G. Stelmachowicz, and D.J. Taylor. 1974. Acoustic reflex relaxation to identify sensorineural hearing impairment. *Archives of Otolaryngology* 99:197.

Nozza, R.J., C.D. Bluestone, D. Kardatzke, and R. Bachman. 1992. Toward the validation of aural acoustic immittance measures for diagnosis of middle ear effusion in children. *Ear and Hearing* 13:442–453.

Olsen, W.O., D. Noffsinger, and S. Kurdziel. 1975. Acoustic reflex and reflex decay: Occurrence in patients with cochlear and eighth nerve lesions. *Archives of Otolaryngology* 101:622–625.

Osterhammel, D., and P. Osterhammel. 1979. Age and sex variations for the normal stapedial reflex thresholds and tympanometric compliance values. *Scandinavian Audiology* 8:153–158.

Ovesen, T., P.B. Paaske, and O. Elbrond. 1993. Accuracy of an automatic impedance apparatus in a population with secretory otitis media: Principles in the evaluation of tympanometrical findings. *American Journal of Otolaryngology* 1:100–104.

Paradise, J.L., C.G. Smith, and C.D. Bluestone. 1976. Tympanometric detection of middle ear effusion in infants and young children. *Pediatrics* 58:198–210.

Peterson, J.L., and G. Lidén. 1972. Some static characteristics of the stapedial muscle reflex. *Audiology* 11:94–114.

Popelka, G.R., ed. 1981. *Hearing assessment with the acoustic reflex*. New York: Grune and Stratton.

Popelka, G.R., R.H. Margolis, and T.L. Wiley. 1976. Effect of activating signal bandwidth on acoustic reflex thresholds. *Journal of the Acoustical Society of America* 59:153–159.

Porter, T.A. 1974. Otoadmittance measurements in a residential deaf population. *American Annals of the Deaf* 119:47–52.

Robertson, P.O., J.L. Peterson, and L.E. Lamb. 1968. Relative impedance measurements in young children. *Archives of Otolaryngology* 88:162–168.

Roush, J., A. Drake, and J.E. Sexton. 1992. Identification of middle ear dysfunction in young children: A comparison of tympanometric screening procedures. *Ear and Hearing* 13:63–69.

Shanks, J.E. 1984. Tympanometry. *Ear and Hearing* 5:268–280.

Shanks, J.E., and R.H. Wilson. 1986. Effects of direction and rate of ear-canal pressure changes on tympanometric measures. *Journal of Speech and Hearing Research* 29:11–19.

Silman, S. 1976. The growth function of the stapedius reflex in normal ears and ears with hearing loss due to cochlear dysfunction. Ph.D. diss., New York University, New York.

———. 1988. The applicability of the modified bivariate plotting procedure to subjects with functional hearing loss. *Scandinavian Audiology* 17:125–127.

———. 1990. Detection of middle-ear effusion. Short course presented at the Annual Convention of the American Speech-Language-Hearing Association, November 1990, Seattle.

Silman, S., and S.A. Gelfand. 1979. The effects of aging on the acoustic reflex thresholds. *Journal of the Acoustical Society of America* 66:735–738.

———. 1981. The relationship between magnitude of hearing loss and acoustic reflex threshold levels. *Journal of Speech and Hearing Disorders* 46:312–316.

Silman, S., S.A. Gelfand, and T.H. Chun. 1978. Some observations in a case of acoustic neu-
    roma. *Journal of Speech and Hearing Disorders* 43:459–466.
Silman, S., S.A. Gelfand, J.C. Howard, and T.J. Showers. 1982. Clinical application of the bi-
    variate plotting procedure in the prediction of hearing loss with the bivariate plotting
    procedure. *Journal of Speech and Hearing Research* 27:12–19.
Silman, S., S.A. Gelfand, N. Piper, C.A. Silverman, and L. Van Frank. 1984. Prediction of
    hearing loss from the acoustic reflex threshold. In *The acoustic reflex: Basic principles
    and clinical applications*, ed. S. Silman. New York: Academic Press.
Silman, S., G.R. Popelka, and S.A. Gelfand. 1978. Effect of sensorineural hearing loss on
    acoustic stapedius reflex growth functions. *Journal of the Acoustical Society of America*
    64:1406–1411.
Silman, S., and C.A. Silverman. 1991. *Auditory diagnosis: Principles and applications*. San
    Diego: Academic Press.
Silman, S., C.A. Silverman, and D.S. Arick. 1992. Acoustic-immittance screening for detec-
    tion of middle-ear effusion in children. *Journal of the American Academy of Audiology*
    3:262–268.
———. 1994. Pure-tone assessment and screening of children with middle-ear effusion. *Jour-
    nal of the American Academy of Audiology* 5:173–182.
Silman, S., C.A. Silverman, S.A. Gelfand, J. Lutolf, and D.J. Lynne. 1988. Ipsilateral acoustic-
    reflex adaptation testing for detection of facial-nerve pathology: Three case studies. *Jour-
    nal of Speech and Hearing Disorders* 53:378–382.
Silman, S., C.A. Silverman, T.J. Showers, and S.A. Gelfand. 1984. The effect of age on predic-
    tion of hearing loss with the bivariate plotting procedure. *Journal of Speech and Hearing
    Research* 27:12–19.
Silverman, C.A., S. Silman, and M.H. Miller. 1983. The acoustic reflex threshold in aging
    ears. *Journal of the Acoustical Society of America* 73:248–255.
Smith, P.S.U., T.L. Wiley, and G.M. Pyle. 1993. Efficacy of ASHA guidelines for screening
    middle-ear function in children. Poster session presented at the Annual Convention of the
    American Speech-Language-Hearing Association. November, Anaheim.
Sprague, B.H., T.L. Wiley, and R. Goldstein. 1985. Tympanometric and acoustic-reflex stud-
    ies in neonates. *Journal of Speech and Hearing Research* 28:265–272.
Terkildsen, K. 1964. Clinical application of impedance measurements with a fixed frequency
    technique. *International Audiology* 3:123–128.
Van Camp, K.J., R.H. Margolis, R.H. Wilson, W.L. Creten, and J.E. Shanks. 1986. *Principles
    of tympanometry*. ASHA Monograph no. 24. Rockville, MD: American Speech-Language-
    Hearing Association.
Vanhuyse, V.J., W.L. Creten, and K.J. Van Camp. 1975. On the W-notching of tympano-
    grams. *Scandinavian Audiology* 4:45–50.
Weatherby, L., and M. Bennett. 1980. The neonatal acoustic reflex. *Scandinavian Audiology*
    9:103–110.
Wiley, T.L., D.L. Oviatt, and M.G. Block. 1987. Acoustic immittance measures in normal
    ears. *Journal of Speech and Hearing Research* 30:161–170.
Wilson, R.H., J.E. Shanks, and D.J. Lilly. 1984. Acoustic-reflex adaptation. In *The acoustic
    reflex: Basic principles and clinical applications*, ed. S. Silman. New York: Academic
    Press.

7

Auditory Evoked Responses

Herbert Jay Gould and Maurice I. Mendel

INTRODUCTION

AUDITORY evoked responses (AERs) or auditory evoked potentials (AEPs) have been available for audiologic assessment for several decades. During that time, they have evolved from crude measures of gross neurophysiologic responses to sound to sophisticated measures capable of delineating anatomic areas and psychophysiological function. For audiologists, AER diagnostic procedures now look at two different areas. The first area—one that receives a significant amount of research—is the use of AERs for neurologic assessment. Does the patient have a lesion? This area is important in many otologic and audiologic practices dealing with adults but is less germane to the typical pediatric population. The second area of diagnosis, highly relevant to pediatric audiology, is estimation of auditory threshold. This second area is the focus of this chapter.

We strongly recommend that the reader examine the other areas on behavioral assessment of auditory function before reading this chapter. The authors believe that AERs are the test of last resort in evaluating any infant or child who may be testable by other means. It should be kept in mind that AERs do not evaluate hearing, but rather, estimate hearing based on neural integrity of the auditory system. Given technical limitations, the entire auditory system is typically not evaluated. Therefore, errors in the estimate can arise. In addition, some of the AERs, notably the quite popular auditory brainstem response (ABR), not only reflect a limited anatomic area but also a limited frequency range. This chapter shows methods for evaluation that are applicable to providing reasonable estimates of auditory function, aimed primarily at the pediatric population.

OVERVIEW OF AUDITORY EVOKED POTENTIALS

IT is not the purpose of this chapter to review extensively the basis of auditory evoked potentials as there are texts and review articles available for that purpose (ASHA 1987; Hall 1992; Kraus, Kileny, and McGee 1994; Moore 1983; Weber 1994). However, as terminology sometimes varies among authors, we briefly review the various responses that are used. As shown in Figure 7.1, the auditory evoked potential is a continuous response that is arbitrarily subdivided into time domains based on historical precedent and technological limitations.

Electrocochleogram

The electrocochleogram (ECochG), shown at the bottom of Figure 7.1, is the earliest set of waves recorded from the auditory system. It reflects the cochlear microphonic and summating potential, which are waves generated in response to local cochlear activity. In addition, the N1 wave (labelled AP for action potential) is generated from the eighth nerve. The ECochG is recorded by either extratympanic or transtympanic electrodes. The recording quality falls off dramatically as the distance of the active electrode from the tympanic membrane increases in extratympanic recordings.

Auditory Brainstem Response

The auditory brainstem response (ABR) also is known as the brainstem electric response (BSER) and the brainstem auditory evoked response (BAER). The response is often represented as a series of five vertex positive waves (labeled I through V in Figure 7.1) occurring within 10 to 12 msec of signal presentation. The waves reflect activity within the auditory system up to the level of the inferior colliculus. The ABR is an extremely robust response using modern recording techniques. Typical electrode placement locates the active electrode on the forehead or vertex with the referent electrode on the earlobe or mastoid ipsilateral to the stimulus. Placing the active electrode on either the vertex or high forehead does not have an appreciable effect on latency or amplitude as the ABR is a far field potential.

Middle Latency Response

The middle latency response (MLR) was also known as the early response in the literature of the late 1960s and early 1970s. This terminology, as the early response, created confusion at the time the ABR was discovered and became the new early response. Thus, after the mid-1970s, this response became known as the middle latency response. The MLR is recorded using a vertex active to ipsilateral earlobe or mastoid referent. It is a series of four waves occurring primarily within 50 msec of a stimulus and is labeled Po-Nb in Figure 7.1. The MLR is most likely generated from midbrain and primary auditory cortex of the brain.

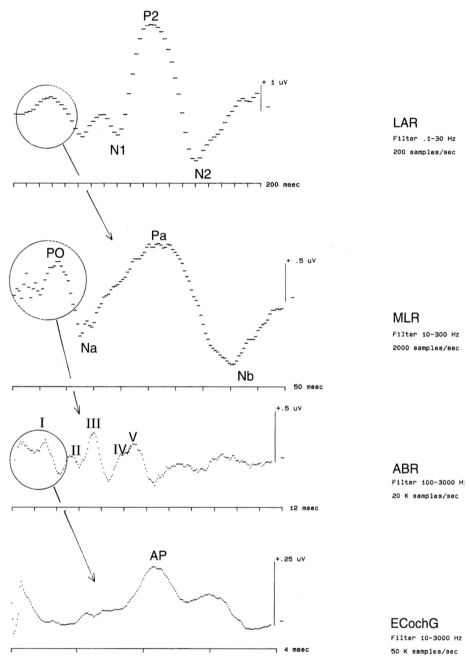

Figure 7.1. The auditory evoked potential is a continuous response starting at the stimulus and progressing to over 200 msec. The responses in the figure are represented as a series of short, unconnected lines that represent the sample time and discrete data as represented in the computer. The circled area in each response is the enlarged area represented as the next lower response in the figure. The entire ECochG response at the bottom is represented by one data point in the LAR tracing at the top of the figure.

The amplitude of the MLR appears to be significantly affected by sleep state, and the morphology may be affected by age in children.

Late Response

The late auditory response (LAR) was the first recorded auditory evoked potential. It is a large response and, at times, can be seen in the unaveraged EEG tracing. The response is recorded in the same manner as the ABR and MLR, with a vertex active electrode and referent electrode ipsilateral to the stimulus. The LAR is believed to originate in auditory cortical areas. The classic response is a negative wave at approximately 90 msec followed by a positive wave at approximately 120 msec, labelled N1 and P2 in Figure 7.1. The response is highly influenced by the subject's general physiologic and psychologic state.

P300

The P300 or P3 response, not shown in Figure 7.1, is a positive wave occurring about 300 msec after the onset of a stimulus. It is generated at a cortical level in response to a difference detection. Electrode arrangement is similar to that for other auditory evoked potentials from the central nervous system. The presence or absence of the P300 wave is determined by the subject's perception of difference between a frequently occurring standard stimulus and an intermittently occurring stimulus that is different. The different stimulus is often referred to as the oddball stimulus. The response is not widely used in the assessment of auditory threshold. The P300 requires an alert subject who is attending to the listening task. In addition, the P300 is highly dependent on age. Jirsa and Clontz (1990) have used this response in the evaluation of central auditory processing. Their results indicate that children with processing problems have smaller amplitude and longer latency than normal controls. They have further demonstrated that P300 response latency and amplitude approach normal values with appropriate therapy.

Mismatched Negativity

The mismatched negativity (MMN) is similar to the P300 in that it is generated in response to a difference detection between two stimuli. However, the MMN appears to be unaffected by subject state and may be less affected by subject age than the P300. Unlike the P300, MMN appears to be a strictly auditory phenomenon generated in temporal and frontal lobe areas. The use of the MMN for auditory threshold assessment has not been reported. Preliminary reports suggest that age may not affect response latency. However, response magnitude is generally greater in children than in adults (Kraus et al. 1992, 1993). For an extensive review of MMN, see Näätänen (1992).

CONTINGENT NEGATIVE VARIATION

THE contingent negative variation (CNV) is also generated by the detection of two signals. The stimulus generation is different from that for MMN and P300. For the CNV, the two stimuli must be paired and have precise timing relationships for occurrence. The response is a negative shift in potential that is initiated by the first stimulus and terminates upon presentation of the second stimulus. The CNV is generated in cortical areas and has been reported as a measure of auditory threshold in adults and children (Prevec, Ribaric, and Butinar 1984). Responses from children were significantly affected by the child's attentiveness, stimulus repetition rate, and duration.

Exogenous vs. Endogenous Potentials

Of the responses listed above, the four shown in Figure 7.1 are classified as exogenous responses (ECochG, ABR, MLR, Late), and the last three are endogenous responses (P300, MMN, CNV). Exogenous responses are affected more by stimulus variables such as level, rate, and frequency than by internal subject variables such as attention. Endogenous responses, however, are more affected by internal state and less by the external attributes of stimuli.

RESPONSE DETECTION

WHAT is required for threshold estimation using AERs? There are several reports that discuss the shape of the various waveforms and the latencies of the components within a waveform (ASHA 1987; Davis 1976; Picton et al. 1974). However, as the intensity of the stimulus is reduced, the structure of the waveform typically diminishes in amplitude and definition. There is also a prolongation in latency of each of the components. Finally, when the examiner can no longer determine that a wave is present, auditory threshold is declared as the lowest level that elicited the expected waveform. This is the crux of the problem in auditory threshold estimation: When is a response present, and when is it absent?

The goal of improving response detection and determining detection reliability has been pursued from the earliest recordings of auditory evoked potentials (Derbyshire and McCandless 1964; Palmer, Derbyshire, and Lee 1966; Schimmel 1967; Schimmel, Rapin, and Cohen 1974; Wong and Bickford 1980). Response detection takes one of two forms. The first is a correlational method or template matching. At its simplest (or most complex, depending on the point of view) is visual detection of a response. Through experience, we have learned that the AERs have typical wave shapes. For example, as shown in Figure 7.1, the ABR is a five-wavelet series occurring within the first six msec after a signal; the MLR is a four-wave series within 50 msec; and the Late waveform has a negative peak at approximately 90 msec (N1) and a positive peak at approximately 120 msec (P2). We also have learned to accept a certain amount of variation and attribute it to noise.

We first match the waveform that we collect against the internal representation of the wave and then repeat the trace and match the original to the replication. Several attempts have been made to use template matching in the computer (Arnold 1985; Elberling 1979; McClellend and Sayers 1984; Palmer, Derbyshire, and Lee 1966; Picton et al. 1983). Some of the methods are: (1) cross correlation with a known signal shape; (2) correlation with a response collected at a higher signal presentation level; and (3) difference between replication correlation and correlations performed with the no-stimulus condition.

The second method of detection is to estimate both the signal level and the noise level. To help understand these techniques, a quick review of the composition of an evoked response is necessary. Figure 7.2 is a schematic of a hypothetical evoked response test session. Each row in the figure represents a single epoch evoked by a click stimulus. Each column in the figure represents a latency after the stimulus presentation. Therefore, each cell in the figure represents a particular latency in a given epoch. Each cell is composed of a signal (S), which is constant, and a noise (N), which varies. In the ideal AER, the noise cancels itself out because of its random distribution around 0. So, when the average is made, the signal is recreated. Using signal-to-noise ratio measures to determine the presence of a response requires that an estimate of the noise be obtained. One method for estimating the noise level was the +/− average of Wong and Bickford (1980). In this technique, two averages were created for any evoked potential. In one, a simple average was performed; in the other, every other epoch was multiplied by −1, so that, when the response was summed, the signal was eliminated, leaving residual noise. The variance of the residual noise was computed and compared to the variance of the first average. This technique, which is computationally intensive, has been modified for online use and reported as the F_{sp} or F ratio for a single point (Don, Elberling, and Waring 1984; Elberling and Don 1984, 1987; Elberling and Walgreen 1985; Sininger 1993; Zapala 1993).

The F_{sp} is a method for evaluating the probability that the average is different from the background noise. The F_{sp} uses a single latency (i.e., a single column in Figure 7.2) to estimate the noise level in the average by computing the variance at that time. This assumes that the signal is stationary and the variance is an estimate of noise strength. Once the noise variance is estimated, the signal+noise variance in the average is computed. The two variances, signal+noise and noise, are then compared with an F_{max} statistic.

This technique is helpful with children for two reasons. First, it can help shorten the length of test administration. This is accomplished by averaging to a given probability of wave occurrence rather than to a fixed number of sweeps. Second, the examiner has a probability measure of response presence. Probability measures for an adult are shown in Table 7.1.

LATENCY

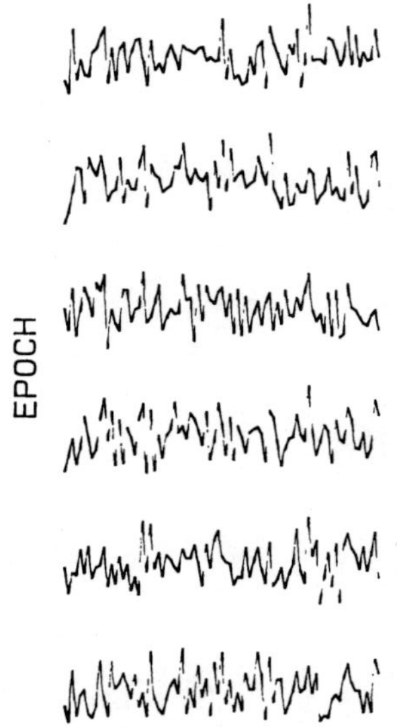

	1	2	3	4	5	6	7	8	9	10		n
	S+N	1+0	5+2	3-1	-1+0	-5+3	-3-1	2+2	0+1	1+1	. . . . .	S+N
	S+N	1-2	5+0	3+4	-1-1	-5+1	-3-1	2+1	0+1	1-2	. . . . .	S+N
	S+N	1-5	5-3	3-1	-1+2	-5-5	-3+5	2-3	0-3	1+1	. . . . .	S+N
	S+N	1+4	5-1	3-5	-1-3	-5+3	-3-1	2-5	0-2	1-2	. . . . .	S+N
	S+N	1+2	5+0	3+2	-1+2	-5+1	-3+2	2+0	0+6	1+3	. . . . .	S+N
	S+N	1+1	5+2	3+1	-1+0	-5-1	-3-4	2+5	0-3	1-1	. . . . .	S+N
SUM	ΣS+N	6	30	18	-6	-30	-18	12	0	6		
AVERAGE	S	1	5	3	-1	-5	-3	2	0	1		

EPOCH

Figure 7.2. For any evoked potential, each response to a single stimulus (as represented by each of the EEG traces on the left of the figure) is collected by the computer as a series of numbers. Each number represents the voltage on the surface of the head at a given time (latency) after the stimulus onset. The individual numbers consist of the electrical signal (S) that is evoked by the stimulus plus the ongoing EEG background noise (N). The entire evoked potential data collection can be envisioned in the computer as a two-dimensional spreadsheet. Each row represents one response to a stimulus (epoch), and each column represents a period of time after the stimulus (latency). As shown, the signal at each time point is constant while the noise varies around zero. Therefore, given a sufficient number of samples, the noise will average out of the response, leaving just the original signal.

Table 7.1. Probability of Presence of ABR

F_{sp}	Probability
3.1	99%
2.3	95%
1.9	90%
1.4	75%
.88	50%

Note: The F_{sp} procedure is a statistical method of expressing the variability of a response in relation to the estimated variability of the background noise. It is based on the F_{max} statistic, and the resulting value provides the probability that a signal is present in a given average.

The measures shown in Table 7.1 may or may not be reasonable for infants and neonates. The probability table was generated using resting adult EEG activity collected within a specific time frame (2 to 12 msec poststimulus) and with a specific filter setting (100–3000 Hz). The assumption is made that the infant and child will have statistically similar activity if the tester is using the same time and filter parameters. If time and filter parameters are changed, the table should be recomputed. Gould et al. (1992) reported on the F_{sp} technique for the middle latency response in adults and provided information using 50 and 100 msec time domains as well as several different high-pass filter settings. Only minor differences were seen in the cumulative distributions for the no-signal condition, suggesting that, although not precise, the probabilities in Table 7.1 may be reasonable estimates of response probability.

NORMAL DEVELOPMENT

Anatomic and Physiologic Changes

THE human auditory system develops rapidly during the first and second years of life. During the third prenatal trimester and the infantile period, there is a decrease in the density of the nerve cells in the cochlear nucleus and inferior colliculus. Myelination, however, is increasing in the lateral lemniscus (Inagaki et al. 1987). The cochlear traveling wave is also affected by maturation. Significant decreases in delay are seen for the basal end of the cochlea with age, whereas the apical end is relatively unaffected (Eggermont et al. 1991). These changes in traveling wave are probably related to the changes seen in cochlear maturation (Rubel et al. 1984).

The external auditory meatus (EAM) is also developing during the first year. The EAM development is reflected in a resonant frequency pattern different from that for the normal adult ear (Lurquin et al. 1989). This suggests that stimulus calibration values should be considered in evaluating the neonate and young infant.

ABR

Because of its extensive use for auditory screening and estimation of threshold, ABR has been extensively investigated with regard to its normal and abnormal development. In contrast, other responses, such as the MLR and Late Auditory Response, have received considerably less attention. Nevertheless, ABR literature is often confusing because of a host of factors including, but not limited to, the different age ranges studied, whether the subject was full term or premature, and stimulus characteristics (Hall 1992).

ABR Morphology Changes with Maturation

The ABR is profoundly affected by the maturation process from birth to approximately eighteen months of age. The consensus is that waves III through V are delayed. There is some speculation as to the status of wave I at birth. Several studies of newborns have shown a delayed wave I that is from 0.3 to one msec longer than adult values (Cox, Hack, and Metz 1981; Goldstein et al. 1979; Jacobson, Morehouse, and Johnson 1982; Stockard, Stockard, and Coen 1983). However, there is suggestion that wave I is relatively well developed in the neonate (Morgan, Zimmerman, and Dubno 1987). Gorga et al. (1989) report little to no change in wave I latency between three months and three years of age. However, a significant change was noted in wave V latency. ABR latency and amplitude data showing maturation effects from several studies have been collected and published (Hall 1992).

Of primary concern, given the shorter hospital stays of many neonates, are the rapid alterations in the response during the first three days of life. Maurizi et al. (1986) looked at the ABR wave pattern during the first fifty-eight hours after birth in full-term newborns. In two thirds of the cases, wave I was absent in the first nine hours of life. Latency values for wave I tend to decrease in a statistically significant way; this decrease is almost complete by the second recording session at thirty hours. Contralaterally recorded potentials are often absent at birth but evident fifty-eight hours later. The wave II-III complex seen in the neonate by contralateral recording is reported to be separated into individual waves by seven months of age (Hatanaka et al. 1988).

As the contralateral response can be recorded in the infant, care must be taken to avoid response recording by stimulating the nontest ear. Sobhy and Gould (1993) recommended masking for levels greater than 50 dB used in adults. Hatanaka et al. (1990) recorded a response from a dead ear to an 85-dB HL click in an infant. They report that a 45 dB HL masker will eliminate such responses.

AUDITORY BRAIN STEM RESPONSE

THE ABR has been the hearing screening test of choice in the neonatal nursery. Unfortunately, the expense and time required for testing has limited its use primarily to the neonatal intensive care unit (NICU). Because a higher percentage of these infants experiences a hearing loss than normal newborns do, this limitation is cost efficient. Other available screening tools, such as the high risk register or otoacoustic emissions, should be applied to all neonates; ABR should then be used as a follow-up tool in those who fail.

Electrode Application

Electrode application is similar to that for adults, with the noninverting electrode applied to vertex or forehead and the inverting electrode applied to the mastoid ipsilateral to the stimulus. The ground can be applied to the mastoid contralateral to the stimulus. Using a three-electrode configuration requires switching the ground and inverting electrodes when the stimulus ear is changed. However, this method is advantageous in that one less electrode is applied, which saves time and may avoid waking a sleeping infant. Electrodes in the neonatal nursery should not be moved between infants unless they have been properly sterilized. An alternative to sterilization is disposable electrodes, which are available from most supply houses.

Electrical Safety

Grounding is critical in the intensive care situation (Grass 1978) because the recording is made in an electrically "hostile" environment. Most NICUs are brightly lit with fluorescent lighting and have numerous electrical sources generating ambient electrical noise. If the infant is connected to other equipment, be sure that amplifiers and other equipment maintain a common AC ground path. If not, potentially dangerous electrical current can be induced in the leads. A good ground that is common to the other sources will also help in this situation by preventing a ground loop that would introduce 60-Hz interference.

It is required that you know the electrical outlets you will be using. If going into a new area, take a socket tester to be sure that the hot, neutral, and ground leads are appropriately wired. Never assume that the leads of any socket are correct. In a check of 734 outlets in a 100-bed hospital, 11% had improper wiring, and 67% did not exert proper tension on the ground plug (Grass 1978).

Stimulus

As most neonates are seen in a screening situation, a click is used to elicit the response. Although the click creates a wideband signal, the response reflects primarily the 2000–4000 Hz range in the cochlea. The use of a click is beneficial in that it has the highest potential for eliciting a response. The fast rise time of the click creates a synchrony in neural discharge that is optimum for recording a response. Tonal stimuli are rarely, if ever, used in the NICU because they do not provide as clear a response and still reflect the basal region of the cochlea as click stimuli.

Latency Intensity Function

The latency intensity function for the neonate (see Figure 7.3) is longer when compared to the adult (see Figure 7.4). In addition, infants, such as those with craniofacial malformations, may have abnormal wave shapes, so care must be taken in using either a specific latency or shape of waveform to determine threshold. Here the F_{sp} technique or some other method for determining signal-to-noise ratio is beneficial; correlational methods may have less validity.

Normative data for click-evoked ABRs have been published by several authors (Cevette 1984; Eggermont and Salamy 1988; Fawer and Dubowitz 1982; Goldstein et al. 1979; Gorga et al. 1989; Jacobson, Morehouse, and Johnson 1982; Lary et al. 1985; Stockard, Stockard, and Coen 1983; Weber 1982). Unfortunately, the data are on different age ranges, using different recording parameters and stimulus transducers. This disparity in techniques makes it virtually impossible to compare studies. When evaluating ABRs, local norms should be established. Published data should be consulted to determine whether your latency and amplitude measurements are comparable. When using published data, be sure to use the same age measure—gestational, conceptional, or chronologic. Figure 7.3 provides information on wave V maturation from four studies. Data in the figure that were reported using conceptional age have been corrected to gestational age by subtracting two weeks from the reported date.

Screening procedures often use one or two stimulus levels to determine the presence of a response. A higher level stimulus provides a waveform to which the lower level response may be compared.

In the NICU, approximately 1–3% of the population is hearing impaired; for every child identified, approximately six will fail the ABR screening test. In the normal newborn nursery, approximately 0.1% of the population is impaired, and for every child identified, 100 will fail the screening test (National Institutes of Health 1993).

MIDDLE LATENCY RESPONSE

MLR Morphology Changes with Maturation and Recording Parameters

THE MLR appears to be less affected by the maturation process than the ABR (Mendel 1985). The MLR waveform in neonates, infants, and children resembles that of adults (McRandle, Smith, and Goldstein 1974; Mendel, Adkinson, and Harker 1977; Mendelson and Salamy 1981). Recording parameters for the MLR (electrode application, electrical safety, stimulus) are essentially those described for the ABR above, with the following differences: The time window is usually set to 50 or 100 msec; filter settings vary among laboratories, but 10–1000 Hz is common (see below); and the repetition rate is between 10 and 20 per second, depending on whether the 50- or 100-msec window is used. However, slower rates may provide better waveform morphology.

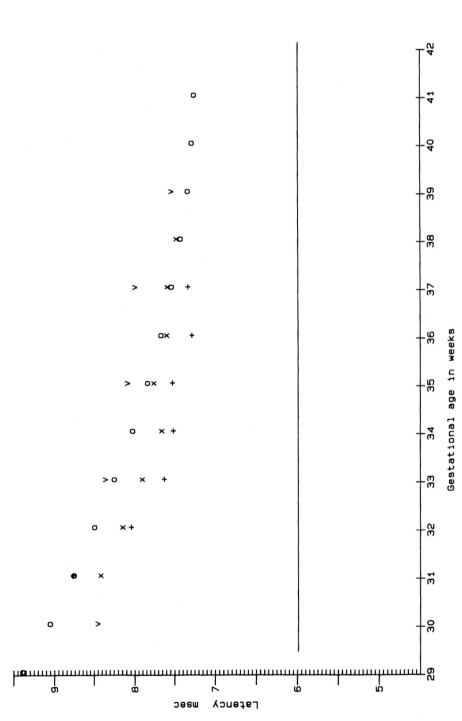

Figure 7.3. The latency of the wave V response decreases with increasing age. The data are from four studies that used a 60- or 65-dB HL click stimulus (Fawer and Dubowitz 1982 (o); Goldstein et al. 1979 (+); Cevette 1984 (x); and Weber 1982 (v)). Ages that were reported as conceptional were corrected by two weeks to gestational. It should be noted that the studies used a number of different stimulus delivery and recording methods that could lead to different response latencies. However, all studies show a consistent reduction of wave V latency with increasing age.

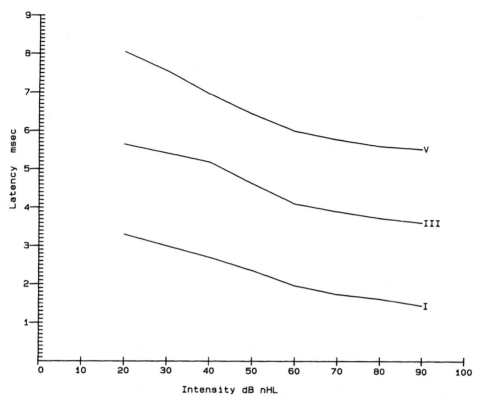

Figure 7.4. Adult normative data collected on 120 adult subjects using an earphone producing a rarefaction click. Subjects ranged from 20 to 60 years of age, and both male and female data are represented.

A principal use of the MLR is with the use of tone pips or tone bursts in the determination of low frequency threshold at 500 or 1000 Hz. Initial studies using frequency-specific stimuli were reported by McFarland, Vivion, and Goldstein (1977) and Thornton, Mendel, and Anderson (1977). A study by Sobhy (1993) indicates that high level click stimuli tend to produce responses from more basal regions of the cochlea in a manner similar to the ABR.

Neonates

The middle latency response is not often seen in newborn infants. This may be due to a number of recording factors as well as physiologic differences. As demonstrated in the initial studies, the response is reduced in amplitude during deep sleep in adults (Mendel and Goldstein 1971), and a similar effect may occur in the neonate. Recording parameters play a meaningful role in MLR identification. Before six months of age, N_a and P_a are significantly less detectable than in adults. Kraus et al. (1987) suggest that 40% of children younger than six months of age will not have a detectable N_a. Further, over 80% of those children may not have a detectable P_a.

Filtering

The high-pass filter appears to have a profound effect on the detectability of the response. Filtering of the MLR has received a significant amount of attention, and optimal filter settings remain controversial (Lane et al. 1974; Ozdamar and Kraus 1983). Raising the high-pass filter of the response reduces the low frequency components of the response and phase-shifts energy from the ABR into the MLR response window (Kavanagh and Domico 1986). This phase-shifting can be reduced by using digital filters or slopes with very low rolloffs. However, from a clinical viewpoint of threshold detection, the energy shift of ABR information into the MLR time domain is of little consequence, provided locally established norms are used that were obtained with the same stimulus and recording parameters.

Sleep State Determination

Initial studies have shown that the middle latency response is reduced in amplitude during deep sleep in adults, whereas latency remains essentially stable regardless of stage of sleep (Mendel and Goldstein 1971). Monitoring of sleep stage in neonates may be necessary while recording the MLR (Crawford 1991; Kraus, Kileny, and McGee 1994).

PATHOLOGIC CONDITIONS

ALTHOUGH threshold identification is a primary function in pediatric evoked potential testing, a knowledge of pediatric neurologic disorders is helpful in interpreting the test results. Evoked potential abnormalities have been reported for a number of pathologic entities. Fortunately, many of these entities are rare. Unfortunately, because of the small number of patients, results are often presented as anecdotal case reports. As evoked potential testing is site specific and not pathology specific, results will be similar in many of these entities. These cases demonstrate that the ABR results must be interpreted in light of the overall medical status of the patient.

Acquired Immune Deficiency Syndrome (AIDS)

AIDS is on the rise in newborn populations as a congenital pathology. Infants and children with AIDS may exhibit prolonged absolute and interpeak latencies. Increasing stimulation rate will show a larger latency shift for the AIDS patient than for a normal cohort (Frank et al. 1992). A case report of one infant suggests that zidovudine may improve latency measures over a course of twelve months (Brivio et al. 1991).

Adrenoleukodystrophy (ALD)

Adrenoleukodystrophy is a sex-linked genetic disorder leading to progressive destruction of adrenal cortex and white matter in the nervous system. Children with ALD show prolonged absolute and interpeak wave latencies. Wave I-III has been reported as showing the greatest incidence of abnormality (Shimizu, Moser, and Naidu 1989). In a single case report, Iinuma et al. (1989) reported normal ABR and SSEP (Somatosensory Evoked Potential) at an early stage with VEP (visual evoked potential) being abnormal.

Angelman Syndrome

Angelman syndrome is characterized by abnormal facies with protruding tongue, paroxysmal laughter, and jerky movements. Patients often have frequent epileptic seizures and optic nerve and cerebral atrophy (Niedermeyer and Lopes da Silva 1987). The syndrome is associated with chromosome DNA deletion (Sugimoto et al. 1992). Sugimoto et al. report elevated ABR thresholds with normal interpeak latency in three siblings.

Apert Syndrome

Apert syndrome is characterized by craniosynostosis, midface hypoplasia, relative prognathism, bony fusion of the middle three digits of the hands and feet with soft tissue fusion of the other digits, and limitation of joint movement. Children with Apert syndrome are at a greatly increased risk for conductive hearing loss, primarily due to otitis media (Gould and Caldarelli 1982). There are reports of middle ear malformation (Bergstrom, Neblett, and Hemenway 1972; Gould and Caldarelli 1982; Lindsay, Black, and Donnelly 1975). ABR results indicate increased absolute latency consistent with the conductive pathology and an increased wave I-III interpeak latency. The I-III change may be related to the cranial configuration.

Atresia

Congenital aural atresia is a prime reason to perform ABR testing. These children often have an intact cochlea; identification of cochlear reserve is therefore critical for early habilitation. Two approaches are possible for assessing the infant with congenital atresia. In the first approach, a high level air conduction stimulus is used, and a maximum conductive loss is assumed. Obviously, supraaural or circumaural earphones would be used; inserts would be impossible. If thresholds of 70–80 dB HL are seen, a normal cochlea is most likely present.

The second approach uses bone conduction stimuli in an attempt to directly assess cochlear function. Use of this approach may provide a better estimate of cochlear reserve. However, the examiner must remember that the skull structure of the neonate and infant maintains a different energy transfer function from that of the adult. Significantly shorter wave V latency has been seen in infants younger than one year of age than in adults with temporal bone placement of the bone vibrator (Yang et al. 1987). This difference in energy transfer may be compounded in children who have congenital craniofacial malformations as well as atresia. Durrant and Hyde (1993) report on temporal aspects of bone conducted clicks in normal adolescents and adults. They indicate low frequency filtering effects and propagation delays. Finally, care must be exercised to reduce vibrator-produced electrical artifacts that can obscure a response.

Cleft Palate

Cleft palate is a common malformation leading to a high incidence of conductive hearing impairment. ABR results typically exhibit prolonged absolute wave I and V latencies that coincide with the conductive impairment. An increased I-V interpeak latency was reported for six of ten normal gestation infants with cleft palate studied between one and twenty months chronologic age (Gould 1980). The trend in these data suggested normal I-V latency by twenty months. Clefting is often associated with other syndromes. This necessitates a careful examination to rule out other possible abnormalities.

Charcot-Marie-Tooth Syndrome

Charcot-Marie-Tooth syndrome comprises a group of hereditary motor and sensory neuropathies. It is characterized by sensitivity disorders, areflexia, and atrophy of leg muscles and was first reported in 1967 by Lemieux and Neemeh. Approximately 28% of cases will exhibit hearing loss associated with VIII nerve and brain stem disorder (Perez et al. 1988). Absolute and interpeak wave latencies may be affected. Cassandro et al. (1986) report no ABR abnormalities in five cases. The vestibular system may be affected, as caloric responses were reported absent in one individual case (Hanson, Farber, and Armstrong 1970).

Chiari Syndrome

Chiari or Arnold-Chiari syndrome is characterized by displacement of the medulla and cerebellum into the basilar part of the occipital bone. It is associated with hydrocephalus, spina bifida, and meningomyelocele. There may be an increased interpeak latency. In three cases with malformed pons and tegmen, an increased III-V latency was noted on one side (Kamuro, Inagaki, and Tomita 1992).

Cocaine Exposure

In 1990 there were 158,000 infants born in the United States who were known to have been exposed prenatally to cocaine. This figure excludes, of course, those in whom the exposure is not known. Exposure to cocaine causes vasoconstriction of vessels delivering nutrients and oxygen to a fetus. This exposure may affect neurobehavioral development. Shih, Cone-Wesson, and Reddix (1988) investigated ABRs of eighteen neonates born to women who had used cocaine. These infants were compared to eighteen from the normal newborn nursery. The cocaine-exposed infants *all* had prolonged ABR interpeak latencies as compared to controls. These prolongations were believed to "reflect abnormalities in brainstem conduction times rather than a deficit in the auditory periphery" (p. 250). Moreover, five of the eighteen infants appeared to have hearing thresholds poorer than 20 dB, suggesting a possibility of moderate hearing impairment. Salamy et al. (1990) also found prolonged brain transmission times in cocaine-exposed infants.

Down Syndrome

Down syndrome, also known as trisomy 21, is a chromosomal disorder resulting in short stature, short hands with simian crease, abnormal dermatoglyphics, congenital heart disease, muscular hypotonia, and characteristic facies. The facial characteristics are flat face, downward sloping epicanthal folds, oblique palpebral fissures, protruding tongue, and open mouth posture. The auricle tends to be small and somewhat square with small external ear canals. Conductive, sensorineural, and mixed hearing impairment is frequently reported. ABR results have been reported as shortened I-V latency, although this may not occur in older patients who have Down syndrome (Arao and Niwa 1991; Kaga and Marsh 1986; Maurizi et al. 1985).

Friedreich Ataxia

Friedreich ataxia—an autosomal recessive disorder—is characterized as progressive CNS degeneration with preadolescent onset. The posterior and lateral columns of the spinal cord exhibit the most marked degeneration. The syndrome is characterized by gait disturbance, truncal ataxia, nystagmus, dysarthria, and impaired muscular power and sensation. Approximately 25 to 50% of those affected develop cardiomyopathy. A report of fifteen cases with Friedreich ataxia (Cassandro et al. 1986) indicated normal pure tone and immittance findings. The ABR waveforms were absent in eleven patients and abnormal in the remaining four at elevated stimulus levels; cortical responses were normal in all cases. Other hereditary ataxias tend not to show central ABR abnormalities (Taylor, Chan-Lui, and Logan 1985).

Hyperbilirubinemia

Increased bilirubin, at levels requiring exchange transfusion in the infant, has been identified as a risk factor for hearing loss (Joint Committee on Infant Hearing 1991). Because neurotoxic as well as cochleotoxic events are occurring, ABR testing is advocated for these infants. Prolonged absolute and interpeak latencies have been noted and are strongly correlated with serum bilirubin levels (Gupta, Raj, and Anand 1990). Caution is required in the interpretation of ABR results, however, as a number of infants have demonstrated marked improvement in responses after treatment (Hall, Brown, and Mackey-Hargardine 1985). Post blood exchange ABR testing should show improved amplitude and latency values in affected infants (Hung 1989). Esbjorner et al. (1991) found that wave latency was inversely related to the serum reserve albumin concentration for monoacetyldiaminodiphenyl sulphone (MADDS). They suggest that the neurotoxicity of bilirubin may be related to binding properties of the serum albumin. At least the initial changes in ABR with hyperbilirubinemia appear to be associated with reversible neurotoxic effects.

Hydrocephalus

Hydrocephalus, which is related to abnormal CSF circulation and absorption, is a result of increased CSF accumulation in the ventricles. The increased CSF causes an increased intracranial pressure resulting in brain and skull abnormalities. For the neonate, waves I-V appear to have longer absolute latencies and smaller amplitudes. The I-V interpeak latency is within normal limits, and there is a smaller V/I amplitude ratio. The elevated threshold value may be related to intracranial pressure rather than sensory hair cell loss (Edwards, Durieux-Smith, and Picton 1985). Shunt placement to reduce CSF pressure results in improved ABR response patterns (McPherson, Amlie, and Foltz 1985).

Congenital Hypothyroidism

In patients with congenital hypothyroidism, the ABR results are dependent upon age of evaluation. In infants, wave I can be delayed but interpeak latencies are generally normal (Laureau et al. 1986). Beginning at about the age of three years, reports of shortened I-V IPL occur (Hebert et al. 1986). Shortened IPL has been partially correlated with thyroxine serum levels at diagnosis and thyrotopin levels at the time of recording. Thyroxine therapy has been reported to result in a more normal I-V IPL in hypothyroid cases secondary to long-term anticonvulsant therapy (Kodama et al. 1989).

Neurofibromatosis (Von Recklinghausen Disease)

Neurofibromatosis is an autosomal dominant hereditary disease characterized by multiple tumors associated with the peripheral nervous system, CNS tumors, and cafe-au-lait spots (Niedermeyer and Lopes da Silva 1987). There is great variability of expression in this disorder. The most common intracranial tumor is acoustic neurinoma, which often presents as bilateral tumors. Although usually occurring in early adulthood, acoustic tumors may be present during childhood. Regular ABRs are recommended to establish a baseline and then screen for possible developing acoustic neurinomas.

Rett Syndrome

Rett syndrome is a disease confined to females that becomes evident at six to eighteen months of age. There is progressive dementia and loss of language. Purposeful hand motion diminishes, and a stereotypical hand washing movement appears. Gait apraxia is present. Epileptic seizures are present in 80% of the population between one and eight years of age. Most symptoms abate by adolescence, leaving a residual dementia and scoliosis (Niedermeyer and Lopes da Silva 1987). EEG abnormalities are present. ABR abnormality of wave V latency and the III-V interval was noted in a study of eleven subjects with Rett syndrome compared to two normal control groups (Pelson and Budden 1987). MLR and Late responses also have been noted to be abnormal (Bader, Witt-Engerstrom, and Hagberg 1989). In a more recent study of thirty-six subjects with Rett syndrome, normal results were seen 100% of the time for ABR, 50% for MLR, and 36% for late responses (Stach et al. 1994).

Sickle Cell Anemia

Sickle cell anemia is a recessively inherited blood disorder that results in a change in hemoglobin shape during periods of physiologic stress or emotional change. The abnormal hemoglobin shape results in blockage of blood vessels leading to localized ischemia. Auditory function can be impaired in individuals in which blockage to the cochlea results. Individuals can either fully or partially recover from these losses. Central auditory processing has been shown to be affected in some children with sickle cell disease (Forman-Franco et al. 1982; Friedman et al. 1980; Sharp and Orchick 1978). Increased interpeak latency, IT5 (Selters and Brackman 1977), and delta V (Prosser et al. 1983) measures of ABR have been noted in older sickle cell patients when ischemic events involve the central nervous system (Gould et al. 1991).

HEARING AID FITTING

ALTHOUGH evoked auditory potentials have been used primarily to evaluate auditory threshold in infants and children, their potential as a means for fitting amplification has been explored (Beauchaine and Gorga 1988; Beauchaine et al. 1986; Bergman, Beauchaine, and Gorga 1992; Davidson, Wall, and Goodman 1990; Gerling 1991; Gorga, Beauchaine, and Reiland 1987; Hall and Ruth 1985; Hecox 1983; Kiessling 1982; Kileny 1982; McPherson and Clark 1983; Rackliffe and Musiek 1983; Thornton, Farrell, and McSporran 1989; Thornton, Yardley, and Farrell 1987). In the speech and hearing sciences, a basic assumption is that good hearing is necessary for normal development of speech and oral language. Therefore, detection of an auditory deficit calls for the intervention of an audiologist, who selects correct amplification and directs aural rehabilitation when medical or surgical management is precluded.

As in determining auditory threshold, infants and young children pose a problem for testing to determine the best amplification fit. Not only must a general hearing level be estimated, but thresholds must be precisely determined at various frequencies. In addition, most comfortable loudness (MCL) (McPherson and Clark 1983) and the loudness discomfort level (LDL) need to be determined. Finally, many individuals believe that it is important to determine the hearing aids' effects on speech recognition.

In fitting amplification, two main approaches have been employed using the ABR. The first assesses auditory function with the hearing aid in place. A number of pitfalls is associated with this approach, primarily with the electroacoustic characteristics of the hearing aid and its interaction with the acoustic requirements of the ABR stimulus (Kileny 1982).

A second approach evaluates threshold and dynamic range of hearing using unaided responses and then applying prescriptive formulas to fit the hearing aid. This approach, too, has limitations. First, prescriptive formulas require accurate frequency-specific auditory threshold information. As previously noted both in this chapter and by other authors (Hall 1992), the click-evoked response permits only high-frequency threshold estimation. Several techniques have been developed to estimate frequency-specific threshold. Notched noise masking (Picton et al. 1979), derived band response (Don, Eggermont, and Brackmann 1979), and gated tone pips (Gorga and Thornton 1989) have been recommended for this purpose. The first two techniques—notched noise and derived bands—rely on modification of the cochlear response. These techniques desynchronize neural activity in unwanted areas of the cochlea, thus preventing them from contributing to the evoked response. The third technique—gated tone pips—limits the frequency spectrum of the signal being delivered to the cochlea. Several studies have demonstrated that high level, low frequency tone pips have a significant spread into the higher frequency, basal region of the cochlea (Sobhy 1993). Nevertheless, clinical studies suggest that tone bursts at several frequencies can estimate threshold within 20 dB (Hall 1992).

Estimation of LDL by evoked potentials poses a unique challenge. Several authors have examined amplitude-intensity and latency-intensity functions for the ABR in attempts to obtain this information. Kiessling (1982) assumes that the amplitude of V-N5 is a correlate of loudness perception. He uses the amplitude-intensity curve of the subject in conjunction with the normative latency-amplitude curve to project gain and compression functions for the hearing aid. In a follow-up study, Davidson et al. (1990) tested Kiessling's assumption of ABR amplitude and loudness perception correlation. They found that single measures of the amplitude-intensity function were insufficient to judge loudness perception. However, averaging the amplitude-intensity functions for four trials with a one-week separation provided a good correlate with perceived loudness.

Because amplitude is a more variable measure than the latency of wave V in the ABR, other investigators have tried using latency as an estimate of LDL. Thornton et al. (1987, 1989) report on using the slope of the latency-intensity function for LDL estimation. They found that the subjective LDL was equal to the point at which the latency-intensity function became 0.1 ms/10dB plus 15 dB, when using a 10-dB step size in obtaining the ABR. Employing this formula, ABR estimates were within 5 dB of subjective LDL in 66% of subjects and within 11 dB for the remaining 33% of the subjects. When a 5-dB step size was used for ABR measurement, the formula LDL $= I_5 + 10$, where $I_5 =$ 0.08ms/5dB, estimated subjective LDL within five dB for all subjects.

Both of these methods attempt to link parameters of the ABR waveform to a subjective estimate of loudness, specifically LDL. Darling and Price (1990), in a study of loudness and ABR, found that measurement of loudness could not be derived from ABR measurements because of the influence of rate and absolute intensity on the latency and amplitude of the response.

SUMMARY

AUDITORY evoked potentials are valuable tools in the audiologist's armamentarium for diagnosing hearing loss in children. Nonetheless, as with any tool, they are limited in scope. The potentials currently elicited in the diagnosis of hearing loss provide information on subsets of the auditory nervous system. This information is often confounded with numerous variables such as maturation, general health, psychologic state, and stimulus factors. The diagnostician must remain cognizant of these difficulties and not extend interpretation beyond the physiologic constraints of the test. Before utilizing electrophysiologic measures, the reader is well advised to attempt other behavioral testing of the auditory system if at all possible.

REFERENCES

Arao, H. and H. Niwa. 1991. Auditory brain stem responses in Down's syndrome. *Nippon Jibiinkoka Gakkai Kaiho* 94:1673–82.

Arnold, S. 1985. Objective versus visual detection of the auditory brainstem response. *Ear and Hearing* 6:144–149.

American Speech-Language-Hearing Association. 1987. *The short latency auditory evoked potentials.* Rockville, MD: American Speech-Language-Hearing Association.

Bader, G.G., I. Witt-Engerstrom, and B. Hagberg. 1989. Neurophysiological findings in the Rett syndrome, II: Visual and auditory brainstem, middle and late evoked responses. *Brain Development* 11:110–114.

Beauchaine, K., and M. Gorga. 1988. Applications of the auditory brainstem response to pediatric hearing aid selection. *Seminars in Hearing* 9:61–74.

Beauchaine, K., M. Gorga, J. Reiland, and L. Larson. 1986. Application of ABRs to the hearing-aid selection process: Preliminary data. *Journal of Speech and Hearing Research* 29:120–128.

Bergman, B., K. Beauchaine, and M. Gorga. 1992. Application of the auditory brainstem response in pediatric audiology. *The Hearing Journal* 45:19–25.

Bergstrom, L., M. Neblett, and W. Hemenway. 1972. Otologic manifestations in acrocephalosyndactyly. *Archives of Otolaryngology* 96:117–123.

Brivio, L., R. Tornaghi, L. Musetti, P. Marchisio, and N. Principi. 1991. Improvement of auditory brainstem responses after treatment with zidovudine in a child with AIDS. *Pediatric Neurology* 7:53–55.

Cassandro, E., F. Mosca, L. Sequino, F. De Falco, and G. Campanella. 1986. Otoneurological abnormalities in Friedreich's ataxia and other inherited neuropathies. *Audiology* 25:84–91.

Cevette, M. 1984. Auditory brainstem response testing in an intensive care unit. *Seminars in Hearing* 5:57–69.

Cox, L., M. Hack, and D. Metz. 1981. Brainstem evoked response audiometry in the premature infant population. *International Journal of Pediatric Otorhinolaryngology* 3:213–224.

Crawford, M. 1991. The effects of sleep stage on the signal to noise ratio of the middle components. Ph.D. diss., Memphis State University.

Darling, R., and L. Price. 1990. Loudness and auditory brain stem evoked response. *Ear and Hearing* 11:289–295.

Davidson, S., L. Wall, and C. Goodman. 1990. Preliminary studies on the use of ABR amplitude projection procedure for hearing aid selection. *Ear and Hearing* 11:332–338.

Davis, H. 1976. Principles of electric response audiometry. *Annals of Otology, Rhinology, and Laryngology.* (Supplement 28) 85:1–96.

Derbyshire, A., and G. McCandless. 1964. Template for EEG response to sound. *Journal of Speech and Hearing Research* 7:96–98.

Don, M., J. Eggermont, and D. Brackmann. 1979. Reconstruction of the audiogram using brain stem responses and high-pass masking. *Annals of Otology, Rhinology, and Laryngology* (Suppl. 57):1–20.

Don, M., C. Elberling, and M. Waring. 1984. Objective detection of averaged auditory brainstem responses. *Scandinavian Audiology* 13:219–228.

Durrant, J., and R. Hyde. 1993. Observations on temporal aspects of bone-conduction clicks: Real head measurements. *Journal of the American Academy of Audiology* 4:213–219.

Edwards, C., A. Durieux-Smith, and T. Picton. 1985. Auditory brainstem response audiometry in neonatal hydrocephalus. *Journal of Otolaryngology* (Suppl. 14):40–46.

Eggermont, J.J., C.W. Ponton, S.G. Coupland, and R. Winkelaar. 1991. Frequency dependent maturation of the cochlea and brainstem evoked potentials. *Acta Oto-Laryngologica* 111:220–224.

Eggermont, J.J., and A. Salamy. 1988. Development of ABR parameters in a preterm and a term-born population. *Ear and Hearing* 9:283–289.

Elberling, C. 1979. The use of template and cross correlation functions in analysis of brainstem potentials. *Scandinavian Audiology* 8:187–190.

Elberling, C., and M. Don. 1984. Quality estimation of averaged auditory brainstem responses. *Scandinavian Audiology* 13:187–197.

———. 1987. Detection functions for the human auditory brainstem response. *Scandinavian Audiology* 16:89–92.

Elberling, C., and O. Walgreen. 1985. Estimation of the auditory brainstem response (ABR) by means of a Bayesian inference. *Scandinavian Audiology* 14:89–96.

Esbjorner, E., P. Larsson, P. Leissner, and L. Wranne. 1991. The serum reserve albumin concentration for monoacetyldiamino-diphenyl sulphone and auditory evoked responses during neonatal hyperbilirubinaemia. *Acta Paediatrica Scandinavica* 80:406–412.

Fawer, C., and L. Dubowitz. 1982. Auditory brainstem responses in neurologically normal preterm and fullterm newborn infants. *Neuropediatrics* 13:200–206.

Forman-Franco, B., G. Karayalin, D. Mandel, and A. Abramson. 1982. The evaluation of auditory function in homozygous sickle cell disease. *Otolaryngology—Head and Neck Surgery* 89:850–856.

Frank, Y., S.M. Vishnubhakat, and S. Pahwa. 1992. Brainstem auditory evoked responses in infants and children with AIDS. *Pediatric Neurology* 8:262–266.

Friedman, E., N. Luban, G. Herr, and I. Williams. 1980. Sickle cell anemia and hearing. *Annals of Otolaryngology* 89:342–347.

Gerling, I. 1991. In search of a stringent methodology for using ABR audiometric results. *The Hearing Journal* 44:26–30.

Goldstein, P., A. Krumholz, J. Felix, D. Shannon, and R. Carr. 1979. Brainstem evoked responses in neonates. *American Journal of Obstetrics and Gynecology* 135:622–631.

Gorga, M., K. Beauchaine, and J. Reiland. 1987. Comparison of onset and steady-state responses of hearing aids: Implications for use of auditory brainstem response in the selection of hearing aids. *Journal of Speech and Hearing Research* 30:130–136.

Gorga, M., J. Kaminski, K. Beauchaine, W. Jesteadt, and S. Neely. 1989. Auditory brainstem responses from children three months to three years of age: II. Normal patterns of response. *Journal of Speech and Hearing Research* 32:281–288.

Gorga, M., and A.R. Thornton. 1989. The choice of stimuli for ABR measurements. *Ear and Hearing* 10:217–230.

Gould, H. 1980. Early auditory evoked potentials in infants with craniofacial malformation. *Journal of Auditory Research* 20:244–248.

Gould, H., and D. Caldarelli. 1982. Hearing and otopathology in Apert syndrome. *Archives of Otolaryngology* 108:347–349.

Gould, H., M. Crawford, M. Mendel, and S. Dodson. 1992. Quantification technique for the middle latency response. *Journal of the American Academy of Audiology* 3: 153–158.

Gould, H., M. Crawford, W. Smith, N. Beckford, W. Gibson, L. Pettit, and L. Bobo. 1991. Hearing disorders in sickle cell disease: Cochlear and retrocochlear findings. *Ear and Hearing* 12:352–354.

Grass, E. 1978. Electrical safety specifically related to EEG. *Grass Technical Bulletin* #X757C78. Quincy, MA: Grass Instrument Co.

Gupta, A.K., H. Raj, and N.K. Anand. 1990. Auditory brainstem responses (ABR) in neonates with hyperbilirubinemia. *Indian Journal of Pediatrics* 57:705–711.

Hall, J.W. III. 1992. *Handbook of auditory evoked responses.* Boston: Allyn and Bacon.

Hall, J.W. III, D. Brown, and J. Mackey-Hargadine. 1985. Pediatric applications of serial auditory brainstem and middle-latency evoked response recordings. *International Journal of Pediatric Otorhinolaryngology* 9:201–218.

Hall, J.W. III, and R. Ruth. 1985. Acoustic reflexes and auditory evoked responses in hearing aid evaluation. *Seminars in Hearing* 6:251–277.

Hanson, P., R. Farber, and R. Armstrong. 1970. Distal muscle wasting, nephritis, and deafness. *Neurology* 20:426–434.

Hatanaka, T., H. Shuto, A. Yasuhara, and Y. Kobayashi. 1988. Ipsilateral and contralateral recordings of auditory brainstem responses to monaural stimulation. *Pediatric Neurology* 4:354–357.

Hatanaka, T., A. Yasuhara, A. Hori, and Y. Kobayashi. 1990. Auditory brainstem response in newborn infants: Masking effects on ipsi and contralateral recording. *Ear and Hearing* 11:233–236.

Hebert, R., E. Laureau, M. Vanasse, J.E. Richard, J. Morrissette, J. Glorieux, M. Desjardins, J. Letarte, and J.H. Dussault. 1986. Auditory brainstem response audiometry in congenitally hypothyroid children under early replacement therapy. *Pediatric Research* 20:570–573.

Hecox, K. 1983. Role of auditory brain stem response in the selection of hearing aids. *Ear and Hearing* 4:51–55.

Hung, K. 1989. Auditory brainstem responses in patients with neonatal hyperbilirubinemia and bilirubin encephalopathy. *Brain Development* 11:297–301.

Iinuma, K., K. Haginoya, I. Handa, A. Kojima, N. Fueki, J. Aikawa, M. Ito, J. Hatazawa, and T. Ido. 1989. Computed tomography, magnetic resonance imaging, positron emission tomography, and evoked potential at early stage of adrenoleukodystrophy. *Tohuku Journal of Experimental Medicine* 159:195–203.

Inagaki, M., Y. Tomita, S. Takashima, K. Ohtani, G. Andoh, and K. Takeshita. 1987. Functional and morphometrical maturation of the brainstem auditory pathway. *Brain Development* 9:597–601.

Jacobson, J.T., C.R. Morehouse, and M. Johnson. 1982. Strategies for infant auditory brainstem response assessment. *Ear and Hearing* 3:263–270.

Jirsa, R.E., and K.B. Clontz. 1990. Long latency auditory event-related potentials from children with auditory processing disorders. *Ear and Hearing* 11:222–232.

Joint Committee on Infant Hearing (1991). 1990 position statement. *Asha* (suppl. 5) 33:3–6.

Kaga, K., and R. Marsh. 1986. Auditory brainstem responses in young children with Down's syndrome. *International Journal of Pediatric Otorhinolaryngology* 11:29–38.

Kamuro, K., M. Inagaki, and Y. Tomita. 1992. Correlation between morphological abnormalities of Chiari malformation and evoked potentials. *No-To-Hattatsu* 24:554–558.

Kavanagh, K., and W. Domico. 1986. High-pass digital filtration of the 40-Hz response and its relationship to the spectral content of the middle latency and 40-Hz responses. *Ear and Hearing* 7:93–99.

Kiessling, J. 1982. Hearing aid selection by brainstem audiometry. *Scandinavian Audiology* 11:269–275.

Kileny, P. 1982. Auditory brainstem responses as indicators of hearing aid performance. *Annals of Otolaryngology* 9:61–64.

Kodama, S., K. Tanaka, H. Konishi, K. Momota, H. Nakasako, S. Nakayama, J. Yagi, and K. Koderasawa. 1989. Supplementary thyroxine therapy in patients with hypothyroidism induced by long term anticonvulsant therapy. *Acta Paediatrica Japan* 31:555–562.

Kraus, N., P. Kileny, and T. McGee. 1994. Middle latency auditory evoked potentials. In *Handbook of clinical audiology*, 4th ed., ed. by J. Katz. Baltimore: Williams and Wilkins.

Kraus, N., T. McGee, A. Micco, A. Sharma, T. Carrell, and T. Nicol. 1993. Mismatch negativity in school-age children to speech stimuli that are just perceptibly different. *Electroencephalography and Clinical Neurophysiology* 88:123–130.

Kraus, N., T. McGee, A. Sharma, T. Carrell, and T. Nicol. 1992. Mismatch negativity event-related potential elicited by speech stimuli. *Ear and Hearing* 13:158–164.

Kraus, N., N. Reed, I. Smith, L. Stein, and C. Cartee. 1987. High-pass filter settings affect the detectability of MLRs in humans. *Electroencephalography and Clinical Neurophysiology* 68:234–236.

Lane, R., M. Mendel, G. Kupperman, M. Vivion, L. Buchanan, and R. Goldstein. 1974. Phase distortion of the AER imposed by analog filtering. *Archives of Otolaryngology* 99:428–432.

Lary, S., G. Briassoulis, L. deVries, L. Dubowitz, and V. Dubowitz. 1985. Hearing threshold in preterm and term infants by auditory brainstem response. *Journal of Pediatrics* 107:593–599.

Laureau, E., M. Vanasse, R. Hebert, J. Letarte, J. Glorieux, M. Desjardins, and J. Dussault. 1986. Somatosensory evoked potentials and auditory brain-stem responses in congenital hypothyroidism. I: A longitudinal study before and after treatment in six infants detected in the neonatal period. *Electroencephalography and Clinical Neurophysiology* 64:501–510.

Lemieux, G., and J. Neemeh. 1967. Charcot-Marie-Tooth disease and nephritis. *Canadian Medical Association Journal* 97:1193–1198.

Lindsay, J., F. Black, and W. Donnelly. 1975. Acrocephalosyndactyly Apert's syndrome: Temporal bone findings. *Annals of Otolaryngology* 84:174–178.

Lurquin, P., P. Magera, S. Hassid, and D. Hennebert. 1989. Evolution du seuil auditif durant les premiers mois de la vie liee aux modifications de la physiologie du conduit auditif externe. [Development of the auditory threshold during the first months of life related to modifications of the physiology of the external auditory canal.] *Acta Otorhinolaryngologica Belgica* 43:417–426.

Maurizi, M., G. Almadori, L. Cagini, E. Molini, F. Ottaviani, G. Paludetti, and F. Pierri. 1986. Auditory brainstem responses in the full-term newborn: Changes in the first 58 hours of life. *Audiology* 25:239–247.

Maurizi, M., F. Ottaviani, G. Paludetti, and S. Lungarotti. 1985. Audiological findings in Down's children. *International Journal of Pediatric Otorhinolaryngology* 9:227–232.

McClellend, R., and B. Sayers. 1984. Evaluation of the cross correlation method for detection of auditory threshold for brainstem auditory evoked potentials. In *Evoked potentials II*, ed. R.H. Nodar and C. Barber. The Second International Evoked Potentials Symposium. Boston: Butterworth.

McFarland, W., M. Vivion, and R. Goldstein. 1977. Middle components of the AER to tone-pips in normal-hearing and hearing-impaired subjects. *Journal of Speech and Hearing Research* 20:781–798.

McPherson, D., R. Amlie, and E. Foltz. 1985. Auditory brainstem response in infant hydrocephalus. *Child's Nervous System* 1:70–76.

McPherson, D., and N. Clark. 1983. ABR in hearing aid utilization: Simulated deafness. *Hearing Instruments* 34:12–15, 66.

McRandle, C., M. Smith, and R. Goldstein. 1974. Early averaged electroencephalic responses to clicks in neonates. *Annals of Otology, Rhinology, and Laryngology* 83: 695–702.

Mendel, M. 1985. Middle and late auditory evoked potentials. In *Handbook of clinical audiology*, 3d ed., ed. J. Katz. Baltimore: Williams and Wilkins.

Mendel, M., C. Adkinson, and L. Harker. 1977. Middle components of the evoked potentials in infants. *Annals of Otology, Rhinology, and Laryngology* 86:293–300.

Mendel, M., and R. Goldstein. 1971. Early components of the averaged electroencephalic response to constant level clicks during all-night sleep. *Journal of Speech and Hearing Research* 14:829–840.

Mendelson, T., and A. Salamy. 1981. Maturational effects on the middle components of the averaged electroencephalic response. *Journal of Speech and Hearing Research* 24: 140–144.

Moore, E. 1983. *Bases of auditory brain-stem evoked responses*. New York: Grune and Stratton.

Morgan, D., M. Zimmerman, and J. Dubno. 1987. Auditory brainstem evoked response characteristics in the full-term newborn. *Annals of Otology, Rhinology, and Laryngology* 96:142–151.

Näätänen, R. 1992. *Attention and brain function*. Hillsdale, NJ: Lawrence Erlbaum and Associates.

National Institutes of Health. 1993. *Early identification of hearing impairment in infants and young children*. NIH Consensus Statement 11:1–24. Washington, D.C.: National Institutes of Health.

Niedermeyer, E., and F. Lopes da Silva. 1987. *Electroencephalography: Basic principles, clinical applications, and related fields*. 2d ed. Baltimore: Urban and Schwarzenberg.

Ozdamar, O., and N. Kraus. 1983. Auditory middle-latency responses in humans. *Audiology* 22:34–49.

Palmer, C., A. Derbyshire, and A. Lee. 1966. A method for analyzing individual cortical responses to auditory stimuli. *Electroencephalography and Clinical Neurophysiology* 20: 204–206.

Pelson, R.O., and S.S. Budden. 1987. Auditory brainstem response findings in Rett syndrome. *Brain Development* 9:514–516.

Perez, H., J. Vilchez, T. Sevilla, and L. Martinez. 1988. Audiologic evaluation in Charcot-Marie-Tooth disease. *Scandinavian Audiology* (Suppl. 30):211–213.

Picton, T.W., S.A. Hillyard, H.J. Kraus, and R. Galambos. 1974. Human auditory evoked potentials, I: Evaluation of components. *Electroencephalography and Clinical Neurophysiology* 36:179–190.

Picton, T., R. Linden, G. Hamel, and J. Maru. 1983. Aspects of averaging. *Seminars in Hearing* 4:327–341.

Picton, T., K. Oulette, G. Hamel, and A. Smith. 1979. Brainstem evoked potential to tone pips in notched noise. *Journal of Otolaryngology* 8:289–314.

Prevec, T., K. Ribaric, K., and D. Butinar. 1984. Contingent negative variation audiometry in children. *Audiology* 23:114–126.

Prosser, S., E. Arslan, G. Conti, and S. Michelini. 1983. Evaluation of the monaurally evoked brainstem response in the diagnosis of sensorineural hearing loss. *Scandinavian Audiology* 12:103–106.

Rackliffe, L., and F.E. Musiek. 1983. An introduction to ABR in hearing aid evaluation. *Hearing Instruments* 34:9–10.

Rubel, E., D. Born, J. Deitch, and D. Durham. 1984. Recent advances toward understanding auditory system development. In *Hearing science*, ed. C. Berlin. San Diego: College Hill Press.

Salamy, A., L. Eldridge, J. Anderson, and D. Bull. 1990. Brainstem transmission time in infants exposed to cocaine in utero. *The Journal of Pediatrics* 117:627–629.

Shih, L., B. Cone-Wesson, and B. Reddix. 1988. Effects of maternal cocaine abuse on the neonatal auditory system. *International Journal of Pediatric Otorhinolaryngology* 15:245–251.

Schimmel, H. 1967. The +/–reference: Accuracy of estimated mean components in average response studies. *Science* 157:92–93.

Schimmel, H., I. Rapin, and M. Cohen. 1974. Improving evoked response audiometry. *Audiology* 13:33–65.

Selters, W., and D. Brackman. 1977. Acoustic tumor detection with brainstem electric response audiometry. *Archives of Otolaryngology* 103:181–187.

Sharp, M., and D. Orchick. 1978. Auditory function in sickle cell anemia. *Archives of Otolaryngology* 104:322–324.

Shimizu, H., H. Moser, and S. Naidu. 1989. Auditory brainstem response and audiologic findings in adrenoleukodystrophy: Its variant and carrier. *Otolaryngology—Head and Neck Surgery* 98:215–220.

Sininger, Y. 1993. Auditory brain stem response for objective measures of hearing. *Ear and Hearing* 14:23–30.

Sobhy, O. 1993. Frequency specificity of the auditory middle latency response. Ph.D. diss., Memphis State University.

Sobhy, O., and H. Gould. 1993. Interaural attenuation using insert earphones: Electrocochleographic approach. *Journal of the American Academy of Audiology* 4:76–79.

Stach, B., W. Stoner, S. Smith, and J. Jerger. 1994. Auditory evoked potentials in Rett syndrome. *Journal of the American Academy of Audiology* 5:226–230.

Stockard, J.E., J.J. Stockard, and R. Coen. 1983. Auditory brain stem response variability in infants. *Ear and Hearing* 4:11–23.

Sugimoto, T., A. Yasuhara, T. Ohta, N. Nishida, S. Saitoh, J. Hamabe, and N. Niikawa. 1992. Angelman syndrome in three siblings: Characteristic epileptic seizures and EEG abnormalities. *Epilepsia* 33:1078–1082.

Taylor, M., W. Chan-Lui, and W. Logan. 1985. Longitudinal evoked potential studies in hereditary ataxias. *Canadian Journal of Neuroscience* 12:100–105.

Thornton, A., M. Mendel, and C. Anderson. 1977. Effects of stimulus frequency and intensity on the middle components of the averaged auditory electroencephalic response. *Journal of Speech and Hearing Research* 20:81–94.

Thornton, A.R.D., G. Farrell, and E. McSporran. 1989. Clinical methods for the objective estimation of loudness discomfort level (LDL) using auditory brainstem responses in patients. *Scandinavian Audiology* 18:225–230.

Thornton, A.R.D., L. Yardley, and G. Farrell. 1987. The objective estimation of loudness discomfort level using auditory brainstem evoked responses. *Scandinavian Audiology* 16:219–225.

Weber, B.A. 1982. Comparison of auditory brain stem response latency norms for premature infants. *Ear and Hearing* 3:257–262.

———. 1994. Auditory brainstem response: Threshold estimation and auditory screening. In *Handbook of clinical audiology*, 4th ed., ed. by J. Katz. Baltimore: Williams and Wilkins.

Wong, P., and R. Bickford. 1980. Brain stem auditory evoked potentials: The use of noise estimate. *Electroencephalography and Clinical Neurophysiology* 50:25–34.

Yang, E.Y., A.L. Rupert, and G. Moushegian. 1987. A developmental study of bone conduction auditory brain stem response in infants. *Ear and Hearing* 8:244–251.

Zapala, D. 1993. Statistical quantification of auditory brain-stem response waveshape quality and its relation to peak latency measurement accuracy. Ph.D. diss., Memphis State University.

8

Testing Otoacoustic Emissions in Newborns, Infants, Toddlers, and Children

Brenda L. Lonsbury-Martin, Glen K. Martin,
Margaret J. McCoy, and Martin L. Whitehead

OTOACOUSTIC emissions (OAEs), or sounds generated by the hearing (or cochlear) portion of the healthy inner ear, can be measured objectively and noninvasively from a microphone sealed in the outer ear canal (Kemp 1978). The results of considerable research indicate that OAEs are produced by the cochlea as part of the normal hearing process. Outer hair cells (OHCs) are extremely vulnerable to injury from agents that commonly impair hearing (e.g., systemic pathogens such as bacteria and viruses, and certain external agents such as excessively intense sound and ototoxic drugs). Isolated (in vitro) from the cochlea, OHCs change shape when activated with alternating electrical current (Brownell et al. 1985). The discovery of this phenomenon has spawned the popular notion that the stimulus-induced cyclic lengthenings and shortenings of this very abundant type of sensory cell generate OAEs (Brownell 1990).

The apparent ability of OAEs to specify the fine vibromechanical movements of the OHC system has resulted in considerable research aimed at assessing the clinical utility of these objective tests. These investigations have consistently indicated that OAE measures show excellent promise as an objective, noninvasive method for establishing the differential diagnosis of sensorineural hearing loss. They may be used for screening hearing and for serial monitoring of hearing capability in individuals suspected of exhibiting progressive changes in hearing status. These include individuals with a family history, known progressive ear pathologies such as Ménière disease, congenital cytomegalovirus

Portions of this work were supported by grants from the Public Health Service (DC00613, DC01668, ESO3500). The authors thank B.B. Stagner for technical assistance, and M.T. Ruiz for secretarial services.

infection, noise-induced hearing loss, and so on. Although much of the investigative work so far has been conducted in adult populations representing both normal-hearing and hearing-impaired patients, an impressive number of studies has focused on evaluating the usefulness of OAE testing in various subpopulations of children.

The primary purpose of the present review is to summarize our current knowledge of the applicability of OAE methods to the examination of hearing in newborns, infants, toddlers, and preschool and school-aged children. With this goal in mind, we discuss the practical features of OAE testing with regard to their benefits and limitations for these special patient groups; we also address the details necessary for establishing procedures to measure evoked emissions in pediatric audiology settings.

To provide a background for considering this growing body of literature and the adaptation of OAE testing to the special needs of infants and children, we present (a) the particular advantages of emitted responses in assessing the hearing capability of these sometimes difficult-to-test patients; (b) the specific types of OAE testing available; (c) a summary of our basic knowledge of OAEs and developing humans; (d) factors that influence the quality and quantity of the emitted response (including acoustic noises from the patient and ambient setting); and (e) the status of middle-ear function.

Background

Advantages of OAEs as a Clinical Test

WHEN OAEs were first described, Kemp (1978) recognized that the beneficial features of this response measure would make it an important new component of the audiometric test battery. One principal advantage of OAEs is their objectivity as an unbiased evaluator of cochlear function. Also, the noninvasive feature of OAEs yields simple set-up procedures that do not require highly trained technicians, resulting in a relatively inexpensive and rapidly administered test.

The typical devices used to measure OAEs are described below for two common commercial instruments. These devices combine a sound source and a sensitive microphone into a miniature probe sealed into the outer ear canal. In addition, the specificity of OAEs for assessing the functional status of the OHCs (i.e., the cochlear component most vulnerable to many of the diseases and disorders that damage hearing) implies that these methods can compose a sensitive test that detects problems at an early onset stage. This selective OHC-testing property also suggests that OAEs can function as an objective means of assessing certain aspects of central auditory processing because of the known connections between a major component of the cochlear efferent system, the medial olivocochlear bundle pathway, and OHCs.

Finally, results from the OAE assessment of OHC function can be combined with those provided by conventional and special purpose audiometric tests to establish the sensory versus neural nature of a sensorineural impairment. This latter capability has furnished new information on the primary site of otopathologies that underlie some of the more puzzling ear ailments. These include Ménière's disease (Harris and Probst 1992) and sudden idiopathic sensorineural hearing loss (Sakashita et al. 1991), although these afflictions rarely affect children.

In addition, the frequency specificity of OAE testing permits a precise definition of normal compared to abnormal regions of OHC function with respect to the frequency pattern. This feature may lead to improved approaches to habilitation with amplification based on a detailed knowledge of the frequency extent of the impairment. Moreover, the amenability of the objectively measured OAEs to computer control results in measures that can be thoroughly, accurately, and rapidly performed. The ease of computer-based measures of OAEs also promises to lead to methods that permit an automatic interpretation of the resulting information (see newborn screening section below). A final advantage of OAE testing is that emitted responses can be elicited from essentially all normal ears, whereas they are reduced or absent in impaired ears. The relationship between the presence vs. absence of OAEs and hearing ability provides a metric against which the performance of an unknown ear can be rigorously assessed based on statistically defined degrees of abnormality. This characteristic of OAE testing also promises that some aspect of their specific quantitative features (e.g., detection threshold, level in response to suprathreshold stimulation, onset latency) will eventually be used to predict an accurate hearing level.

Together, these positive features support the expectation that OAEs will become an important new clinical assessor of hearing capability. These benefits have been primarily responsible for stimulating a great deal of research, resulting in the publication of more than 800 reports since their discovery. Figure 8.1 indicates that, as OAEs have become more recognized, the publication rate of studies on adults (solid circles) has been augmented from a yearly increase of about five per year (1978–1987) to approximately twenty-two per year more recently. Because the data point for 1993 represents only the first six months of that year, it is probable that up to 200 reports on OAEs would have been published in 1993 alone.

This overview of the strengths of OAE testing demonstrates that many of these beneficial properties (including their objectivity, simple and brief set-up procedures, and potential ability to predict hearing level) are especially applicable to young patients. Such useful attributes support the development of OAEs into special-purpose tests (including exams that screen for hearing problems) especially suited for use with infants and young children—in particular, newborns, older infants, toddlers, and preschool children.

Other OAE procedures can be developed to monitor cochlear status in the young patient subpopulations who are at risk for developing hearing problems. Among these are patients who have a familial tendency for progressive impairment and children who are undergoing life-saving treatments with drugs or procedures that are potentially harmful to hearing. Finally, the differential diagnosis attribute of OAE testing to establish the primary site of pathology in young ears known to be abnormal helps to optimize the selection of an appropriate habilitative strategy. Given the considerable strengths that OAEs contribute to the examination of hearing in young subjects, it is surprising that so few studies have been conducted on the utility of emissions testing in these special patients. The curve in Figure 8.1 represented by the open circles supports this observation in that only about 6% of the total number of OAE studies to date have been conducted in individuals younger than twenty years old. However, the cumulative growth rate indicates that in recent years the number of studies on infants and children has been increasing from none or one per year to about three per year. Given the current interest in establishing universal screening programs for neonates, the number of studies conducted in children is expected to rise dramatically in the next few years.

Types of OAEs

Otoacoustic emissions are frequently divided into two general categories based on the nature of the acoustic stimulation needed to elicit them (Probst, Lons-

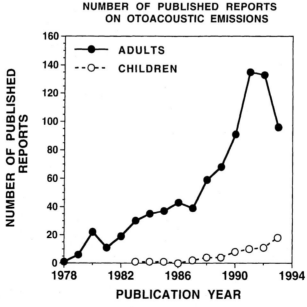

Figure 8.1. Number of published reports on otoacoustic emissions for adults (solid circles) and children (<20 years) as a function of year since their discovery in 1978.

bury-Martin, and Martin 1991). One type, known as *spontaneous OAEs*, consists of low-level, tonal-like signals that occur naturally in the absence of sound stimulation in the ears of over 60% of normal hearing people.

Spontaneous OAEs (SOAEs) are so weak that they are usually imperceptible to the individuals who exhibit them. They are not present in every normal ear, thus making it difficult to judge normality versus abnormality based simply on their presence or absence. When they are present, SOAEs are ear-specific; their frequencies and levels are unique to the ear exhibiting them, making it difficult to develop a normal database against which the status of an unknown ear can be judged. Moreover, SOAEs disappear as hearing levels (HLs) increase beyond 20 dB. For these reasons, it is not expected that this class of emission will ever be clinically useful. However, knowledge of both their presence and level and frequency characteristics helps to explain, for some individuals, focused idiosyncratic enhancements or reductions in the levels of other types of OAEs. The role of SOAEs in the normal-hearing process is unknown, but their presence may indicate the high degree of OHC mechanical activity responsible for the excellent hearing of the persons who exhibit them.

The other main emission class—the evoked OAEs—is elicited from virtually all normal ears by low-to-moderate-level test sounds. The various subclasses of evoked OAEs are defined according to the precise acoustic signal needed to elicit them. These stimuli range from brief tone pips or clicks, which produce transient- or click-evoked OAEs (TEOAEs or CEOAEs, respectively), to more continuous single pure tones, which elicit stimulus-frequency OAEs (SFOAEs) and combinations of two pure tones, which produce distortion-product OAEs (DPOAEs). The straightforward methods used to separate the acoustic energy of the outgoing emitted response in the ear canal from that of the ingoing stimulus results in greater ease in measuring and interpreting TEOAEs and DPOAEs; thus, these measures have received the most investigative attention. In essence, TEOAEs represent a time-delayed response to brief acoustic stimuli. In contrast, DPOAEs, which routinely are measured at a frequency that is particularly robust in the human ear (i.e., at the $2f_1$-f_2 frequency with $f_2 > f_1$), are an intermodulated distortion response to two simultaneously applied pure-tone stimuli.

The review of OAE applications in infants and children below makes it evident that by far the majority of the studies performed in these young subjects have used the transient form of the OAE elicited by clicks (i.e., the CEOAE). Less than one-quarter of the currently known OAE studies in children have used DPOAEs to examine cochlear function. The instrumentation and associated protocols now available for testing both CEOAEs and DPOAEs are comparable in terms of the total time needed for preparing the subject, performing the test, and generating the report; therefore, preference for click-based OAE testing in young patients cannot be wholly explained by the test-time factor. Thus, it appears that the primary reason for preferring click-evoked over bitonally-evoked OAEs is the similarity of the transiently based response to other physiological tests of the hearing process, including the auditory brainstem response (ABR).

Understandably, then, the method of evoking transient responses with brief acoustic stimulation would be more familiar to audiologists, otologists, and neurotologists than administering complex, long-lasting bitonal stimuli that elicit an unpleasant-sounding response, which is called "distorted." In truth, as clinical evaluators of the peripheral ear, both types of evoked OAEs have benefits and limitations, and much research has been aimed at establishing the circumstances that are optimal for applying each test.

It is noteworthy that the CEOAE, in particular, has been used to study the influence of the medially based cochlear-efferent system on peripheral processing. The procedure commonly used to investigate the so-called efferent effect measures the level-reducing consequences of a contralaterally applied broadband-noise stimulus on the ipsilaterally recorded CEOAE response (Collet et al. 1990). The beginning knowledge base concerning the effects of efferent stimulation on cochlear emissions for adult ears has established that the resulting CEOAE (Collet et al. 1990) or DPOAE (Moulin, Collet, and Duclaux 1993) is reduced about one dB on average. However, there is no comparable information for infants or children. Despite the seemingly minimal effect of efferent activation on evoked OAEs and the clear deficiency in forming a similar knowledge base for young subjects, it is likely that a clinical test of OAE-based efferent function will eventually be developed. Such a test may provide an important means of evaluating the role of central auditory-system processing, particularly in young school children with learning difficulties.

Recording OAEs

For measuring evoked OAEs in infants and young children, typically one of two subclasses of emitted responses previously noted is measured. Because the primary goal in testing young individuals is to screen hearing, the most common OAE method utilized by far for this patient subpopulation has been the CEOAE. A few investigators have been testing the feasibility of screening with DPOAEs. For either technique, the available commercial instrumentation makes use of noise rejection and signal averaging—principles that are commonly used in electrophysiological measures of hearing-related processes for improving the signal-to-noise ratio.

Because CEOAEs are separated in time from the acoustic transient, conventional, time-based, signal-averaging techniques are used to detect them. In contrast, DPOAEs are measured in the presence of either long-lasting tone bursts or continuous sounds. However, because they are separated in frequency from the higher-frequency evoking tones (i.e., the primary frequencies f_1 and f_2), they are typically examined by spectral analysis (i.e., very narrowband filtering), after time-based, phase-locked averaging has minimized background noises. Both types of evoked OAEs are recorded using a specially constructed, conical probe with a detachable, soft rubber immittance ear tip sealed snugly in the outer ear canal. Both to elicit and measure the evoked OAEs, the probe contains several miniature components developed for the hearing-aid industry as either one (for CEOAEs) or two (for DPOAEs) earspeakers and a microphone, respectively.

To measure DPOAEs, rather than incorporate the sound-generators within the ear probe, several commercially available instruments (see more details below) incorporate two separate plastic tubes within the probe for delivering sound from the two external speakers. These are attached by Velcro to a headband or are mechanically clipped onto the patient's apparel or swaddling clothes. In all cases, the DPOAE stimuli are mixed acoustically in the outer ear canal before being conducted to the inner ear via the middle ear transmission system. Both types of evoked-OAE test are computer-based. The stimuli are synthesized digitally, and the emitted responses are measured and analyzed with either an on-board digital signal processor (DSP) mounted within a personal microcomputer or with the programmed capability of the computer's central processing unit (CPU).

TEOAEs and CEOAEs

Although several groups of investigators of TEOAEs in young subjects have developed their own customized microcomputer-based approaches to screening hearing with click stimuli (e.g., Cope and Lutman 1988; Johnsen, Bagi, and Elberling 1983; Stevens et al. 1987), CEOAEs are most commonly recorded and processed using procedures developed and commercialized by Kemp and Bray (Bray 1989; Bray and Kemp 1987) in several generations of instruments (Otodynamics Ltd., United Kingdom) developed at the Institute of Laryngology and Otology (ILO). The original model of this device, the Otodynamic Analyser or ILO88, is shown in the left portion of Figure 8.2. The ILO88 has been modified, updated, and incorporated into both the ILO92 version, with the capability of performing DPOAE testing, and the more newly developed infant-screening device. The hardware components of the ILO instrument consist of a personal microcomputer (IBM compatible) system (microcomputer with keyboard, video monitor, data-storage medium, hard-copy printer), which is provided by the user. Other hardware components are an assortment of acoustic probes configured to fit the outer ear canal (infant, child, adult), an interface analog box for impedance matching the probe unit to the computer and amplifying the signal, one or two (depending on the ILO model) plug-in circuit boards (analog/digital and digital/analog converters), calibration unit, and software (Version 3.9x, depending on the ILO model) provided by the manufacturer.

The plastic ear probe, shaped like an ear speculum, contains a microphone and an earspeaker (Knowles 1843 and BP1712, respectively) that are embedded in a clear, plastic resin. For infants and small children, the stimulus is reduced by 20 or 10 dB, respectively, to compensate for their small ear canals. The software of the ILO system generates and controls the presentation of the click stimulus.

It records important details of the data including certain stimulus and response properties (see Kemp and Ryan [1993] for a clear explanation of the displayed information), averages the responses, and spectrally processes the averaged response and the eliciting stimulus. The click stimulus is produced by a non-filtered, rectangular electrical pulse of 80 μs duration. The resulting acoustic transient is typically about 80 dB peSPL, and it is presented at a rate of fifty per second.

With the instrument set to the "nonlinear mode" of operation, time-based averaging is done alternately by two separate buffers (A and B), resulting in two distinct measurements, each in response to 260 sets of clicks. In this default setting, each stimulus set consists of four clicks (i.e., each A and B response average is generated by 1,040 clicks). The polarity of one of the four transients is reversed, and its level is three times greater when compared to the remaining three stimuli. This strategy decreases the likelihood that a particular averaged response is contaminated by linearly based artifacts including ringing of either the middle ear or transmitter components.

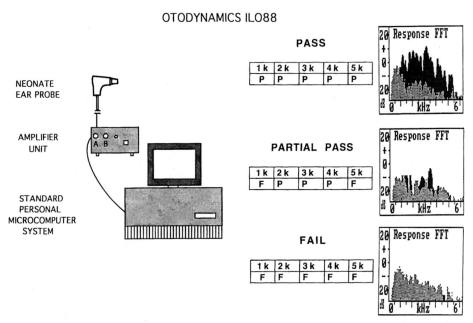

Figure 8.2. Schematic diagram at left of the commercially available ILO88 equipment used to record CEOAEs using a PC-based system. The right portion of the figure illustrates a typical scoring system used to ascertain pass (P)/fail (F) determinations for screening newborn hearing using CEOAEs. For example, an overall "pass" (upper right) is defined as displaying clear TEOAE activity (dark shaded area) above the level of background noise (stippled area) within at least four of the five 1-kHz frequency bands (i.e., evoked emissions over a frequency range of 500 Hz within each band) between 1 and 6 kHz; a "partial pass" (middle right) consists of a pattern of TEOAE activity over three of the five frequency regions of interest; and a "fail" (lower right) is designated as evoked TEOAEs within fewer than three of the noted frequency regions.

The standard poststimulus analysis time of the ILO devices is twenty milliseconds, with the first 2.5 ms nullified to eliminate typical stimulus-ringing problems. The acquired data are filtered with a passband of 500 to 6,000 Hz. Presence or absence of the CEOAE is determined according to the criterion of the reproducibility of the two A and B averages, which is computed from their cross-correlation and converted to a percentage. Reproducibility is determined over the entire CEOAE spectrum (i.e., 0.5–6 kHz) and for the 1-kHz bands centered at 1, 2, 3, 4, and 5 kHz. Typically, a reproducibility criterion of 50% or more is used to ascertain the presence or absence, respectively, of a response (Bray and Kemp 1987).

Additional criteria sometimes include the requirement(s) that (a) the total level of the emission be greater than three or five decibels above the background noise level, (b) the level of the stimulus be within a few dB of the ideal intensity of 80 dB peSPL, (c) the stimulus stability be greater than 70%, and (d) the frequency extent of the resulting amplitude spectrum be present in greater than 50% of each of the three 1-kHz bands between one and four kHz. Some important features of the ILO88 and 92 commercial systems are the interactive artifact-rejection level, which is adjustable on-line by the test giver, and the "check fit" capability, which ensures that the probe unit is properly placed in the patient's ear.

For recording DPOAEs from young subjects, customized systems are typically used (e.g., Bonfils et al. 1992; Lasky, Perlman, and Hecox 1992; Owens et al. 1992; Smurzynski et al. 1993). However, three commercial devices are now available for measuring DPOAEs. These are the Otoacoustic Emissions Test Instrument (Model 330, Virtual Corporation, Portland OR), the CUBᵉDIS (Etymotic Research, Elk Grove Village, IL), and the Otoacoustic Analyser (Model ILO92, Otodynamics Ltd., United Kingdom). An example of a DPOAE-test instrument is shown in the left portion of Figure 8.3: the Virtual Model 330. All three marketplace instruments have user-selected options governing all the significant stimulus and response variables to DPOAE testing. Typically, however, the $2f_1$-f_2 DPOAE is measured, which is the most robust acoustic-distortion product in humans. The f_2/f_1 ratio is set to an optimal value around 1.22 (Harris et al. 1989); the levels of the lower (f_1) and higher-frequency (f_2) primary tones are equivalent (L=L). Each spectrally averaged DPOAE is a time average of several measurements (e.g., n = 16 or 32) for the 330 and ILO92DP models or an average of about four amplitude spectra for the CUBᵉDIS. The DPOAE is plotted with respect to either the geometric mean (i.e., $[f_1 \times f_2]^{0.5}$) of the two primaries (Model 330) or to f_2 (ILO92, CUBᵉDIS). Similar to the response definition for CEOAEs, DPOAEs are considered measurable if their level is at least 3 or 5 dB above the noise floor at an adjacent frequency.

In all three commercial DPOAE systems, stimulus-calibration software compensates for the level (in dB SPL re 20 μPa) of the primary signals at each frequency for the particular ear-canal volume under test. In addition, noise

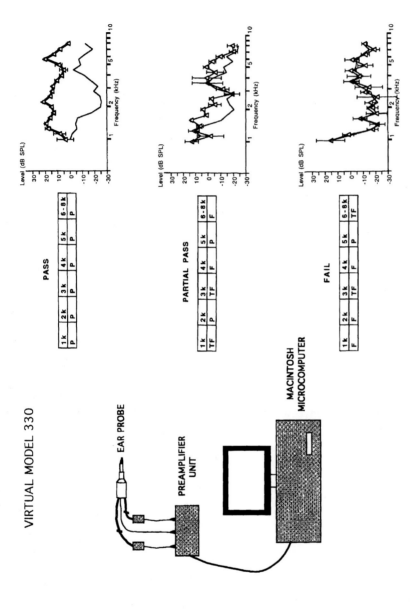

Figure 8.3. Schematic diagram at left of the commercially available Virtual Model 330 equipment used to record DPOAEs using a Macintosh-based microcomputer system. The right portion of the figure illustrates a common scoring system used to assign pass/fails in newborn hearing-screening programs based on this subclass of evoked emission. For example, an overall "pass" (upper right) is defined as displaying clear DPOAE activity (line with open triangles) above the level of background noise (uninterrupted line) within at least four of the six specified frequency bands (i.e., evoked emissions over a frequency range greater than or equal to one-half of the number of frequencies tested within each band) between 1–8 kHz; a "partial pass" (middle right) consists of a pattern of DPOAEs within three or fewer of the six frequency regions of interest; and a "fail" (lower right) is designated as no DPOAEs within three or fewer of the noted frequency regions. (See text for a more complete explanation of this system for scoring DPOAEs as pass/fails.)

rejection is typically effected by the test software comparing the ambient noise in the ear canal (at a frequency or frequencies around the DPOAE) to an averaged sample of pretest values; as a result, the emission is not measured until the noise floor is within a criterion amount of the prelevel.

Acoustic-distortion products are commonly measured in one of two forms: either as a level-versus-frequency function (DPOAE "audiogram" [see Figure 8.3] or DP-gram) or as a response/growth or input/output (I/O) function. Although user-selectable to a certain extent, the frequency function is typically measured between 0.5 and 8 kHz with respect to the geometric-mean (Model 330) or f_2 (CUB^{c}DIS) frequency, or between 0.7 and 6 kHz with respect to the f_2 frequency (Model ILO92), at frequency intervals of a set number of points per octave (usually four or six). All the commercial devices also measure I/Os in a user-designated series of step sizes (e.g., 2, 3, 5, 6 dB) between approximately 30 and 75 dB SPL and frequencies that are commonly related to the standard audiometric frequencies (i.e., 0.5, 1, 2, 3, 4, 6, 8 kHz). The lowest primary-tone level for which a response is detected at the criterion level above the noise floor is specified as the detection threshold.

Factors Affecting the Measurement of OAEs

It is well recognized that the nature of OAEs as an acoustic signal makes it exceedingly susceptible to the adverse influences of loud sounds generated both environmentally and by the patients themselves. Excessive environmental sound can originate from many sources, depending on the setting in which the recording is made. These include noises from nearby individuals (relatives or healthcare workers who are conversing with one another) or the youngsters themselves, who talk or cough. The recording device may contain an internal ventilation fan, or there may be other adjacent instrumentation, including air-conditioning equipment. Other subject-generated noises also contaminate the recording of OAEs because they are converted to acoustic stimuli by the same recording microphone that measures the OAEs. Thus, limb movements against the body, loud respiratory sounds (e.g., sucking), crying, and jaw motions, for example, are subject noises that need to be controlled because of their adverse effects on the evoked-OAE recording.

Because the conduction pathway involving the middle-ear apparatus is required to transmit both eliciting stimuli from the tympanic membrane to the inner ear and the emitted response from the cochlea to the outer ear canal, its functional status is of primary importance to the measurement of OAEs. Pathological conditions involving negative pressure or fluid in the middle-ear space have dire consequences (see examples below) on not only the frequency and level features of OAEs but also their recordability (i.e., whether they are present or absent). This influence of middle ear factors on the measurement of OAEs is especially important in young-patient populations, in which middle-ear disease is most frequently observed. Moreover, it is the youngest patients (i.e., new-borns) who still have pre- and perinatal fluids and debris present in both the middle ear space and the outer canal for the first hours after birth.

Finally, newborns in the neonatal intensive-care unit are considered at risk for developing hearing loss. Hence, they are ideal candidates for hearing screening because of the nature of the relevant life-saving procedures, many of which involve the administration of potentially ototoxic drugs. However, at-risk neonates, who often have nasogastric feeding or airway tubes in place, are especially prone to middle ear problems because of the direct transmission route to the middle ear that such tubes provide for disease-causing pathogens (Balkany et al. 1978). Thus, the child populations who would optimally benefit from OAE testing are the ones most susceptible to middle ear difficulties and their accompanying adverse effects on our ability to record emissions.

GENERAL DEVELOPMENTAL FEATURES OF OAEs, TEOAEs, AND CEOAEs

TEOAEs

IN their early studies of OAEs, Kemp et al. (1986) recognized that infants and children generated CEOAEs that were different from those of adults. Specifically, the pattern of CEOAE-elicited activity in adults is primarily restricted to the 0.5–4 kHz frequency range. In contrast, the frequency distribution of CEOAEs in newborns and young children is broader, typically 0.5–6 kHz, with more narrow band peaks than exhibited by the adult ear. However, with regard to the frequency range over which CEOAEs can be measured, frequencies <1 kHz are usually immeasurable in newborns and especially infants. This is due to both subject-generated noises (e.g., sucking, crying) and the insufficient sound-damping properties of the external features of the thin bone of the skull and delicate skin of the external ear and canal with respect to ambient noise in the test environment.

In a demonstration of the changes in OAE features with age, Johnsen, Parbo, and Elberling (1989) showed that the frequency content in the CEOAEs of four-year-olds elicited with 2-kHz, half-sinusoidal clicks was lower than those obtained from the same subjects as newborns. In a later study, Kemp, Ryan, and Bray (1990) demonstrated that the CEOAE levels in neonates were greater than those of the average adult by about 10 dB. Norton and Widen (1990) assessed CEOAEs in a series of infants, children, and young adults ranging from about three weeks to thirty years old. They established systematic and statistically significant decreases in CEOAE level with increasing age.

These differences between adult and child CEOAEs have been attributed to the smaller volume of the child's ear canal (Johnsen, Bagi, and Elberling 1983). However, other possible explanations are that (a) children have a more efficient middle-ear conduction system (i.e., better acoustic coupling or impedance matching between the microphone and young ear); (b) age-related alterations in active cochlear mechanisms exist (Bonfils, Uziel, and Pujol 1988; Norton and Widen 1990); or (c) technical factors involving the different microphone probe units used to record OAEs in younger versus older ears contribute to the observed differences.

DPOAEs

The ability of young ears to exhibit emissions has been more intensely studied for CEOAEs and TEOAEs than for DPOAEs. However, Kim, Smurzynski, and their colleagues reported detailed information concerning the features of DPOAEs elicited by 65-dB SPL primaries in normal-hearing young children (Spektor et al. 1991) and healthy newborns with no suspected or documented hearing problems (Lafrenière et al. 1991; Smurzynski et al. 1993). These studies showed that, although the CEOAEs showed the expected stronger high-frequency spectral components in the 4- to 6-kHz region (based on the earlier observations reviewed above) and an average level over 6 dB higher than in adults, the DPOAEs of neonates and young children were qualitatively similar to those of adults; they showed the identical frequency distribution between 0.5 and 8 kHz. DPOAEs were higher in level only within two specific frequency regions: They were about 5 dB greater in the 1.2 kHz range, yet only a few dB greater around 6 kHz.

Chuang, S.W., Gerber, and Thornton (1993) showed that CEOAEs could be acquired from preterm infants who were well otherwise. Smurzynski and his colleagues (1993) demonstrated the feasibility of recording DPOAEs and CEOAEs in preterm infants. By quantifying and comparing both evoked-OAE types regarding their half-octave RMS (root-mean-square) levels, these investigators showed for preterm neonates that the average magnitudes of their emissions were above the ninetieth percentile of those recorded for full-term newborns. It will be interesting to learn whether the evoked-OAE levels for preterm babies correspond more closely to the magnitudes of well babies at postnatal times when the former infants reach postconceptional ages similar to those of the full-gestation newborns. In other words, the emission levels of full-term neonates may also be enhanced at corresponding prenatal periods. Satisfactory resolution of the observed differences in the magnitudes of evoked OAEs between pre- and full-term neonates awaits the time when it is technically feasible to record OAEs from the latter patients using in utero procedures.

Remaining OAEs

Whereas there is virtually no published information concerning the primary features of SOAEs in subjects younger than about twenty years old (Lonsbury-Martin et al. 1990), Burns and associates (Burns, Arehart, and Campbell 1992; Strickland, Burns, and Tubis 1985) have studied the prevalences, frequencies, and levels of SOAEs in newborns, infants, and young children. They discovered that the occurrence of SOAEs in young subjects is similar to that observed in adults, with the same strong gender preference (about twice as many females demonstrate these emissions as do males). Moreover, in infants and young children, the levels and particularly the preferred frequency range tend to be higher than in their adult counterparts: for adults, 8.5 vs. −3 dB SPL; for infants, 1–2 vs. 2.5–5 kHz (Burns, Arehart, and Campbell 1992). Similar to the qualifications regarding the differences between the quantitative features of evoked OAEs in adults and children, it is unknown whether developmental or technical factors cause these unique level and frequency effects.

In a study of SOAEs in newborns ranging in age from one to ten days, Kok, van Zanten, and Brocaar (1993) noted a prevalence of 78%, which is higher than previously reported for adults and full-term, healthy neonates. To measure SOAEs, these investigators used the stimulus-synchronizing technique inherent to the commercial equipment manufactured Ä˝†OtodynamiÅ˝†Ltd. (i.e., the ILO88). This SOAE-recording software spectrally analyzes the ear-canal sound activity recorded from twenty-one to eighty ms following the presentation of standard click stimuli. It is likely that the presence of click stimuli in the immediate premeasurement period enhances, in some unknown manner, the number of SOAEs detected with the ILO88 technique. Thus, in measuring SOAE prevalence and features in young ears, the most accurate method is to record these emissions in the absence of any sound stimulation.

CLINICAL APPLICATIONS OF EVOKED OAEs IN YOUNG EARS

BY 1993 there were more than sixty published accounts in either abstract or full-report form describing the results of OAE testing in young ears; most of these, however, had been conducted in either newborns and young infants (birth to three months of age) or older children (i.e., four to ten years old). There are only isolated descriptions of emissions in older infants, toddlers, and preschool-aged children. Because of such a nonmethodical approach, the review below summarizes our published knowledge about evoked OAEs in children by concentrating the available information into two general categories: (1) the neonate and young infant and (2) essentially school-aged children, with only limited mention of their properties in the remaining age categories.

In reviewing the literature on evoked OAEs and children, it is clear that the primary goal of objective testing of neonates and young infants (with the CEOAE being the test of choice) has been to screen newborn hearing. In contrast, the principal aim of evaluating evoked OAEs in older children, predominantly of school age, has been to document the confounding effects on emissions of the middle-ear problems commonly experienced by these young patients. Such investigations have tended to compare the effects of middle ear disease on both CEOAEs measured with the ILO88 and DPOAEs analyzed with either a customized version of the CUBᶜDIS system (e.g., Spektor et al. 1991) or laboratory-based equipment (e.g., Owens et al. 1992) similar to the Model 330.

Newborns (birth to 28 days) and Young Infants (29 days to 3 months)

Newborn Hearing Screening

Screening the hearing of a newborn is an important goal of pediatric audiology. Because the conventional ABR is time-consuming and requires highly trained technical staff and supervisors, it has been impractical for screening every live birth. Thus, the major strategy in screening newborns for hearing impairment has focused on testing only neonates at risk for hearing loss, that is, those for whom at least one of the following is relevant: abnormal prenatal history, aberrant bilirubin value, anatomic head or neck malformation, history of bacterial meningitis, ototoxic drug use, asphyxia, or family history of childhood hearing impairment (Joint Committee on Infant Hearing 1994). However, several professional societies composing the Joint Committee on Infant Hearing (e.g., American Academy of Audiology [AAA], American Academy of Otolaryngology–Head and Neck Surgery [AAO-HNS], American Academy of Pediatrics [AAP], American Speech-Language-Hearing Association [ASHA], Council on Education of the Deaf [CED], and directors of speech pathology and audiology programs in state health and welfare agencies) have recently endorsed the idea of universal hearing screening of infants before three months of age.

The purpose of this expanded position statement on infant hearing was "to ensure that all neonates with hearing loss are identified and intervention is initiated by six months of age" (Joint Committee on Infant Hearing 1994). Because OAEs can be conducted quickly and have relatively low test administration costs, they can provide for the universal screening of newborns. A panel of experts convened by the National Institutes of Health to discuss the early identification of hearing impairment in infants and young children recommended that evoked OAEs be implemented as the initial method for screening newborns for hearing problems (NIH 1993).

Johnsen, Bagi, and Elberling (1983) were first to report the recording of half-cycle based, 2-kHz CEOAEs at levels between 50 and 70 dB peSPL from every ear of a small number (n = 20) of healthy newborns. These earlier TEOAE findings were replicated later in another 100 well babies by the same investigators (Johnsen et al. 1988). After the initial demonstration of neonatal TEOAEs, several researchers have reported CEOAEs in both full-term newborns and graduates of neonatal intensive care units (Bonfils, Uziel, and Pujol 1988; Bonfils et al. 1990, 1992; Chuang K.W. et al. 1993; Kennedy et al. 1991; Kok, van Zanten, and Brocaar 1992, 1993; Lafrenière et al. 1991; Plinkert et al. 1990; Salomon et al. 1992; Stevens et al. 1987, 1989, 1990, 1991; Uziel and Piron 1991; Webb and Stevens 1991; White et al. 1992; White, Vohr, and Behrens 1993;

Zorowka 1993). The various aspects of these studies (e.g., the approach to sub-ject selection; their numbers, ages, and risk factors; type of follow-up evaluation if relevant) have been summarized by White et al. (1993) and Norton (1994).

In an earlier study of CEOAEs in neonates and young infants, Bonfils and his colleagues (1988) made a particularly noteworthy observation about the presence or absence of evoked OAEs and the prediction of hearing level. By comparing CEOAEs and ABRs from the same infants aged three months or younger (n = 46), they discovered that those with ABR wave-V thresholds <30 dB HL had an emission present. Those with ABR thresholds >40 dB HL did not exhibit CEOAEs. Other investigators have been less successful in determining the precise magnitude of the hearing level (e.g., 30, 35, 40, 45 dB HL) at which CEOAEs are immeasurable. Overall, it appears that the absence of a CEOAE cannot quantify the degree of hearing loss (Kemp et al. 1986). However, certain properties of emissions—including their reproducibility or their absolute or relative CEOAE levels with respect to the magnitude of the noise floor—can be reliably used to define the presence (pass) or absence (fail) of an evoked OAE (Prieve et al. 1993).

Most of the early studies used custom, laboratory-based microcomputer sys-tems to measure neonatal CEOAEs, with the primary goal of validating the evoked-emissions test by using the outcome of conventional ABR screening as a reference. The studies performed by Stevens and his colleagues (1987) on over 700 newborns (with follow-up behavioral hearing tests in over half of these pa-tients at six months to one year old) represent the most comprehensive CEOAE data set yet available.

Lutman and his colleagues (Cope and Lutman 1988) developed their own laboratory-based system to conduct comparative studies of ABR and CEOAE screening in newborns. These investigators discovered results that were as im-pressive as those of the Stevens group. The failure rate for the emitted responses and both conventional and automated ABR testing were quite similar at about 3% (Kennedy et al. 1991).

With the commercial availability of the ILO88, essentially all the studies in the published literature have made use of this CEOAE method of screening hear-ing in newborns. The largest newborn database using ILO88-based CEOAEs originated from the Rhode Island Hearing Assessment Project. In this project, almost 10,000 infants were evaluated to determine whether emitted responses can be used for the universal screening of all live births. An entire issue of the *Seminars in Hearing* (1993, vol. 14) was devoted to reporting the methods and results of this ongoing clinical trial of a CEOAE-based, universal screening pro-gram. The Rhode Island project has been so successful that it is being used as a model for similar universal screening programs in several other states, including Hawaii (Johnson et al. 1993). Indeed, the NIH study group used data from this neonate screening project as the basis for recommending evoked OAEs for the early identification of hearing difficulties in newborns, infants, and young chil-dren. One important practical strategy implemented by the Rhode Island investigators and others to minimize subject-based acoustic artifacts is to perform these measurements after feeding when neonates are typically in natural sleep.

Several studies have also discovered that newborn CEOAEs are easier to detect when measured at least 24 to 48 hours after birth (Chuang S.W., Gerber, and Thornton 1993; Kok, van Zanten, and Brocaar 1992). This problem—an example of which is shown in Figure 8.4—also surfaced in our own research. The original CEOAE and DPOAE measures (6/22) were obtained when the female infant, BT, was only ten hours old. Note that for both the right (above) and left (below) ears, neither evoked-OAE test resulted in an identifiable response above the level of background noises. For this neonate, the emissions' testing was repeated several days later (6/25), and the results of both evaluations show the presence of evoked OAEs. These subsequent data demonstrate generally lower background noise levels than the ones measured a few days earlier. Clearly, however, if the OAEs had been as large during the initial test session as they were during the later one, they would have been recordable over some portion of the frequency range during the earlier examination period.

A common explanation for this tendency in newborn ears for OAEs to increase in level and thus become easier to detect over the first few postnatal days is that sufficient time is required for prenatal fluids to clear from the middle-ear space. This notion is consistent with the observations referred to previously and illustrated below that fluid in the middle ear decreases the likelihood of measuring OAEs. However, Chuang K.W. et al. (1993) found no evidence of middle-ear effusions in over eighty newborn ears they examined otoscopically. Rather, they noted that intrauterine material (in the form of vernix caseosa and other prenatally related debris) contaminated the external ear canals of many of their newly born subjects. The accepted explanation is that the difficulties in recording evoked OAEs in a significant proportion (possibly up to 25%) of neonates immediately after birth are more related to the presence of debris in the outer ear canal as well as to an extremely pliant ear canal that tends to collapse near the tympanic membrane. A "floppy" ear canal contaminated with debris would clearly block the propagation pathway of the ingoing acoustic stimuli and the outgoing emitted response.

As reported earlier, Kim, Lafrenière, Smurzynski, and their colleagues (e.g., Lafrenière et al. 1991; Smurzynski et al. 1993) were the first to characterize DPOAEs in both healthy, full-gestation newborns between two and six days old and in preterm neonates with an average gestational age at birth of about 29 weeks. So far, however, there is no published information illustrating the application of DPOAEs as a newborn hearing-screening procedure.

IMPLEMENTING AN EVOKED-OAE-BASED NEWBORN HEARING-SCREENING PROGRAM

IN establishing a newborn-screening program, the type of evoked OAE to measure (TEOAE or DPOAE) and, for DPOAEs, the equipment manufacturer

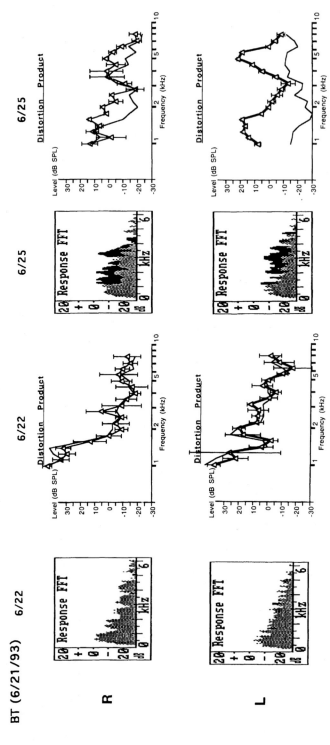

Figure 8.4. Evoked OAEs for the right (R) and left (L) ears of a ten-hour-old neonate (6/22) and for the same newborn at three days of age (6/25). Note the absence of CEOAEs and DPOAEs in the earlier recording sessions and their clear presence three days later.

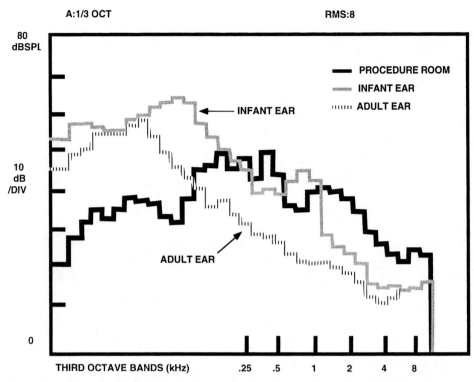

Figure 8.5. A spectral analysis in one-third octave bands of the sounds in a procedure room adjacent to a well-baby nursery showing features of the ambient noise as measured from the emissions' microphone under three conditions: open to the room noise (bold line), in the ear of an infant (shaded line), and in the ear of an adult (hatched line).

must be selected. One important aspect of OAE screening in hospitals is the importance of designating a quiet test area, preferably separate from the relatively loud noises associated with busy neonatal services. In urban hospitals, a procedure room separate from the nursery may not be an option due to the high utilization of physical space in such settings.

The data in Figure 8.5 illustrate the shortcomings of the newborn skull compared to an adult's with respect to providing some natural attenuation of the background noises associated with a well-baby nursery. Full-term, healthy-baby nurseries usually do not include the high sound levels associated with noisy monitoring instrumentation outfitted with auditory-feedback features and with the frequent verbal interactions of the medical staff. The amplitude spectrum of the environmental sounds in the nursery (Figure 8.5) indicates that the thin meatal tissues of a baby's ear provide little impedance to the transmission of low-frequency sounds. They do not begin to attenuate room noises effectively until about 1 kHz and reach the full range of an adult's capability only for stimuli above 4 kHz.

One of several techniques can be used to overcome the disadvantages of testing in such noisy environments. One viable approach is to obtain a sound-treated isolette (Acoustic Isolette, Acoustic Systems, Austin, TX) that has been

Table 8.1. Baby Pass/Fail Criteria

	PASS		TECHNICAL FAIL
_↑_	DPOAE ≥10th percentile normal DPOAE ≥3 dB noise floor	_↑_	DPOAE ≥10th percentile normal DPOAE <3 dB noise floor
.... 10TH PERCENTILE NORMAL DPOAE			
	FAIL		FAIL
_↑_	DPOAE <10th percentile normal DPOAE ≥3 dB noise floor	_↑_	DPOAE <10th percentile normal DPOAE <3 dB noise floor

specially constructed to accommodate the requirements for recording OAEs and satisfying the stringent infection-control procedures of hospitals. Another option is to adopt software-based procedures that have been specially developed to reduce the influence of extraneous sounds on measured acoustic signals (e.g., Lonsbury-Martin et al. 1994).

In addition to the physical aspects of the evoked-OAE testing of newborns, a strategy for assigning passes and fails must be determined. Because the application of otoacoustic emissions is relatively new, there is no standardized approach to scoring these data. Examples that help guide the user can be found in the literature for both CEOAEs derived from commercially available systems (Kemp and Ryan 1993; Lafrenière et al. 1991; White, Vohr, and Behrens 1993) and for DPOAEs measured with customized equipment (Bonfils et al. 1992; Lafrenière et al. 1991; Smurzynski et al. 1993).

To illustrate this aspect of OAE screening, several examples from our own newborn hearing screening program are presented. A primary emphasis of our newborn screening research is the investigation of the benefits and limitations of DPOAEs in determining how best to interpret the data. The example in Figure 8.6 illustrates the scoring procedure for DPOAEs from both ears of a two-day-old neonate. In our approach, the interpretation of DPOAEs from a test ear is based on the emission level with respect to the magnitude of DPOAEs measured in a population of healthy newborns (hereafter called "normal" DPOAEs) and with respect to their own related noise floor, according to the rules summarized in Table 8.1.

As shown in the table inset at the top of Figure 8.6, the data are obtained initially between 1 and 8 kHz in intervals of six points per octave. The DPOAE frequency-level functions on each side of this table show plots for the right (R) and left (L) ears of the levels of the emissions (open triangles) and their related noise floors (bold line) in dB SPL. For each frequency interval, a comparison of the DPOAE (DP) level to a database of normal amplitudes at the same frequency

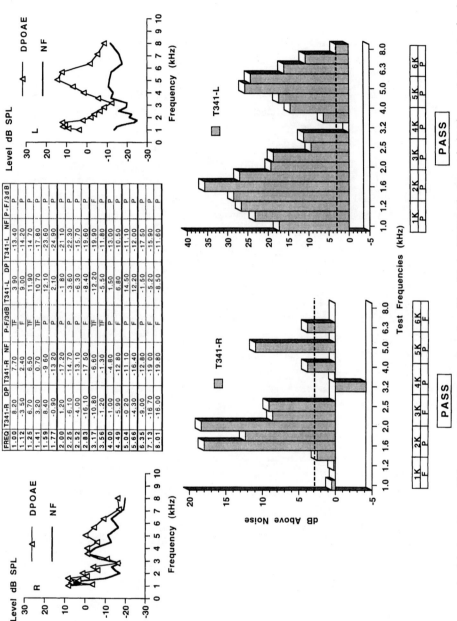

FREQ	T341-R DP	T341-R NF	P-F/3dB	T341-L DP	T341-L NF	P-F/3dB
1.00	8.20	7.70	TF	3.90	-13.40	P
1.12	-3.50	2.40	F	9.90	-14.20	P
1.25	6.70	6.50	TF	11.90	-14.70	P
1.41	3.20	0.70	TF	10.70	-17.80	P
1.59	8.40	-9.60	P	12.10	-23.60	P
1.77	-0.90	-13.20	P	2.10	-24.90	P
2.00	1.20	-17.20	P	-1.80	-21.10	P
2.25	-6.10	-14.70	P	-3.60	-22.30	P
2.52	-4.00	-13.10	P	-6.30	-15.70	P
2.83	-16.10	-17.50	F	-8.40	-19.60	P
3.17	-10.80	-6.60	TF	-12.20	-19.90	F
3.56	-1.20	-1.30	TF	-5.50	-11.80	P
4.00	-1.00	-4.80	P	-13.00	-13.00	P
4.49	-5.90	-12.80	F	1.50	-10.50	P
5.04	-0.20	-11.10	P	6.80	-11.10	P
5.66	-4.30	-16.40	P	12.20	-12.00	P
6.35	-9.00	-12.80	P	14.50	-17.50	P
7.13	-16.70	-19.00	F	-1.50	-15.90	P
8.01	-16.00	-19.80	F	-8.50	-11.60	P

1K	2K	3K	4K	5K	6K
F	P	P	P	P	F

PASS

1K	2K	3K	4K	5K	6K
P	P	P	P	P	P

PASS

Figure 8.6. An example of designating pass/fail scores to DPOAEs for a two-day-old well baby (T341). The "smoothed" (three-point) emission levels in the form of DPOAE frequency/level functions are shown at the top for right (R) and left (L) ears. The numeric form of these data for both the DPOAEs (DP) and noise floors (NF) along with the assigned pass/fails (P/F) and technical fails (TF) are indicated in the center table. At the bottom of the figure, the resulting scores for each of the six frequency regions of interest and the global result are indicated, with the graphical representations of the assigned Ps, Fs, and TFs displayed above. (See text for a detailed explanation of this particular scoring system.)

and to the level of its corresponding noise floor (NF) is automatically performed by an Excel-based (Microsoft, V4.0) subroutine.

A pass (P) is assigned to a frequency interval if its DPOAE level is equal to or greater than the tenth percentile of normal DPOAEs at that frequency. Conversely, a fail (F) is designated if either one of two conditions is met. These are that (1) the DPOAE level is below the 10th percentile of normal DPOAEs and is also at or above 3 dB above the related noise floor for that ear, or (2) the DPOAE level is below the 10th percentile of normal activity and is also less than 3 dB above the corresponding noise floor. Finally, a technical fail (TF) is denoted if the DPOAE is below the 10th percentile of normal emissions and is also less than 3 dB above the noise floor. The table in the upper part of Figure 8.6 notes the pass/fail designations (P-F/3dB) for each DPOAE measured in this infant's ears. The plots in the center of the figure show graphical representations of the comparative data (DP-NF) for each of the nineteen frequency intervals. In these plots, the three possible outcomes are defined as follows: (1) the pass intervals are indicated as gray columns extending above the 3 dB noise line (dashed); (2) the fails are shown as open areas at the 0 dB line; and (3) the technical fails are indicated as gray columns between −5 and +3 dB above the 0 dB noise level.

Next, an additional software-based subroutine sums the six-point/octave data into six arbitrary frequency intervals (indicated on the table by the bold horizontal lines) consisting of the 1, 2, 3, 4, 5, and 6–8 kHz regions. For each of these six frequency bands, a pass/fail score (indicated in the small table near the bottom of the figure) is assigned based on the rule that the designation agrees with the majority (i.e., >50%) of the scores for the component bands. When a frequency band consists of only two bands (e.g., 3, 4, 5 kHz) and one is a pass and the other a fail or technical fail, the rule is to designate it a pass. Finally, a global pass/fail is determined in a similar manner: The general designation is based on the majority of scores, with passes again determining the final assignment in "tie" instances. Thus, in Figure 8.6, for the left ear, the findings of six out of a potential of six passes indicates a total or global pass for this ear. This assignment clearly agrees with the visual impression provided by both the raw-data plot at the top right of the figure and their quantitative representation located directly below. The global outcome is a little more difficult to discern for the right ear. However, because three of the six frequency bands are scored as passes, a global pass is assigned to this ear based on the >50% majority rule that favors passes in instances of a tie (i.e., in the presence of three fails).

Older Infants and Young Children: Infants (3 to 12 months), Toddlers (13 to 30 months), and Preschool Aged Children (2.5 to 4 years)

The published literature describing the features of evoked OAEs in young ears contains only occasional illustrations of the clinical utility of recording emissions in older infants, toddlers, and the younger preschool aged children. For example, Owens et al. (1992, 1993) and Prieve (1992) illustrate the distorting effects of tympanostomy tubes on the parametric properties of DPOAEs or CEOAEs for children between about one and three years of age. Clearly, a systematic study of evoked OAEs in these specific subpopulations is needed to establish their usefulness and to determine the average features of TEOAEs or CEOAEs and DPOAEs during these particular age intervals.

OLDER CHILDREN: PRESCHOOL-AGED CHILDREN (4 TO 5 YEARS) AND SCHOOL-AGED CHILDREN (5.1 TO TEENS)

SEVERAL survey studies of evoked OAEs have been completed on children between about two and 14 years of age, with most of the children being more than four years old. Spektor et al. (1991), in a study comparing the outcomes of CEOAE and DPOAE testing, were first to establish normal levels of DPOAEs in children from four to ten years old (average age = 7.5 years). These results were used to judge the normality of CEOAEs and DPOAEs for the ears of an additional fourteen hearing-impaired youngsters of similar age. A major finding of Spektor and his colleagues was the agreement between the pure-tone audiogram and the DPOAE frequency-level function in delineating the regions of hearing difficulties for these children.

The principal aim of other investigations into the application of evoked-OAE testing in young children has been to document the effects of middle-ear pathology on the detectability of emissions in a population of subjects who are most prone to problems involving the sound-conduction pathway of the peripheral ear. For example, the studies of Owens et al. (1992, 1993) examined OAE production in young patients between two and eight years of age who exhibited various degrees of conductive loss due to inflammation of the middle ear. As in the earlier Spektor et al. (1991) investigation, the status of these unknown ears was evaluated based on average levels of DPOAEs from a group of normal-hearing children of comparable age.

In normal-hearing children with hearing levels of 20 dB or better, CEOAE levels are well above the related noise floor, and the frequency range typically extends between about 0.5 and 5 kHz. In addition, the "repro" value, on average, is about 90%. Similarly, DPOAE levels for healthy youngsters customarily range between 10 and 20 dB SPL from 0.7 to 8 kHz. However, in young patients with middle-ear impairment, the emitted responses are drastically affected by the disease state because of the critical importance of the middle-ear system in measuring evoked OAEs.

For example, an otoscopic examination of RA, the six-year-old male of Figure 8.7, revealed a reddened and retracted tympanic membrane on the right side, with a visible fluid line on the left tympanic membrane. These observations

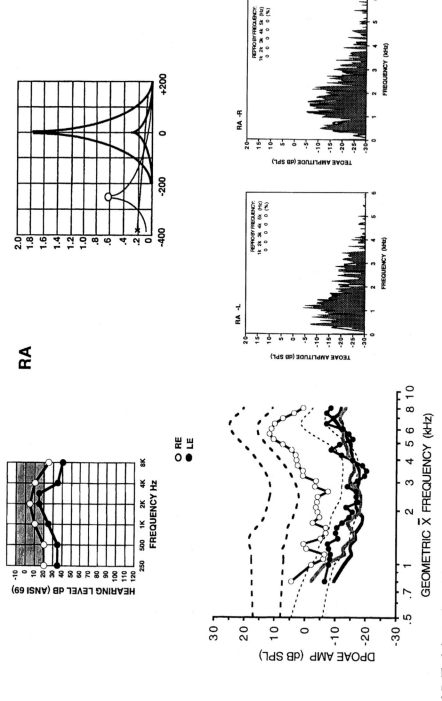

RA

Figure 8.7. The behavioral (top left), standard tympanometric (top right), DPOAE (bottom right), and CEOAE (bottom left), findings for RA, a six-year-old male child exhibiting signs of an acute episode of otitis media. Note the essentially normal hearing for the right ear (open circles), displaying a negative middle-ear pressure of about −250 daPa. No CEOAEs and only below-average amplitude DPOAEs (open circles) were recordable from this ear. In contrast, the left ear (solid circles) showed a pattern of mild hearing loss affecting the low and high frequencies, along with a flat tympanogram (x) that was associated with an oto-scopically observable fluid line on the tympanic membrane. Below, the evoked-OAE measurements indicate that neither CEOAEs nor DPOAEs were recordable under these fluid-filled middle ear conditions.

were consistent with the working diagnosis of acute serous otitis media. The immittance findings for this patient shown in the upper right portion of Figure 8.7 reveal the presence of negative pressure in the right ear (open circles) in the form of a type C tympanogram and a flat type B tympanogram for the left ear (cross). The related acoustic reflexes were absent (not shown). The remaining functional findings of Figure 8.7 show that, whereas pure-tone hearing thresholds were relatively unaffected on the right side (open circles), the left ear (solid circles) exhibited mild threshold elevations (no air-bone gap). It is clear from the amplitude spectra in the lower right portion of Figure 8.7 that CEOAEs were immeasurable bilaterally. Similarly, for the left ear exhibiting visible signs of a middle-ear effusion, DPOAEs (lower left) were not recordable (solid circles). However, for the right ear where there was negative pressure in the middle ear, DPOAEs were reduced from normal levels but were clearly measurable. This pattern of evoked-OAE findings consisting of reduced DPOAEs and absent CEOAEs in the presence of negative middle ear pressure and absent DPOAEs and CEOAEs associated with a fluid-filled middle ear are typical findings in young patients experiencing an acute episode of otitis media.

The plots of Figure 8.8 exemplify the results for another situation commonly observed in young patients. In this case, three-and-a-half-year-old JG (male) has a long history of recurrent ear and throat infections consisting of three to four incidents yearly. Although JG's hearing is in the normal range, the shape of his tympanograms indicates the presence of a slight amount of negative middle-ear pressure bilaterally. Although not shown here, threshold testing of the uncrossed and crossed acoustic reflexes showed either elevated thresholds or absent reflexes, respectively, for both ears. The CEOAE results show activity present from about 2 to 5 kHz for the left ear and a more focused pattern between 2 and 4 kHz for the right ear. From the DPOAE-frequency functions, the classic observation of negative middle-ear pressure affecting low more than high frequencies is evident. Here, DPOAEs become measurable above about 1 kHz for both ears but remain essentially below normal levels until about 6 kHz. This pattern of evoked-OAE activity involving reduced or partially present emitted responses, especially for the low test frequencies, is commonly observed for ears with recurrent episodes of middle-ear infection.

Finally, the data of Figure 8.9 illustrate another finding that is commonly observed in older children who exhibit recurrent middle-ear problems. For AR, an eight-year-old male, the moderate high-frequency hearing loss shown for the left side is reflected by the absent CEOAEs and DPOAEs for frequencies >3 kHz. Whereas the tympanometric findings indicate only a slight amount of negative pressure in the left middle ear, the acoustic reflexes were absent, and the otoscopic examination revealed some scarring of the ear drum.

These findings indicate that evoked-OAE testing in ears exhibiting middle-ear disease provides an invalid assessment of the functional status of the cochlea's outer hair cell system. Clearly, however, such testing can be used as a

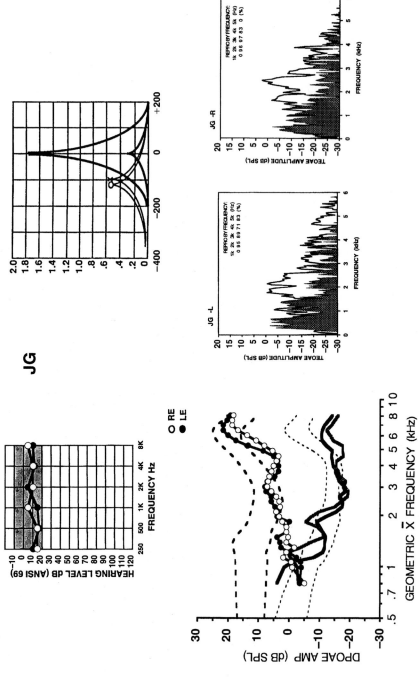

Figure 8.8. The behavioral, standard tympanometric, and emissions-testing results for JG, a 3.5-year-old male child who has experienced recurrent ear and throat infections over the past three years. This child was reported to speak less fluently than his peers and, at the time of testing, was not under medical treatment for his recurrent-infection condition. Note the normal hearing in the presence of a slight negative middle ear pressure that was exhibited bilaterally. Although not shown here, the ipsilateral acoustic reflexes tested at both 1 and 2 kHz showed elevated thresholds. Similar findings were noted for the crossed reflexes that were tested at 0.5, 1, and 2 kHz, with thresholds being indeterminable for 4 kHz. Essentially low-level (for this patient's age group) CEOAEs were measured, primarily in the mid-frequency region, extending from about 1.5 kHz to 4 kHz, whereas the DPOAE pattern of below-average to normal levels showed a classic configuration indicating the adverse influence of the increased middle-ear mass on the low- to mid-frequencies.

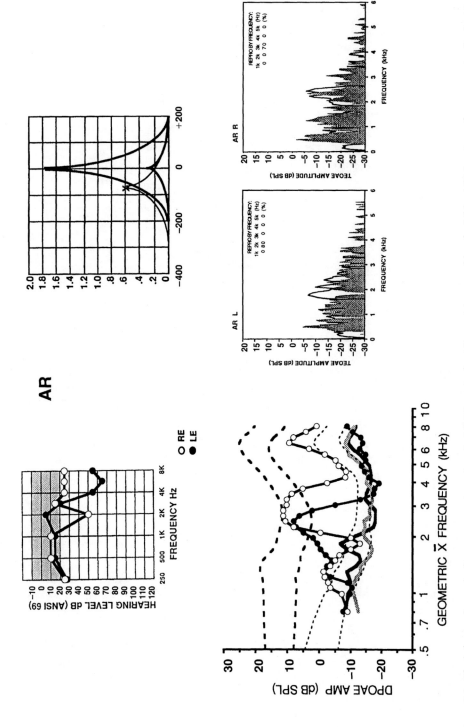

Figure 8.9. The behavioral, standard tympanometric, and evoked-OAE results for AR, an eight-year-old male child exhibiting signs of an acute episode of otitis media. Note the essentially normal hearing for the right ear (open circles) displaying a negative middle-ear pressure of about −50 daPa. No CEOAEs and only below-average amplitude DPOAEs (open circles) were recordable from this ear. In contrast, the left ear (solid circles) showed a pattern of mild hearing loss affecting the low and high frequencies, along with a flat tympanogram (x) that was associated with an otoscopically observable fluid line on the tympanic membrane. Below, the evoked-OAE measurements indicate that neither CEOAEs nor DPOAEs were recordable under these fluid-filled middle-ear conditions.

simple indicator of the presence or absence of conditions affecting the signal-conducting function of the middle ear. The findings illustrated in Figures 8.7 through 8.9 demonstrate the extreme sensitivity of OAEs to the integrity of middle-ear function. Other work has shown that this feature can be used advantageously to monitor the efficacy of subsequent treatment strategies involving either the administration of systemic antibiotics or antihistamines or the surgical placement of tympanostomy tubes through the tympanic membrane. The data in Figure 8.9 for the right ear of AR show that evoked OAEs can be measured, although with rather atypical patterns of activity in the presence of ventilating tubes, thus indicating the status of their patency. In this case, both the DPOAEs and CEOAEs show some focused emitted-response activity, particularly around 3 kHz.

FUTURE DIRECTIONS

FROM this review of OAEs in young patients, it is clear that several practical aspects of emissions testing should be addressed rather immediately if this procedure is to be optimized for clinical utilization. For example, for newborn screening, the optimal timing of the postnatal test session must be firmly established. Further, if the initial observations of Kok et al. (1993) are confirmed (i.e., that the likelihood of detecting evoked OAEs improves for postnatal days greater than one), safe strategies for cleaning birth-related debris from the outer ear canal need to be developed. Establishing such preparatory, pretest methods would be essential because the length of stay in U.S. hospitals for healthy babies is rapidly becoming one day or less due to the escalating cost of medical care. In the absence of effective pretest procedures that can be implemented during the first postnatal day, hearing screening for healthy babies may be delayed until, perhaps, a three-month immunization appointment or the first well baby check.

Another practical problem for applying OAE testing to young children is the difficulty of assessing ears with middle ear infections. It is clearly difficult to imagine the development of an acceptable procedure for combating the effects of middle ear effusions under acute-testing conditions. However, preliminary evidence indicates that negative middle-ear pressure can be corrected by introducing compensatory pressure into the outer ear canal to achieve equal pressure across the tympanic membrane (Trine, Hirsch, and Margolis 1993). In this manner, CEOAEs that were immeasurable under the negative-pressure condition became detectable.

Standardization of such compensatory methods will obviously increase the usefulness of evoked-OAE testing in young children. A final practical problem that needs immediate solving for the successful application of OAE testing to young patients is the development of effective noise-reduction methods. It is common with such subjects that their own vocalizations and body noises contaminate, particularly, the low-frequency response region (i.e., <2 kHz). Clearly, many techniques used in the signal-processing field can be applied effectively to OAE instrumentation to improve the signal-to-noise ratio.

To facilitate the clinical application of evoked-emissions testing to young patient populations, it is also important to develop quantitative means for assessing the normality of OAE properties obtained from unknown ears. Comparing the statistical distributions of certain features (e.g., detection threshold, slope of the growth of OAE level with increasing stimulus level, and the amplitude of the OAE at a given stimulus level in the normal and hearing-impaired ears of neonates, infants, toddlers, and young children) will permit us to determine the degree to which emissions can accurately predict the hearing ability of a previously untested ear. Developing algorithms for relating OAE properties to audiometric status is clearly the ultimate aim of the clinical application of evoked OAEs to these special patient populations.

In addition, the usefulness of measures of other OAE types (e.g., SFOAEs, toneburst-TEOAEs as well as other distortion products, $2f_2$-f_1, $3f_1$-$2f_2$, and so on) for the same ear needs to be determined in order to increase the capability for detecting cochlear abnormalities. Finally, the parametric-test set that is most sensitive to hearing level as measured by the pure-tone audiogram must also be determined, especially for DPOAEs.

SUMMARY

ONE of the health promotion and disease-prevention objectives identified in the report on "Healthy People 2000" (Health and Human Services 1991) concerns the disclosing of hearing problems in newborns and infants. Measures of OAEs showed great promise as an objective, noninvasive technique for screening hearing in these very special and acknowledged difficult-to-test patient populations. Because of the emphasis on universal screening of newborn hearing, it is certain that much information on this unique application of evoked-OAE testing will be available in the literature.

The OAE attributes of objectivity and rapidity, in particular, can also be put to good use in evaluating cochlear function in toddlers and very young children, who cannot yet provide reliable behavioral indices of hearing capability and who tend to be very active physically. In the published literature so far, there are only sporadic examples of isolated cases illustrating the features of evoked OAEs for these young patients. Clearly, this is one subpopulation of child patient that lacks the necessary focus of a systematic study.

Although a database describing the features of evoked OAEs in school-aged children is beginning to accumulate, the advantages of emissions testing as a hearing screener for the newborn are also applicable to this age group. This specific application of OAE testing has been virtually ignored by researchers in the study of the clinical utility of emissions, and its usefulness for this purpose deserves to be thoroughly investigated.

A number of years have passed since the discovery of otoacoustic emissions (Kemp 1978). It is a tribute to the modern age of technological development and instantaneous communications that a basic discovery has progressed so rapidly to an advanced stage of development. Clearly, the availability of commercial products and the performance of many on-going clinical trials provide strong evidence of the importance of OAEs to the screening of hearing and the diagnosis of hearing problems in children.

References

Balkany, T.J., S.A. Berman, M.A. Simmons, and B.W. Jafek. 1978. Middle ear effusions in neonates. *Laryngoscope* 88:398–405.

Bonfils, P., P. Avan, M. Francois, J. Trotoux, and P. Narcy. 1992. Distortion-product otoacoustic emissions in neonates: Normative data. *Acta Oto-Laryngologica* 112: 739–744.

Bonfils, P., A. Dumont, P. Marie, M. Francois, and P. Narcy. 1990. Evoked otoacoustic emissions in new-born hearing screening. *Laryngoscope* 100:186–189.

Bonfils, P., A. Uziel, and R. Pujol. 1988. Screening for auditory dysfunction in infants by evoked oto-acoustic emissions. *Archives of Otolaryngology: Head and Neck Surgery* 114:887–890.

Bray, P. 1989. Click evoked otoacoustic emissions and the development of a clinical oto-acoustic hearing test instrument. Ph.D. diss., London University.

Bray, P., and D.T. Kemp. 1987. An advanced cochlear echo technique suitable for infant screening. *British Journal of Audiology* 21:191–204.

Brownell, W.E. 1990. Outer hair cell electromotility and oto-acoustic emissions. *Ear and Hearing* 11:82–92.

Brownell, W.E., C.R. Bader, D. Bertrand, and Y. Rabaupierre. 1985. Evoked mechanical responses of isolated outer hair cells. *Science* 227:194–196.

Burns, E.M., K.H. Arehart, and S.L. Campbell. 1992. Prevalence of spontaneous otoacoustic emissions in neonates. *Journal of the Acoustical Society of America* 91:1571–1575.

Chuang, K.W., B.R. Vohr, S.J. Norton, and M.D. Lekas. 1993. External and middle ear status related to evoked otoacoustic emission in neonates. *Archives of Otolaryngology: Head and Neck Surgery* 119:276–282.

Chuang, S.W., S.E. Gerber, and A.R.D. Thornton. 1993. Evoked otoacoustic emissions in preterm infants. *International Journal of Pediatric Otorhinolaryngology* 26:39–45.

Collet, L., D.T. Kemp, E. Veuillet, R. Duclaux, A. Moulin, and A. Morgon. 1990. Effect of contralateral auditory stimuli on active cochlear micromechanical properties in human subjects. *Hearing Research* 43:251–262.

Cope, Y., and M.E. Lutman. 1988. Oto-acoustic emissions. In *Pediatric audiology 0–5 years*, ed. B. McCormick. London: Taylor and Francis.

Harris, F.P., B.L. Lonsbury-Martin, B.B. Stagner, A.C. Coats, and G.K. Martin. 1989. Acoustic distortion products in humans: Systematic changes in amplitude as a function of f_2/f_1 ratio. *Journal of the Acoustical Society of America* 85:220–222.

Harris, F.P., and R. Probst. 1992. Transiently evoked oto-acoustic emissions in patients with Meniere's disease. *Acta Oto-Laryngologica* 112:36–44.

Health and Human Services. 1991. *Healthy people 2000: National health promotion and disease prevention objectives.* Washington, D.C.: United States Government Printing Office.

Johnsen, N.J., P. Bagi, and C. Elberling. 1983. Evoked acoustic emissions from the human ear. III. Findings in neonates. *Scandinavian Audiology* 12:17–24.

Johnsen, N.J., P. Bagi, J. Parbo, and C. Elberling. 1988. Evoked acoustic emissions from the human ear. IV. Final results in 100 neonates. *Scandinavian Audiology* 17:27–34.

Johnsen, N.J., J. Parbo, and C. Elberling. 1989. Evoked acoustic emissions from the human ear. V. Developmental changes. *Scandinavian Audiology* 18:59–62.

Johnson, J.L., G.W. Mauk, K.M. Takekawa, P.R. Simon, C.C.J. Sia, and P.M. Blackwell. 1993. Implementing a statewide system of services for infants and toddlers with hearing disabilities. *Seminars in Hearing* 14:105–119.

Joint Committee on Infant Hearing. 1991. 1990 position statement. *AAO-HNS Bulletin* March:15–18.

———. 1994. 1993 position statement. *Audiology Today* 6:6–9.

Kemp, D.T. 1978. Stimulated acoustic emissions from within the human auditory system. *Journal of the Acoustical Society of America* 64:1386–1391.

Kemp, D.T., P. Bray, L. Alexander, and A.M. Brown. 1986. Acoustic emission cochleography: Practical aspects. *Scandinavian Audiology Supplementum* 25:71–96.

Kemp, D.T., and S. Ryan. 1993. The use of transient evoked oto-acoustic emissions in neonatal hearing screening program. *Seminars in Hearing* 14:30–45.

Kemp, D.T., S. Ryan, and P. Bray. 1990. A guide to the effective use of otoacoustic emissions. *Ear and Hearing* 11:93–105.

Kennedy, C.R., L. Kimm, D.C. Dees, P.I.P. Evans, M. Hunter, S. Lenton, and A.R.D. Thornton. 1991. Otoacoustic emissions and auditory brainstem responses in the newborn. *Archives of Disease in Childhood* 66:1124–1129.

Kok, M.R., G.A. van Zanten, and M.P. Brocaar. 1992. Growth of evoked otoacoustic emissions during the first days postpartum. *Audiology* 31:140–149.

———. 1993. Aspects of spontaneous otoacoustic emissions in healthy newborns. *Hearing Research* 69:115–123.

Kok, M.R., G.A. van Zanten, M.P. Brocaar, and H.C.S. Wallenburg. 1993. Click-evoked otoacoustic emissions in 1036 ears of healthy newborns. *Audiology* 32:213–224.

Lafrenière, D., M.D. Jung, J. Smurzynski, G. Leonard, D.O. Kim, and J. Sasek. 1991. Distortion-product and click-evoked otoacoustic emissions in healthy newborns. *Archives of Otolaryngology: Head and Neck Surgery* 117:1382–1389.

Lasky, R., J. Perlman, and K. Hecox. 1992. Distortion-product otoacoustic emissions in human newborns and adults. *Ear and Hearing* 13:430–441.

Lonsbury-Martin, B.L., F.P. Harris, B.B. Stagner, M.D. Hawkins, and G.K. Martin. 1990. Distortion-product emissions in humans: II. Relations to stimulated and spontaneous emissions and acoustic immittance in normally hearing subjects. *Annals of Otology, Rhinology, and Laryngology* (Supplement 147) 99:14–28.

Lonsbury-Martin, B.L., G.K. Martin, M.J. McCoy, and M.L. Whitehead. 1994. Testing young children with otoacoustic emissions: Middle-ear influences. *American Journal of Otology* (Supplement 1) 15:13–20.

Moulin, A., L. Collet, and R. Duclaux. 1993. Contralateral auditory stimulation alters acoustic distortion products in humans. *Hearing Research* 65:193–210.

National Institutes of Health (1993). Early identification of hearing impairment in infants and young children. *NIH Consensus Statement* 11:1–24.

Norton, S.J. 1994. Emerging role of evoked otoacoustic emissions in neonatal hearing screening. *American Journal of Otology* (Suppl. 1) 15:4–12.

Norton, S.J., and J.E. Widen. 1990. Evoked otoacoustic emissions in normal-hearing infants and children: Emerging data and issues. *Ear and Hearing* 11:121–127.

Owens, J.J., M.J. McCoy, B.L. Lonsbury-Martin, and G.K. Martin. 1992. Influence of otitis media on evoked otoacoustic emissions in children. *Seminars in Hearing* 13:63–66.

———. 1993. Otoacoustic emissions in children with normal ears, middle-ear dysfunction, and ventilating tubes. *American Journal of Otology* 14:34–40.

Plinkert, P.K., G. Sesterhenn, R. Arold, and H.P. Zenner. 1990. Evaluation of otoacoustic emissions in high-risk infants by using an easy and rapid objective auditory screening method. *European Archives of Otorhinology* 247:356–360.

Prieve, B.A. 1992. Otoacoustic emissions in infants and children: Basic characteristics and clinical application. *Seminars in Hearing* 13:37–52.

Prieve, B.A., M.P. Gorga, A. Schmidt, S.T. Neelym, J. Peters, L. Schultes, and W. Jesteadt. 1993. Analysis of transient-evoked otoacoustic emissions in normal-hearing and hearing-impaired ears. *Journal of the Acoustical Society of America* 93:3308–3319.

Probst, R., B.L. Lonsbury-Martin, and G.K. Martin. 1991. A review of otoacoustic emissions. *Journal of the Acoustical Society of America* 89:2027–2067.

Sakashita, T., Y. Minowa, K. Hachikawa, T. Kubo, and Y. Nakai. 1991. Evoked otoacoustic emissions from ears with idiopathic sudden deafness. *Acta Oto-Laryngologica* (Suppl. 486):66–72.

Salomon, G., B. Anthonisen, J. Groth, and P.P. Thomsen. 1992. Otoacoustic hearing screening in newborns: Optimization. In *Screening children for auditory function*, ed. F.H. Bess and J.W. Hall III. Nashville: Bill Wilkerson Center Press.

Smurzynski, J., M.D. Jung, D. Lafrenière, D.O. Kim, M.V. Kamath, J.C. Rowe, M.C. Holman, and G. Leonard. 1993. Distortion-product and click-evoked otoacoustic emissions of preterm and full-term infants. *Ear and Hearing* 14:258–274.

Spektor, Z., G. Leonard, D.O. Kim, M.D. Jung, and J. Smurzynski. 1991. Otoacoustic emissions in normal and hearing-impaired children and normal adults. *Laryngoscope* 101:965–976.

Stevens, J.C., H.D. Webb, J. Hutchinson, J. Connell, M.F. Smith, and J.T. Buffin. 1989. Click evoked oto-acoustic emissions compared with brain stem electric response. *Archives of Disease in Childhood* 64:1105–1111.

———. 1990. Click evoked oto-acoustic emissions in neonatal screening. *Ear and Hearing* 11:128–133.

———. 1991. Evaluation of click-evoked oto-acoustic emissions in the newborn. *British Journal of Audiology* 25:11–14.

Stevens, J.C., H.D. Webb, M.F. Smith, J.T. Buffin, and H. Ruddy. 1987. A comparison of otoacoustic emissions and brain stem electric response audiometry in the normal newborn and babies admitted to a special care baby unit. *Clinical Physical and Physiological Measurement* 8:95–104.

Strickland, E.A., E.M. Burns, and A. Tubis. 1985. Incidence of spontaneous otoacoustic emissions in children and infants. *Journal of the Acoustical Society of America* 78:931–935.

Trine, M.B., J.E. Hirsch, and R.H. Margolis. 1993. The effect of compensatory ear-canal pressure on otoacoustic emissions. *Ear and Hearing* 14:401–407.

Uziel, A., and J-P. Piron. 1991. Evoked otoacoustic emissions from normal newborns and babies admitted to an intensive care baby unit. *Acta Oto-Laryngologica* (Suppl. 482): 85–91.

Webb, H.D., and J.C. Stevens. 1991. Auditory screening in high risk neonates: Selection of a test protocol. *Clinical Physical and Physiological Measurement* 12:75–76.

White, K.R., A.B. Maxon, T.R. Behrens, P.M. Blackwell, and B.R. Vohr. 1992. Neonatal screening using evoked otoacoustic emissions: The Rhode Island hearing assessment project. In *Screening children for auditory function*, ed. F.H. Bess and J.W. Hall III. Nashville: Bill Wilkerson Center Press.

White, K.R., B.R. Vohr, and T.R. Behrens. 1993. Universal newborn hearing screening using transient evoked otoacoustic emissions: Results of the Rhode Island hearing assessment project. *Seminars in Hearing* 14:18–29.

Zorowka, P.G. 1993. Otoacoustic emissions: A new method to diagnose hearing impairment in children. *European Journal of Pediatrics* 152:626–634.

9

Central Testing

Gail D. Chermak

MANY children suspected of having central auditory processing disorders (CAPD) are referred to audiologists for evaluation. Thorough assessment of these children is crucial given the potential for communication, learning, and socioemotional problems. The approach to evaluation described in this chapter is consistent with a model of central auditory processing that recognizes the reciprocal relationship between auditory perception and language, and a definition of CAPD that encompasses the concomitant scope of communication and learning deficits. Comprehensive assessment is recommended to determine the neuromaturational status and integrity of the central auditory nervous system and the range of functional difficulties associated with deficits in processing speech and other acoustic signals.

SCOPE AND LIMITATIONS OF THE CHAPTER

AN approach to identifying and assessing CAPD in pediatric populations is described in this chapter. It is divided into sections presenting tests and procedures useful for screening and evaluating specific age groups, from neonates to school-age children. Results of tests and procedures commonly employed in neuroaudiologic assessment of adults with confirmed neurologic lesions are briefly reviewed before describing outcomes obtained from children with CAPD who were administered similar tasks. Current clinical use and future application of electrophysiologic measures and brain imaging procedures are also discussed.

The tests presented do not represent an exhaustive compilation; rather, they offer examples of more widely researched and more frequently used clinical assessment tools. No attempt is made to study the neuroanatomy of the auditory system. The reader is advised to consult sources and become familiar with the anatomy, physiology, and neuromaturation of the auditory system before undertaking assessment of central auditory function. Furthermore, the reader will not find specific instructions regarding administration of the tests reviewed. To obtain these instructions, the reader is referred to the original references in the scientific literature, test manuals, and chapters of text books devoted to this subject (e.g., Katz 1994; Keith 1977; Lasky and Katz 1983; Pinheiro and Musiek 1985).

DEFINITION AND PROFILE OF CAPD

CENTRAL auditory processing disorders "are deficits in the information processing of audible signals not attributed to impaired peripheral hearing sensitivity or intellectual impairment" (ASHA 1992). CAPDs disrupt the continuous auditory processing of acoustic, phonetic, and linguistic information and affect information processing from sound reception to discourse understanding. Given the potential magnitude of disruption, diverse functional deficits are often observed in children with CAPD. These include difficulty comprehending speech in backgrounds of noise or competing speech, distractibility, inattentiveness, difficulty understanding verbal directions, reduced memory, and associated reading difficulties due to auditory-phonetic confusions (ASHA 1992; Chermak and Musiek 1992; Musiek and Geurkink 1980; Willeford 1985; Willeford and Burleigh 1985). In addition to listening and learning problems, children with CAPD often experience social difficulties, ranging from withdrawal to aggression, in adjusting to their everyday environments (Willeford and Burleigh 1985).

Auditory Perceptual Versus Linguistic Deficit

That children with CAPD demonstrate both auditory perceptual and auditory-language processing deficits is undisputed. Besides deficits in dichotic listening, selective attention, and temporal processing, children with CAPD often present deficits in auditory memory and sound blending. Unresolved, however, is whether auditory processing deficits either underlie or reflect language disorders. Research suggests that new assessment strategies may clarify the relationships among auditory processing, cognitive, and linguistic deficits (Campbell and McNeil 1985; Chermak, Vonhof, and Bendel 1989; J. Jerger et al. 1991; S. Jerger, Johnson, and Loiselle 1988; S. Jerger, Martin, and J. Jerger 1987; Tobey and Cullen 1984).

Findings of normal performance on a speech task presented with ipsilateral competition, with depressed performance on the contralateral competing condition, in children with confirmed lesions of the central auditory nervous system, are known in children suspected of CAPD. Hence, S. Jerger, Johnson, and Loiselle (1988) concluded that auditory perceptual processing deficits rather than linguistic processing deficits underlie CAPD. S. Jerger, Martin, and J. Jerger (1987) reported a general pattern of audiologic and language results consistent with an auditory-phonologic processing disorder as opposed to a linguistic-cognitive deficit in a child with learning disability. Similarly, increased susceptibility to masking regardless of linguistic content led Chermak et al. (1989) to posit an acoustic-phonetic basis for auditory-language deficits presented by adults with learning disabilities.

Model of Central Auditory Processing

The suggested approach to assessment, elaborated in a subsequent section, corresponds to an emerging model of central auditory processing that invokes both bottom-up and top-down processes involving parallel and interactive networks (Churchland and Sejnowski 1988; Massaro 1987; Warren 1983). Bottom-up and top-down processes are regarded as complementary; context (top-down) guides acoustic and phonetic analysis with constraints supplied by reciprocal input from bottom-up information sources (Cole and Jakimak 1980; Cutler and Norris 1988; Luce 1986; Marlsen-Wilson 1987; McClellend and Elman 1986). Listening and situational demands generally determine the relative role of bottom-up and top-down processes for message resolution. For individuals with CAPD, internal distortions degrade the auditory signal to the degree that top-down processing typically predominates in most listening situations, particularly those in which complex linguistic and cognitive demands are coupled with background noise.

Historical View

Although central auditory testing of adults with neurologic impairments has a rather extensive history, assessment of central auditory processing in children has gained momentum only in more recent years as efforts to understand and remediate learning disabilities (LD) have intensified. The behavioral profiles of children with CAPD, LD, and Attention-Deficit Hyperactivity Disorder (ADHD) often overlap, as might be expected given the complex interactions among auditory processing, language skills, cognition, and learning. Children with CAPD, LD, and ADHD often exhibit listening and learning problems despite normal intelligence, normal peripheral hearing sensitivity, and characteristically unremarkable neurologic findings. Poor academic performance is the major complaint of parents of children with CAPD (Willeford 1985), and many children with CAPD are enrolled in special education programs (ASHA 1993). CAPD, LD, and ADHD are not necessarily concomitant, however; not all children with language impairment, learning disability, or hyperactivity exhibit CAPD. Thorough assessment can lead to differentiation of these related conditions as well as refine therapeutic efforts.

EVOLVING TEST MATERIALS AND PROCEDURES

MANY investigations have shown less efficient auditory processing in children relative to adults, associated with maturational differences (as well as peripheral processing differences) in neural and linguistic development and response strategies (Allen et al. 1989; Elliott 1986; Elliott and Hammer 1988; Hall and Grose 1990, 1991; Maxon and Hochberg 1982; Musiek, Baran, and Pinheiro 1990; Musiek, Verkest, and Gollegly 1988; Sussman 1991; Werner 1992; Willeford 1977). Depending on the task, significant improvements in performance have been observed through age twelve years, the age at which human auditory pathway maturation is probably completed. Early pediatric evaluative efforts relied on central auditory tests developed for adults, with norms adjusted for normal developmental differences (Keith and Jerger 1991). However, given the multiplicity of factors underlying performance differences between children and adults, it is unlikely that simply renorming tests designed for adults will ensure adequate assessment of central auditory and auditory-language skills in children.

Some evaluative efforts have incorporated central auditory tests developed specifically for the pediatric population (Cherry 1980; S. Jerger and J. Jerger 1984; Keith 1986). These tests are constructed to minimize linguistic-cognitive demands while emphasizing auditory perceptual demands (Keith 1981a). Notwithstanding the use of tests designed for children, maturation and task variables complicate interpretation of central auditory test results obtained from children. Hence, interpreting these results may require invoking a maturational model rather than an adult, neural lesion model.

Objectives of Central Auditory Assessment with Children

A fairly standard test battery is used for assessment of the adult central auditory nervous system; however, a comparable battery of tests proven efficient for assessment of central auditory function in children is less well established. This situation may be related to differences in assessment objectives. Neuroaudiologic assessment with adults is directed to detecting and localizing lesions. The objectives of central auditory assessment in children, however, are to ascertain neuromaturational status and the functional integrity of the central auditory nervous system as it relates to the child's communication, academic, and social skills. Although positive neurologic findings in children with CAPD are uncommon, a small percentage of these children may have diffuse neurological involvement or actual lesions of the central auditory nervous system that may be disclosed through extensive assessment. Indeed, comprehensive central auditory test batteries may elucidate a neural basis for a CAPD as revealed by depressed performance patterns implicating hemispheric, brainstem, or interhemispheric dysfunction (S. Jerger, Johnson, and Loiselle 1988; Musiek, Gollegly, and Baran 1984a, b).

The clinician must not risk overlooking a serious medical problem. Cortical or subcortical dysfunction, secondary to maturational lag or neurodevelopmental morphological abnormality, may underlie CAPD in children (Galaburda et al. 1985; S. Jerger 1987; S. Jerger et al. 1988; Musiek et al. 1984, 1985). Lesion or dysfunction of the efferent system—and, in particular, the olivocochlear bundle—may influence selective listening deficits commonly observed in children with CAPD (Musiek and Chermak 1995). Although the possibility for physiologic abnormality may be small, children suspected of CAPD should receive a medical examination concurrent with the audiologic evaluation.

Comprehensive Assessment

The broad objectives of central auditory assessment in children and the complex interactions among auditory perception, cognition, and language require inclusion of tests of auditory perception and auditory-language processing in the pediatric central auditory battery. These must be preceded by a detailed case history and a basic audiologic evaluation of peripheral function. The range and wide intersubject variability of deficits often involved in CAPD (Ferre and Wilber 1986) warrant a comprehensive test battery to ensure accurate diagnosis and understanding of the functional deficits and to appropriately plan remediation.

Examination of auditory processing in the absence of substantial language processing demands is necessary to determine the integrity of the central auditory nervous system (Keith 1981b). Language variables can complicate interpretation of central auditory test results. Hence, central auditory tests employing nonspeech (e.g., tonal) stimuli or familiar language should be used to challenge the basic functions of the central auditory nervous system. However, the additional inclusion of speech tests is warranted to assess better the range of auditory perceptual and functional deficits and to direct intervention.

Tests involving more substantial language manipulation allow examination of processing of the complex signal that underlies functional deficits in academic and social contexts. Hence, language-based tests should also be administered to more fully understand the impact of CAPD for listening, communication, learning, and social functions. In fact, sensitized speech tests (e.g., low-pass-filtered speech, time-compressed speech, speech in noise) were among the first tools used to detect and localize central auditory lesions in adults. They remain among the more sensitive indicators of central auditory nervous system integrity.

Given the symptoms of CAPD, clients should be referred to the speech-language pathologist for administration of auditory-language tests. An extensive language assessment should be completed because CAPD can affect the general development of language (Sloan 1980). Results of metalanguage tests are particularly relevant to diagnosis and management of children with CAPD. Evaluating metalinguistic skills (e.g., auditory memory, auditory sequencing, auditory association, and phonemic synthesis or sound blending) may reveal a basis for observed or reported functional deficits affecting communicative, academic, and social behaviors (Katz 1983; Willeford and Billger 1985; Willeford and Burleigh 1985). The reader is cautioned that measurement of individual metalinguistic skills in isolation is difficult because many skills share the common underlying processes of attention and discrimination (Keith 1981b; Witkin 1971). However, patterns of performance across metalinguistic tests may indicate underlying deficits pertinent to the global functions of listening and classroom performance.

The audiologist may also request neuropsychological evaluation to estimate the relative contributions of cognitive factors to functional difficulties. Neuropsychological evaluation is particularly relevant to the differential diagnosis of CAPD, LD, and ADHD.

Behavioral tests generally reveal functional processing deficits. In contrast, measures of electrophysiologic function (see chapter 7) reveal the integrity and capacity of the central auditory nervous system and may confirm level or site of lesion (Musiek and Gollegly 1988). Indeed, electrophysiologic tests may be more sensitive to certain lesions of the central auditory nervous system than any available behavioral test (Baran and Musiek 1991). This is the case for the auditory brainstem response (ABR), which is highly sensitive to brainstem lesions (Hall 1992). Reports suggest that P300, an endogenous, late auditory event-related potential reflecting active cognitive processes, may provide a measure of high level auditory processing deficits (Jirsa and Clontz 1990; Musiek, Baran, and Pinheiro 1992; Squires and Hecox 1983).

An unintended consequence of examining various auditory perceptual and auditory-language processes in children presenting heterogeneous manifestations of CAPD may be a considerable degree of overlap in test results for normal subjects and those suspected of CAPD (Berrick et al. 1984; Musiek, Geurkink, and Keitel 1982). No single test has proven efficient in detecting and differentiating CAPD due, in part, to the dispersion and overlap of scores between normal and suspected CAPD subjects (Keith and Jerger 1991). Moreover, given the complexity of the central auditory nervous system, it is unlikely that any one behavioral test can be considered the definitive test of central auditory function. Hence, a comprehensive pediatric central auditory evaluation requires a battery of tests to determine neuromaturational status of the central auditory nervous system, as well as auditory perceptual and auditory-language abilities. This scope of testing requires the coordinated efforts of audiologists and speech-language pathologists, with referral to allied professionals as needed.

Case History

A complete case history with controlled observation in settings associated with difficulties should precede behavioral tests and electrophysiologic measures. Findings of the case history may not only suggest inclusion of particular tests in the battery but also offer a context for interpreting results and suggest management strategies.

Questions posed during history taking should include information about the family; the mother's pregnancy and conditions at birth; the child's growth,

physical development, and medical history; motor coordination and visual perception; speech, language, and social development; hearing and auditory behavior; and educational progress. Questions should reveal the parents' and other in-
formants' primary concerns. The examiner should be alerted to the possibility of
central auditory nervous system dysfunction if high risk factors for neurologic
disorder are revealed (e.g., genetic, biologic, or prenatal factors; trauma, and so
on). Willeford and Burleigh (1985) provide an excellent discussion of information gathering in cases of suspected CAPD and offer a model case history form.

Uses and Limitations of Standardized Tests

Standardized test protocols and normative data facilitate interpretation of the
substantial variability in performance observed across children, even of the same
age. Standardized tests offer the audiologist a means of distinguishing the per-
formances of individuals and determining normality. However, they may not
offer the flexibility needed to assess some difficult-to-test patients. Moreover,
normative data may not be appropriate to a particular patient because of linguistic, cultural, experiential, or other factors (Musiek and Chermak 1995),
thereby precluding the objective interpretation of test results. For example, testing nonnative speakers of English using English language materials is likely to
yield scores reflecting language ability rather than central auditory function.
Local norms should be established for CAPD tests to control for test recording,
equipment, administration, and environmental variables, in addition to differences among patients (Kreul et al. 1968; Musiek and Chermak 1995).

Standardized tests are also limited in that, by design, they are constructed
only to determine the adequacy of an individual's performance relative to the
performance of normal peers (Salvia and Ysseldyke 1981). Determining actual
skill level and gaining more explicit information regarding the ramifications of
CAPD in a particular domain require the use of criterion-referenced tests and
verbal or qualitative descriptions derived from systematic observation or informed report by parents and teachers.

DIFFERENTIAL DIAGNOSIS OF CAPD, ADHD,
AND LEARNING DISABILITIES

CAPDS are often associated with learning disabilities (LD) and ADHD, although visual perceptual deficits may also underlie LD (Boder 1973; Kaufman 1980; Willows, Kershner, and Corcos 1986). Differential diagnosis of these
conditions is challenging given similar deficit profiles, which include inattention,
poor listening skills, distractibility, and inappropriate social behavior (American
Psychiatric Association 1987; Keller 1992; Willeford and Burleigh 1985). Moreover, these conditions are not mutually exclusive: Children may display CAPD,
ADHD, and LD (Katz 1992; Keith 1986; Keller 1992; Newhoff et al. 1992).

Similarities in behavioral manifestations have led some to question whether CAPD, ADHD, and LD reflect a single developmental disorder (Burd and Fisher 1986; Gascon, Johnson, and Burd 1986). Even if these conditions were shown to reflect differences in expression of a common disorder, professionals would still be required to evaluate the integrity of underlying systems and determine the predominant deficits to inform remediation planning. Identification of the primary deficits and conditions underlying academic and social problems is possible through multidisciplinary assessment.

ADHD is a medical diagnosis that is usually confirmed through positive reaction to stimulant medication prescribed to reduce behavioral sequelae. Characteristically, children with ADHD are inattentive, impulsive, and hyperactive. Their attention deficits are pervasive, impacting all sensory modalities. In contrast, children with CAPD typically experience attention deficits restricted to the auditory modality. Further, although children with CAPD and ADHD may experience similar behavioral sequelae, several behaviors are most often restricted to children with ADHD. For example, difficulty waiting one's turn, problems playing quietly, and excessive talking more often characterize children with ADHD rather than CAPD. Similarly, severe socioemotional sequelae (e.g., conduct disorders, juvenile delinquency) are more common among children with ADHD (Newhoff et al. 1992).

Identification of the primary factors underlying listening, learning, and social problems in children requires careful observation of the child, parent and teacher input, and multidisciplinary assessment, including the perspectives of the physician and the psychologist. A comprehensive test battery must be employed to measure the range of behavioral sequelae noted previously, in addition to auditory perception and auditory-language processing. Moreover, appraisal of visual and tactile processing can determine the breadth of processing deficits and potentially reveal a pervasive perceptual deficit that would suggest involvements beyond the auditory system and thereby help in differentiating CAPD and ADHD.

Assessment Strategy

Perception of speech is fairly easy for those with both normal peripheral hearing and central auditory function. Ease of perception is possible due to the redundancy of the speech signal at both acoustic and linguistic levels (Cooper et al. 1952; Liberman 1970). This is coupled with the intrinsic redundancy of the central auditory nervous system due partially to multiple and parallel pathways, interhemispheric communication, and bilateral representation of the auditory system. To expose lesions or processing insufficiencies in this redundant system, materials of low extrinsic (i.e., acoustic or linguistic) redundancy must be presented in ways that tax the auditory system. Tests employing low redundancy stimuli, delivered in formats that strain the central auditory nervous system, are most likely to identify individuals for whom intrinsic neural redundancy has been compromised through lesion or dysfunction (Bocca et al. 1954, 1955; Kimura 1964; Matzker 1962; Teatini 1970). Decreasing the extrinsic redundancy of the speech signal can be done in several ways (e.g., electronic filtering, time compression, presentation with competing signals).

Brain Imaging

In addition to behavioral and electrophysiologic assessment techniques, brain imaging studies hold promise for assessing central auditory processing in children. Given the potential for revealing underlying brain dysfunction and confirming audiologic outcomes, brain imaging technology has been applied to the study of children with CAPD and other conditions presumed related to dysfunction of the central nervous system. This technology may significantly increase our understanding of the brain and transform clinical neurodiagnostic procedures.

Computerized axial tomography (CAT) and magnetic resonance imaging (MRI) reveal the anatomic or structural integrity of the brain. On the basis of CAT scans, Hier et al. (1978) and Rosenberger and Hier (1980) reported—in children diagnosed as dyslexic—reversals of hemispheric asymmetries typically observed in normal right-handed individuals. CAT scans may reveal neoplastic or epileptic disorders associated with a few children with CAPD (Musiek, Gollegly, and Ross 1985).

MRI has quickly become the method of choice for imaging acoustic tumors (Curati et al. 1986; Mikhael, Ciric, and Wolff 1987) and has also been applied in research involving children with learning disabilities (Hynd, Semrud-Clikeman, and Lyytinen 1991). MRI studies revealed that brain regions implicated in language and the regulation of attention and motor control (e.g., corpus callosum, basal ganglia) were smaller in brains of children with dyslexia relative to those of normal children (Hynd and Semrud-Clikeman 1989).

Positron-emission tomography (PET) and single-photon-emission computed tomography (SPECT) offer a window on brain function, mapping of regional cerebral blood flow, metabolic activity, and distribution of specific receptors (Frumkin et al. 1989). Although audiologists and speech-language pathologists will not likely perform or interpret CAT, MRI, PET, or SPECT neurodiagnostic techniques, brain electrical activity mapping (BEAM) may become a clinical tool in the neuroaudiologic test battery. These procedures provide insights regarding CAPD and other conditions with suspected or confirmed involvement of the central auditory nervous system (Finitzo and Pool 1987).

BEAM provides a topographic approach to quantifying electrophysiologic activity in the brain. BEAM allows the visualization of voltage distributions of evoked potentials at specific latencies, providing a dynamic measure of brain metabolism and blood flow (Finitzo and Pool 1987). The topography of the auditory brainstem response and the middle-latency response has been described using brain mapping techniques (Grandori 1986; Kraus and McGee 1988). Using BEAM, Duffy et al. (1980) identified differences in electrical activity in the left temporal, left parietal, and medial frontal regions of the brains of children diagnosed with dyslexia, relative to normal-reading counterparts. Although brain imaging may eventually offer evidence revealing static or active neurologic abnormalities underlying CAPD in some children, behavioral and electrophysiologic measures will continue to provide corroborating evidence. Moreover, behavioral tests will remain essential, offering controlled measures of functional deficits and playing a primary role in bridging between assessment and intervention.

Test Battery

SELECTED tests useful in the identification and assessment of CAPD in children appear in Table 9.1. In contrast to some other tables (Barr 1976; Dempsey 1983; Keith 1988; Willeford and Billger 1985), here tests are categorized according to their primary focus on auditory perception or auditory language. Tests of auditory perception (i.e., tests of binaural integration [synthesis], binaural separation, and resistance to distortion [e.g., speech in noise or selective attention]) are distinguished from tests of metalanguage (e.g., sound blending, auditory association, auditory closure, auditory memory). Application and reporting of results consistent with this distinction should benefit our patients by precisely illuminating underlying capacity of the central auditory nervous system apart from language skills, and clarify our understanding of the relationships among auditory processing, language, and cognition.

Selecting tests for assessing CAPD is a complex matter. The heterogeneous nature of CAPD and the various abilities of children require that a customized battery of tests be chosen to ascertain the neuromaturational status and integrity

Table 9.1. Tests Used to Identify and Assess Central Auditory Processing Disorders

BASIC AUDIOLOGIC EVALUATION: Pure Tone Thresholds; Aural Acoustic Immittance Measurement; Speech Recognition Performance Intensity Functions

ELECTROPHYSIOLOGIC MEASURES: Acoustic Reflex; Auditory Brainstem Response (ABR); Middle-Latency Response (MLR); Late-Latency Response (LLR); Event-Related Evoked Potentials (P300)

AUDITORY PERCEPTION: Brief Tone Audiometry; Competing Environmental Sounds (CES); Dichotic Chords; Dichotic CVs; Dichotic Digits; Dichotic Sentence Identification (DSI); Duration Pattern Perception; Flowers' Auditory Test of Selective Attention; Flowers-Costello Test of Auditory Abilities; Masking Level Differences (MLD); Pediatric Speech Intelligibility (PSI); Pitch Patterns Sequence (PPS); Repetition Test (Tallal); Screening Test for Auditory Processing Disorders (SCAN); Selective Auditory Attention Test (SAAT); Speech Perception In Noise (SPIN); Staggered Spondaic Word Test (SSW); Synthetic Sentence Identification (SSI); Time Compressed Speech (TC); Wepman Auditory Discrimination

METALANGUAGE: Analysis of the Language of Learning; Auditory Conceptualization Test (LAC); Clinical Evaluation of Language Fundamentals—Revised; Denver Auditory Phoneme Sequencing Test; Goldman-Fristoe-Woodcock Auditory Skills Test Battery; Language Processing Test; Phonemic Synthesis; Revised Token Test; Test of Auditory-Perceptual Skills (TAPS); Test of Language Competence; Test of Word Knowledge; Word Test of the central nervous system and clarify functional deficits. Several general issues should be considered in selecting tests.

Test Sensitivity and Specificity

The central auditory test battery should be composed of tests with high efficiency (S. Jerger and J. Jerger 1983; Musiek et al. 1992; Turner and Nielsen 1984). A test's overall efficiency in identifying CAPD is determined by its sensitivity, a measure of a test's ability to reveal abnormality (when abnormality exists of the type the test is designed to detect) and specificity, a measure of a test's ability to reveal normality (when no abnormality exists of the type the test was designed to detect) (S. Jerger 1983; Turner and Nielsen 1984). Unfortunately, data regarding the efficiency of central auditory tests are not always reported in accompanying manuals or in the published literature.

Test Reliability

Test-retest consistency is essential, particularly when monitoring changes in the same patient over time. In children, neuromaturation mediates changes in brain function; therefore, age-appropriate norms must be established.

Ease of Administration

Tests requiring considerable client practice or time to administer and score may not be clinically feasible.

Comprehensive Assessment

Given the complexity and redundancy of the central auditory nervous system, a test battery should consist of sensitive tests assessing a variety of auditory processes. A degree of redundancy offers corroborating evidence. However, two tests that are similar in protocol and task demands are not likely to provide new and clinically useful information needed to confirm a central auditory processing disorder.

Ideally, selected tests should provide insight regarding the processes of binaural separation, binaural integration, and interhemispheric transfer, and incorporate tasks requiring dichotic and temporal processing as well as processing of monotic low-redundancy input (Musiek and Chermak 1995; Musiek and Geurkink 1980). Speech perception depends on precise processing of rapidly presented transient acoustic patterns embedded in the speech signal (Fujisaki, Nakamura, and Imoto 1975; Hirsh 1959). Measures of temporal processing reveal dysfunction at the level of the brainstem (e.g., masking level differences) and the cortex (e.g., pitch and duration patterns) (Bornstein and Musiek 1984; J. Jerger et al. 1969; Musiek and Baran 1987; Pinheiro and Musiek 1985; Swisher and Hirsh 1972). Inclusion of a dichotic listening task can allow differentiation of brainstem from hemispheric dysfunction or lesion. When interpreted in the context of results from a monotic low-redundancy test, it can facilitate differentiation of hemispheric dysfunction or lesion from that of the corpus callosum involving interhemispheric transfer (Musiek, Gollegly, and Baran 1984a, b).

Electrophysiologic measures should also be considered for inclusion in the test battery because they allow examination of central auditory capacity without the confounding influence of linguistic variables. Further, electrophysiologic measures offer the power to detect some lesions with greater sensitivity than behavioral tests.

POPULATION CHARACTERISTICS

TEST batteries should be tailored to the client's age, ability, and suspected dysfunction. Tests must be examined for vocabulary level and complexity of sentence structure as well as cognitive level required to perform the task (S. Jerger and J. Jerger 1984). Similarly, response mode (e.g., verbalization versus picture pointing) must be considered.

Individualized test selection is underscored by the diversity of our case load. Testing nonnative speakers of English and non-English speaking persons requires adaptations such as those requisite to testing children. Thus, an appropriate battery with nonnative and non-English speaking adults must rely on tests involving tonal targets (e.g., frequency and duration patterns, masking level differences) and electrophysiologic measures rather than English speech materials to assess auditory processing skills independently of language skills. Care must be taken to ensure that test instructions are understood before administering tests. If speech materials are to be used, they must be translated and recorded using high quality techniques and normed using an appropriate control population. The importance of renorming is critical: Translated versions may not be equivalent to the original tests in difficulty level or efficiency (Musiek and Chermak 1995).

Peripheral Hearing Sensitivity

CAPD may occur with peripheral hearing impairment. Indeed, the central auditory nervous system and the auditory periphery form a critical interdependency (Musiek 1989). Functional changes in the central auditory nervous system, including tonotopic reorganization and loss of central inhibition, may result from cochlear damage (Robertson and Irvine 1989; Willot, Demuth, and Lu 1984).

Further, studies of transsynaptic degeneration reveal degeneration of fibers in the central auditory nervous system after deprivation of peripheral input (Morest 1983; Webster and Webster 1977).

Interactions between a central auditory processing deficit and peripherally degraded auditory input can influence the outcomes of central auditory tests. Therefore, peripheral impairments must be quantified before central auditory assessment (Baran and Musiek 1991). Immittance measurement must also be included in the basic audiologic test battery due to the presumed relationship between reversible, mild-to-moderate fluctuant hearing loss associated with otitis media and CAPD (Feagans et al. 1987; Gravel and Wallace 1992; Gunnarson and Finitzo 1991; S. Jerger et al. 1983; Roberts et al. 1991).

Evaluation of central auditory processing abilities is more difficult when confounded by peripheral hearing loss, particularly when the hearing impairment is asymmetrical and greater than mild in severity. Frequency and duration pattern tests and dichotic digit, word, and sentence tests, however, are less influenced by sensory hearing loss (Fifer et al. 1983; Speaks, Niccum, and Van Tassel 1985). They may be preferred when assessing central auditory function in clients with peripheral hearing impairment.

Interpretation of Tests

The immature brain demonstrates plasticity and is capable of functional reorganization that may minimize severity of deficits associated with lesions (Aoki and Siekevitz 1988; Musiek, Lenz, and Gollegly 1991). Evidence has accumulated, however, suggesting that the behavioral auditory manifestations of childhood and adult brain lesions may not differ significantly (Bergman et al.1984; Goodglass 1967; S. Jerger 1987; S. Jerger, Martin, and J. Jerger 1987; S. Jerger and Zeller 1989; Nass 1984; Pohl 1979). This similarity suggests that outcomes of central auditory tests administered to children may be interpreted according to principles guiding interpretation of corresponding results in adults, even though the database of auditory test results in children with confirmed central auditory lesions and suspected CAPD is limited (Keith and Jerger 1991). Until this database expands sufficiently to confirm the relationship between central auditory test results and functional deficits that characterize CAPD in children, we are unable to exclude the possibility of active neural lesion (S. Jerger 1987; S. Jerger, Johnson, and Loiselle 1988; Musiek, Gollegly, and Ross 1985), diffuse neuromaturational disorder, or maturational delay (Keith 1983) as the basis for observed functional deficits in children (Keith and Jerger 1991). In interpreting results obtained on the Staggered Spondaic Word (SSW) test, Keith (1983) suggested that central auditory test results obtained from children were more likely an expression of maturational level than neural lesion. Similarly, depressed performance on binaural fusion tasks and reduced masking level differences in children may reflect immaturity of the central auditory nervous system (Hall and

Grose 1990; Roush and Tait 1984). Perhaps brain imaging techniques that offer unique opportunities to visualize brain function will allow differentiation of central auditory nervous system lesions from neurodevelopmental abnormalities or maturational delays.

Use of Test Data

Selection of tests should also be guided by the intended use of the results. In addition to ascertaining the integrity of the central auditory nervous system and quantifying functional deficits requiring treatment, data derived from behavioral tests provide for monitoring of neuromaturational development and recovery of function and also offer a framework for counseling. Particular tests of comparable efficiency may be preferred for differential diagnosis and monitoring disease progression or recovery; other tests may be deemed more useful in revealing functional deficits, guiding intervention planning, and framing counseling efforts. For example, measurement of masking level differences and selective attention may each provide useful diagnostic insight. Masking level differences reveal binaural synthesis and reflect brainstem integrity, whereas tests of selective attention reveal resistance to distortion, which reflects the integrity of the cortex. However, given the abstract nature of the paradigm and the absence of an everyday listening analog, masking level differences offer less useful data for counseling parents. Because selective and divided attention tasks reflect everyday functional problems, results from these tests can aid the counseling process and offer insight for auditory and educational management.

Given the usually unremarkable neurologic findings in pediatric CAPD, the ultimate use of central auditory test results with children is to confirm functional deficits to determine appropriate strategies for management. Remedial programs cannot be formulated based on test results alone, however. Studies report a lack of correlation among depressed performance on tests of auditory perception, metalanguage, and reading skills in learning disabled children (Matkin and Hook 1983; Tobey and Cullen 1984). The reader is referred to Chermak and Musiek (1992) and Katz (1992) for discussions about the use and limitations of central auditory test data for therapeutic intervention.

SCREENING FOR CENTRAL AUDITORY PROCESSING DISORDERS

THE objective of screening is the early identification of a condition in asymptomatic individuals (World Health Organization 1971). Early detection of CAPD is essential to ensure timely intervention to minimize distress and maximize communicative, educational, and social function. Screening for this condition may be redundant, however, because children with CAPD typically experience problems that result in referrals to audiologists and speech-language pathologists and will be administered a comprehensive diagnostic test battery to determine the nature of the processing deficits (Stach 1992). Even so, screening for CAPD may be useful because results are used to direct subsequent assessment efforts. Given the complex relationships among CAPD and attention deficits, language disorders, and learning disabilities (Gascon, Johnson, and Burd 1986), an alternative, but appropriate, use of a screening test for CAPD might be to identify symptoms for further exploration using auditory, language, neuropsychological, and psychoeducational tests. In this way, the influence of nonauditory factors of attention and language may be parceled out, permitting examination of central auditory perceptual function.

ASSESSMENT OF CENTRAL AUDITORY PROCESSING DISORDERS: NEONATE, INFANT, AND TODDLER

EARLY identification and evaluation of CAPD and aggressive intervention are critical given the potentially serious consequences for learning, socioemotional adjustment, and economic potential. Clearly, identification and evaluation of CAPD are important to successful management, as shown by work revealing the functional plasticity of the maturing central nervous system and consequent opportunity for functional change if intervention is initiated early (Aoki and Siekevitz 1988; Hassmannova, Myslivecek, and Novakova 1981; Kalil 1989; Rauschecker and Marler 1987; Schlaggar and O'Leary 1991). Moreover, federal legislation (i.e., PL 94-142, PL 99-457) mandates early education of infants and children with disabilities. Nevertheless, detection and assessment of CAPD in infants and toddlers is not possible.

Ideally, auditory screening should detect abnormalities at all levels of the auditory system. Because neurologic deficits are common among babies born with peripheral hearing impairments (D'Souza et al. 1981; Gerber, Wile, and Hamai 1985; Hubatch et al. 1985), assessing dysfunction at more central levels of the auditory nervous system should be conducted along with peripheral screening. However, accepted neonatal hearing screening methods (e.g., auditory brainstem responses, transient-evoked otoacoustic emissions) are limited to detection of hearing impairment and neural dysfunction up to the level of the brainstem. Moreover, behavioral screening or assessment of neonates, infants, and toddlers is complicated by developmental and maturational limitations, making diagnosis subject to confounding variables including false positive responses and observer bias (Bench et al. 1976; Wilson and Thompson 1984). Commonly employed behavioral tests of central auditory processing (e.g., auditory discrimination and selective auditory attention) and check list and performance scales are inappropriate for infants and toddlers due to task demands and the nature of performance scale probes. Even when techniques become available, access to neonates will remain a problem unless mandated statewide hearing screening programs are implemented across the nation (Blake and Hall 1990; NIH 1993).

Until specific instruments or physiologic measures are developed to identify

CAPD in neonates and infants, any baby deemed at risk for central nervous system damage due to genetic, biological, or prenatal factors as well as adventitious diseases, trauma, or exposure to toxic substances associated with adverse developmental outcomes should be monitored closely for early signs of CAPD, including speech and language developmental delays and other minimal or equivocal (soft) signs of neurologic dysfunction or damage (e.g., delayed motor milestones, awkward gait, difficulties with fine motor coordination). The reader is cautioned, though, that soft signs may also be interpreted as evidence of neurologic immaturity (Schmitt 1975) because they are common in normal children under the age of seven years (Kinsbourne 1973).

Periodic and systematic observation of behaviors of at-risk infants must be conducted throughout early childhood to ascertain whether growth and development are following expected patterns. Integrated assessment of cognition, communication, motor abilities, sensory functions, and socioemotional development should be undertaken if a developmental problem is suspected. Although specific diagnosis of CAPD has not been possible, several behavioral, neurobehavioral, and electrophysiologic measures may suggest immaturity or dysfunction of the central nervous system or central auditory pathways.

Behavioral and Neurobehavioral Approaches to Assessment

Babies who fail behavioral screenings but have normal peripheral hearing may suffer from neurologic deficits that may manifest as a CAPD or learning disability (Mencher 1985). Unusual or abnormal behavioral responses to sound, such as failure to habituate to sound and hypersensitivity to sound, may suggest central auditory dysfunction. Absence of auditory reflexes (e.g., startle reflex, auropalpebral reflex) to sound of moderate intensity, despite normal hearing sensitivity, may also implicate central dysfunction (Northern and Downs 1991).

The Visually Reinforced Infant Speech Discrimination (VRISD) paradigm may offer a behavioral approach to investigating central auditory function in infants and toddlers (Eilers, Wilson, and Moore 1977). The VRISD paradigm applies the operant conditioning paradigm of visual reinforcement audiometry to assess infants' speech perception. Using this paradigm, Diefendorf (1981) found binaural fusion in six- to eight-month-old infants. Because binaural fusion reflects the capacity of the brainstem, the VRISD paradigm may offer clinical possibilities for identifying and assessing potential central auditory processing disorders in infants as young as six months.

Neurobehavioral assessment of newborns and infants provides a window on the maturity and integrity of the central nervous system. The Neonatal Behavioral Assessment Scale (Brazelton 1984) measures a newborn's coping and organizational capacities in interacting with the environment. Attention and orientation, self-regulation, motor status, and autonomic stability are assessed through behavioral and reflexive probes. The Bayley Scales of Infant Development (Bayley

1969) are a standardized measure of development appropriate for infants and toddlers between two and thirty months of age. The BSID probes cognition, motor abilities, and behavioral and temperamental characteristics, furnishing an indication of an infant's current developmental status.

Early language can be assessed using the Sequenced Inventory of Communication Development-Revised, SICD-R (Hedrick, Prather, and Tobin 1984). The SICD-R explores—through parental report and direct observation of the child's responses to test stimuli— receptive and expressive communication milestones attained by normally developing children between four months and four years of age.

Unfortunately, measures derived from these neurobehavioral scales show poor predictive validity. The scales reflect current developmental status rather than predict later development (Bornstein and Sigman 1986; Brooks-Gunn and Lewis 1983; Cohen and Parmelee 1983; Honzik 1976; McCall 1983; Thoman and Becker 1979). The poor predictability of early infant scales may be due to the discontinuity of the developmental process; qualitative differences in the nature of intelligence between infants and children, developing from primarily nonverbal and nonsymbolic to highly verbal and symbolic; and the influence of social and environmental factors on development. Clearly, neurobehavioral assessment does not specifically diagnose CAPD and has limited prognostic value related to later emerging listening, learning, and social problems. Limitations of infant assessment scales underscore the need for periodic follow-up.

Electrophysiologic Assessment

Electrophysiologic investigation of central auditory processing in infants may offer an opportunity to detect and evaluate brain dysfunction underlying later emerging CAPD (Duffy et al. 1979; Hynd et al. 1990; Jirsa 1992; Jirsa and Clontz 1990; Stach, Loiselle, and Jerger 1988). Electrophysiologic responses are independent of the subject's linguistic skill and, except for late-evoked responses, do not demand cognitive processing of sound.

The acoustic reflex (see chapter 6) has proven useful in the adult neuro-audiologic test battery due to the fact that normal stapedius reflex activity in response to acoustic stimuli is contingent upon the integrity of the afferent, brainstem, and efferent pathways (J. Jerger and Northern 1980). Besides its sensitivity to sensory hearing loss, the acoustic reflex can provide information concerning the presence of auditory disorder at the level of the brainstem through comparison of ipsilateral to contralateral acoustic reflex thresholds (Greisen and Rasmussen 1970; J. Jerger, Burney, et al. 1974; J. Jerger and S. Jerger 1977). In the presence of brainstem pathology, crossed (contralateral) reflexes are absent, but uncrossed (ipsilateral) reflexes are present (J. Jerger 1975).

Although acoustic reflexes are absent for low-frequency probe tones in many neonates (McMillan et al 1985; Sprague, Wiley, and Goldstein 1985), neonates' acoustic reflex thresholds approximate those of adults for a 1200-Hz probe tone (Bennett and Weatherby 1982). Recording of contralateral acoustic reflexes for a 660-Hz probe tone can be expected in 38 to 63% of neonates (McMillan et al. 1985). Measurement of the acoustic reflex is also highly dependent upon the state of the middle ear and cochlea; therefore, these factors must be considered before interpreting acoustic reflex results (J. Jerger, Anthony et al. 1974; J. Jerger, Burney et al. 1974). Further, acoustic reflexes should be interpreted within the context of other acoustic immittance measurements (ASHA 1990; J. Jerger, Burney et al. 1974; Northern 1981).

Because contralateral suppression of otoacoustic emissions suggests normal function of the efferent system (Berlin et al. 1993; Collet et al. 1990; Mott et al. 1989; Norton 1993), otoacoustic emissions (see chapter 8) may also prove useful in assessing central auditory processing in infants in addition to their application in monitoring cochlear function (Kemp et al. 1986).

The use of evoked potentials (see chapter 7) to complement behavioral procedures for the assessment of central auditory function in children merits attention (Adams et al. 1987; Jirsa 1992; Jirsa and Clontz 1990). The ABR is the most sensitive audiologic test for detection of intra-axial brainstem pathology in adults (Cohen and Prasher 1988). It has been useful also in confirming brainstem neoplasms in children (Nodar, Hahn, and Levine 1980) and in identifying brain dysfunction in children with autism, minimal brain damage, and psychomotor delay (Gillberg, Rosenhall, and Johansson 1983; Sohmer and Student 1978). However, ABR does not appear particularly sensitive to CAPD in children (Roush and Tait 1984; Shimizu and Brown 1981; Worthington 1981) and should not be relied upon to diagnose CAPD.

The utility of the ABR in the assessment of CAPD in children is quite limited due to the low probability with which central nervous system lesions are found in children, unless specific neurologic symptoms are presented (Ferry 1981; Keith 1983; Musiek and Chermak 1995). Since ABR does not reflect neural synchrony above the brainstem, it cannot reveal neural dysfunction at higher levels thought to be involved in CAPD in children. Moreover, ABR may not be sensitive to diffuse brainstem dysfunction that may be involved in CAPD in children. Protti (1983) reported abnormal ABR tracings in only two of thirteen children whose behavioral test results indicated CAPD. Roush and Tait (1984) reported no difference in ABR results between normal children and children with CAPD.

Because their presence requires the integrity of the higher central auditory centers (Picton et al. 1977), middle-latency and late-latency auditory evoked responses offer greater opportunity than early potentials to discern central auditory dysfunction in children. Late-occurring endogenous potentials have been recorded in infants ranging in chronological ages between one and three months (Tokioka, Crowell, and Pierce 1987). Further research is necessary, however, to determine the eventual role of middle- and late-latency potentials in assessing CAPD in infants and toddlers.

ASSESSMENT OF CENTRAL AUDITORY PROCESSING DISORDERS: PRESCHOOL-AGED CHILD

PRESCHOOL-AGED and older children's greater sophistication and abilities ease evaluation of central auditory function. A clinically accepted criterion for CAPD diagnosis is not available, however, and data regarding the efficiency of available screening tests are sparse (Chermak and Montgomery 1992; Chermak, O'Neill, and Seikel 1992; Stach 1992). Testing speech recognition in the presence of background noise or competing speech is a common approach to identifying children with CAPD and learning disabilities (Katz and Wilde 1985; Keith 1981b). Several commercially available test instruments incorporate speech-in-noise testing or performance-intensity functions in the assessment of central auditory function in young children (Cherry 1980; Keith 1986; S. Jerger and J. Jerger 1984).

Screening Instruments

Limited data are available regarding the reliability and validity of two commercially available screening tests for CAPD: the Selective Auditory Attention Test (SAAT) and the SCAN, a Screening Test for Auditory Processing Disorders.

The Selective Auditory Attention Test is a screening instrument developed by Cherry (1980) to help in the identification of young children (aged four to eight years) "whose selective attention deficits may interfere with academic achievement" (p. 1). The SAAT is a brief and intrinsically interesting task for children and can be administered in less than ten minutes in a quiet, well-lighted room using a high-quality tape recorder (Cherry 1980; Sanderson-Leepa and Rintelmann 1976). The SAAT is a closed-set word identification test that uses new recordings of the four 25-monosyllabic-word lists of the Word Intelligibility by Picture Identification (WIPI) test (Ross and Lerman 1971). The SAAT employs two lists of the WIPI, one list in quiet and one in a competing speech (story) background, under earphones or sound field. The target words and the competing story (message-to-competition ratio of 0 dB) are presented by the same male talker. The child is instructed to point to the picture corresponding to the target word. Performance on the list presented in quiet assesses auditory discrimination; performance on the list presented against the competing speech background reflects selective auditory attention ability (Chermak and Montgomery 1992).

Unfortunately, only limited psychometric data are available for the SAAT. Test-retest and equivalent forms reliability seem adequate as reported by Cherry (1980) and Chermak and Montgomery (1992). Cherry examined the validity of the SAAT based on the performance of 321 four- to eight-year-old children, including some who were diagnosed with or suspected of learning disability. Cherry reported that the SAAT identified 90% of the learning disabled children and 40% of the children judged by teachers as at risk for learning problems. However, 13% of normally-achieving children were incorrectly identified as at risk for learning problems. Moreover, although Dalebout et al. (1991) did not attempt to validate the SAAT, they concluded that it exhibits poor sensitivity to attention deficits in children diagnosed with ADHD and poor specificity in failing to identify normally functioning subjects as normal.

The SCAN: A Screening Test for Auditory Processing Disorders (Keith 1986) was also developed to assist in the identification of children (aged three to eleven years) at risk for auditory-language processing problems and educational difficulties. The SCAN test battery consists of three subtests: auditory figure-ground and low-pass filtered monosyllabic words (both administered monaurally) and a dichotic competing monosyllabic word subtest. The auditory figure-ground subtest provides a measure of selective attention, requiring recognition of monosyllables presented in the presence of a multitalker competing speech background (+8 dB message-to-competition ratio). Performance on the filtered words subtest reflects ability to process minimally distorted, low-pass-filtered (1 kHz) words. The competing words subtest involves dichotic presentation of monosyllabic words and provides insight regarding auditory maturation (Keith 1986). Unlike the SAAT, the child repeats the stimulus word on the SCAN. Because the SCAN can be administered in quiet environments in twenty minutes and requires only a high fidelity portable stereo cassette player and quality headphones, it is particularly appealing for application in the school setting.

The SCAN was standardized on a sample of 1034 children between the ages of three and eleven years, from a variety of geographic regions and racial and economic groups. Keith (1986) reported internal consistency coefficients of moderate to substantial strength. Test-retest reliability coefficients, however, ranged from weak for the filtered word subtest to moderately strong for the competing word subtest and composite score.

Limited data are available corroborating the validity of the SCAN (Chermak, O'Neill, and Seikel 1992; Keith 1986; Keith and Engineer 1991; Keith et al. 1989). In addition to establishing content validity, Keith affirmed the construct validity of the SCAN based upon two lines of reasoning. First, Keith noted that increases in test mean scores with age corroborate the SCAN's ability to reflect auditory maturation. Second, a factor analysis revealed that the SCAN test items represented both a general auditory processing factor and a specific clustering consistent with the assumptions upon which the SCAN was based. Keith also reported a criterion validity study that revealed positive, but weak, correlations between the SCAN subtests and general measures of language. Keith et al. (1989) interpreted a similar pattern of correlation coefficients as evidence that the SCAN is a valid measure of auditory processing. They reasoned that higher correlations with general measures of language should not be seen because the SCAN is focused on a specific aspect of auditory-language processing ability. Besides its reported sensitivity to CAPD, the SCAN appears sensitive to the presence of learning disability and ADHD and reveals improvements in auditory processing following administration of methylphenidate for control of ADHD (Keith and Engineer 1991).

In comparing the SAAT and the SCAN administered to boys with histories of otitis media, and thus at risk for CAPD, Chermak, O'Neill, and Seikel (1992) reported equivalent group means for the two tests. However, individual subject comparisons revealed the SAAT to be more conservative than the SCAN, identifying additional children as at risk for CAPD. Since neither the SCAN nor the SAAT is accepted as the a priori criterion for classifying children with CAPD, they were unable to conclude which of the two tests more efficiently identified CAPD.

The SCAN's apparent sensitivity to CAPD, ADHD, and learning disabilities underscores the pressing need to design pediatric tests of central auditory processing capable of differentiating specific central auditory functions apart from more generalized receptive language deficits, attention deficits, hyperactivity, and other associated, but not necessarily true, disorders of central auditory processing (Stach 1992). Indeed, given the broad conceptualization of CAPD (ASHA 1992), efficient tests must be designed to identify the various levels and types of processing deficits to improve management.

Various checklists and performance inventories have been used to screen and explore the nature of CAPD (Smoski 1990). A more comprehensive scale, the Children's Auditory Processing Performance Scale (CHAPPS) eases quantification of a child's auditory attention span and memory as well as ability to process auditory signals in a variety of settings, including quiet, noise, and with multiple sensory inputs (Smoski, Brunt, and Tannahill 1992). Fisher's Auditory Problems Checklist also purports to identify children at risk for CAPD (Fisher 1980). In addition to identifying CAPD, listening performance scales may also offer a means to measure the effects of therapeutic intervention (Garstecki et al. 1990).

Assessment

Most behavioral tests of central auditory processing require verbal or manual responses (e.g., pointing to pictures depicting stimulus words) and are restricted to use with children in whom language has emerged. The well known influence of receptive language on speech audiometry in young children (Elliott 1979) has prompted the development of speech recognition and central auditory speech tests for these patients (Cherry 1980; Elliott and Katz 1980; S. Jerger and J. Jerger 1984; Keith 1986; Ross and Lerman 1971). Besides controlling vocabulary level, attempts have been made to control the additional influence of nonauditory cognitive factors (e.g., attention, expectation, motivation) through the use of closed message sets, carrier phrases, and vocal contrasts between the primary and competing messages (S. Jerger and J. Jerger 1984).

Performance-intensity functions (i.e., graphic plots of speech recognition performance in percent correct at several sensation levels) using speech recognition materials appropriate for children are useful in the evaluation of central auditory function. They may reveal ear differences that cannot be explained by peripheral sensitivity (J. Jerger and S. Jerger 1975). A significant reduction in performance as presentation levels are raised beyond the level at which the best score is achieved for phonetically balanced word lists (PB max), known as rollover, is frequently observed in the ear ipsilateral to an eighth nerve or brainstem lesion (J. Jerger and S. Jerger 1971). In addition to rollover, a disproportionate word recognition score (PB max) relative to the puretone average suggests retrocochlear involvement (Yellin, Jerger, and Fifer 1983).

Comparing performance-intensity functions for monosyllabic words and sentences, as recommended by Jerger and Hayes (1977), may also differentiate peripheral from central involvement and can be performed using the Pediatric Speech Intelligibility (PSI) test.

Pediatric Speech Intelligibility Test

The Pediatric Speech Intelligibility (PSI) test is modeled on adult diagnostic approaches and was developed for use with children between three and six years of age (S. Jerger and J. Jerger 1984). The PSI consists of monosyllabic words and sentence materials composed by normal children in this age range (S. Jerger 1980; S. Jerger, J. Jerger, and Abrams 1983). The use of stimuli generated by children serves to control vocabulary level, yielding a closed message set. To engage children's attention and minimize cultural differences, sentence materials employ animals rather than people as agents. As with the SAAT, children are required to point to pictures depicted in a closed response set. Although administering the PSI requires more time and more elaborate equipment (i.e., standard two channel speech audiometer) than required for the SAAT or the SCAN, incorporation of two procedures (i.e., performance-intensity functions and message-to-competition ratio functions) shown to be particularly sensitive components of the neuroaudiologic evaluation with adult patients argues for the inclusion of the PSI in pediatric assessment of central auditory processing (S. Jerger 1987). Performance-intensity functions and message-to-competition ratio functions for words (+4 dB) and sentences (0 dB) presented with ipsilateral (ICM) and contralateral (CCM) competition provide multiple measures with diagnostic relevance to CAPD. Normative data are available for six clinical indices derived from performance-intensity and message-to-competition ratio functions.

Good test-retest reliability has been reported for the PSI, with correlation coefficients ranging between 0.82 and 0.96 (S. Jerger and J. Jerger 1984; S. Jerger, Jerger, and Abrams 1983). Validation studies support the efficiency of the PSI in identifying and differentiating children with developmental abnormalities and auditory and nonauditory lesions of the central nervous system (S. Jerger

1987). S. Jerger, Johnson, and Loiselle (1988) found the PSI useful in differentiating three- to eight-year-old children with confirmed lesions from those with suspected CAPD; abnormal PSI results were specific to involvement of the central auditory pathways. Further, comparison of ICM (degraded monotic) versus CCM (dichotic) functions differentiated between brainstem and temporal lobe sites of lesion or disorder. Abnormal CCM results in children suspected of CAPD led them to conclude that these children have neurodevelopmental or pathologic dysfunction at the level of the auditory cortex.

ASSESSMENT OF CENTRAL AUDITORY PROCESSING DISORDERS: SCHOOL-AGED CHILD

ALTHOUGH only a few tests are available to assess central auditory processing in preschool-aged and younger children and infants, a wide variety of tests is available for use with school-aged children, who are generally more cooperative, have greater linguistic sophistication, and are able to meet the listening demands of the more difficult central auditory test battery. Musiek and Chermak recommended specific tests for assessing central auditory function in school-aged children. Dichotic digits, competing sentences, pitch patterns, and the PSI were designated as preferred. The Staggered Spondaic Word (SSW) test, middle-latency evoked response, Tallal's temporal processing tests (Tallal and Piercy 1974), and compressed speech with acoustic modifications (Bornstein and Musiek 1992) were cited as second-order tests, providing additional options if the preferred tests are unavailable or if additional information is needed.

Electrophysiologic Measures

As discussed previously, the acoustic reflex may provide evidence of the integrity of the brainstem. Indeed, acoustic reflex abnormalities have been observed in children with CAPD, despite lack of clinical indication of brainstem involvement (Kraus et al. 1984).

Although ABR may offer only limited utility for assessing CAPD in children (Musiek, Gollegly, and Baran 1984a; Roush and Tait 1984; Shimizu and Brown 1981; Worthington 1981), middle-latency (MLR) and late-latency evoked potentials may offer greater diagnostic potential with school-aged children. Musiek, Gollegly, and Ross (1985) reported the MLR effective in confirming high auditory system dysfunction in a child with a subarachnoid cyst. The P300 auditory late-latency event-related potential appears sensitive to CAPD in children and may serve both screening and diagnostic efforts (Jirsa 1992; Jirsa and Clontz 1990; Stach, Loiselle, and Jerger 1988). School-aged children with CAPD presented delayed P300 latencies and reduced amplitudes relative to control subjects (Jirsa and Clontz 1990). Beyond diagnosis, Jirsa (1992) found P300 capable of documenting changes in clinical status following a treatment program.

Monaural Low-Redundancy Speech Tests

Low-Pass Filtered Speech

Contralateral deficits for low-pass filtered speech have been seen in adult subjects with temporal lobe lesions (Bocca 1958; Bocca, Calearo, and Cassinari 1954; J. Jerger 1960a, b; Lynn and Gilroy 1972). Ipsilateral, contralateral, and bilateral ear effects have been reported for adults with brainstem lesions (Calearo and Antonelli 1968; Lynn and Gilroy 1977).

Although widely used, the low-pass filtered speech subtest of Willeford's (1976) central auditory test battery presents only limited sensitivity to CAPD in children (Baran and Musiek 1991). Willeford and Billger (1978) reported that only 57% of learning disabled children studied obtained abnormal scores. Similarly, other investigators have reported the insensitivity of low-pass filtered speech tests—including filtered versions of the WIPI test and the PBK word lists—in identifying children with suspected or diagnosed CAPD (Martin and Clark 1977; Musiek and Geurkink 1982; Musiek, Geurkink, and Keitel 1982; Pinheiro 1977; Willeford 1980). In contrast, Ferre and Wilber (1986) found a filtered version of the NU-CHIPS able to distinguish learning disabled children with and without presumed auditory impairment. Likewise, Farrer and Keith (1981) found that low-pass-filtered words separated children with normal and abnormal auditory processing abilities. The filtered words subtest of the SCAN offers a standardized, commercially available alternative. However, Chermak, O'Neill, and Seikel (1992) found this subtest least challenging to subjects at risk for CAPD.

Time-Compressed Speech

Although not as sensitive as low-pass-filtered speech, accelerated or time-compressed speech appears moderately sensitive to intracranial lesions, particularly diffuse lesions, involving the temporal lobe (Calearo and Lazzaroni 1957; Kurdziel, Noffsinger, and Olsen 1976; Mueller, Beck, and Sedge 1987). Reduced performance, especially at the 60% compression rate, is typically observed in adults in the ear contralateral to the temporal lobe with diffuse damage.

Beasley, Maki, and Orchik (1975), studying the effect of time compression on four- to eight-year-old children's auditory perception, reported increases in word identification as a function of increases in age and sensation level, and a decrease in percentage of time compression. Beasley and Freeman (1977) and Freeman and Beasley (1978) reported poorer performance on 60% time-compressed speech (PBK-50 and WIPI test) among children with reading problems. Children with learning disabilities performed more poorly than normal peers when rapid rates of compression were used (Manning, Johnston, and Beasley 1977). Contrary to these reports, Ferre and Wilber (1986) were not able to differentiate learning disabled children with and without central auditory impairment using 60% time-compressed NU-CHIPS.

Speech in Noise Competition

The redundancy of the speech signal can also be decreased by adding an ipsilateral competing message or noise. Reduced word recognition has been observed in adults in the ear contralateral to the temporal lobe lesion and in the ipsilateral ear of patients with eighth nerve and extra-axial brainstem lesions (Dayal, Tarantino, and Swisher 1966; Heilman, Hammer, and Wilder 1973; Morales-García and Poole 1972; Noffsinger et al. 1972). Olsen, Noffsinger, and Kurdziel (1975) found marked reductions in speech recognition measured in the presence of ipsilateral competition to be associated with lesions at all levels of the central auditory nervous system. They concluded that speech-in-noise testing may be useful in detecting central auditory nervous system disorders but not in specifying site of lesion.

Recognizing speech in the presence of background competition is among the most common deficits seen among children with learning disabilities (Katz and Illmer 1972; Lasky and Tobin 1973). Many assessment instruments developed for children take advantage of this finding, incorporating a monaural speech-in-noise subtest in the test battery (Cherry 1980; S. Jerger and J. Jerger 1984; Keith 1986). The SAAT, SCAN auditory figure-ground subtest, and the PSI ipsilateral competing message subtest are examples of standardized, commercially available speech-in-noise tests. Although the SAAT and the performance-intensity functions of the PSI may be administered under earphones or sound field, earphone administration allows for comparisons between ears. The Synthetic Sentence Identification (SSI) with ipsilateral competing message subtest (described under Dichotic Speech Tests) may be appropriate for the older school-aged child, as reading is required.

Dichotic Speech Tests

Results Obtained From Adults with Neurologic Lesions

Dichotic speech tasks involve the simultaneous stimulation of both ears with different stimuli and may be classified as binaural integration or binaural separation tasks. Binaural integration tasks (e.g., SSW, SCAN competing word subtest, masking level differences, and dichotic digits, consonant-vowel syllables, and words) require the listener to process stimuli presented to both ears. In contrast, binaural separation tasks require the listener to process stimuli selectively presented to the target ear (e.g., PSI with contralateral competing message, SSI with contralateral competing message, and the Competing Sentence test). The reader is referred to Silman and Silverman (1991) for an excellent discussion of the neural pathways and mechanisms underlying dichotic listening and outcomes expected in persons with central nervous system compromise.

A right ear advantage for dichotic presentations has been reported consistently in normal subjects (Berlin et al. 1973; Kimura 1961a, b). Kimura found depressed recognition performance when digits were presented to the ear contralateral to temporal lobe damage. Many other reports confirm the contralateral deficit on dichotic digits, CVs, words, and sentences in cases of temporal lobe damage (J. Jerger and S. Jerger 1975; Katz, Basil, and Smith 1963; Lynn and Gilroy 1972, 1977; Niccum, Rubens, and Speaks 1981; Speaks et al. 1975).

An ipsilateral-ear (left) effect has been demonstrated in persons with lesions involving the interhemispheric (i.e., corpus callosum) pathways (Baran, Musiek, and Reeves 1986; Milner, Taylor, and Sperry 1968; Musiek and Wilson 1979; Musiek, Wilson, and Pinheiro 1979; Sparks and Geschwind 1968). Beyond the expected contralateral ear effect seen for persons with cortical lesions, Musiek (1983c) reported predominantly ipsilateral ear effects for persons with unilateral brainstem lesions. Further, he found dichotic digits slightly more sensitive to hemispheric rather than brainstem lesions.

Similar outcomes have been obtained for CV syllables (Berlin et al. 1972, 1975) and competing sentences (Lynn and Gilroy 1975; Musiek 1983a) in adult patients. However, many reports reveal dispersion of outcomes—including ipsilateral, bilateral, and contralateral effects—on dichotic tests administered to patients with brainstem lesions (J. Jerger and S. Jerger 1974, 1975; Katz 1970; Musiek 1983a; Musiek and Geurkink 1982; Pinheiro, Jacobson, and Boller 1982; Rintelmann and Lynn 1983). The variability in outcomes probably results from the intricate and compact nature of the brainstem (Musiek 1983c). J. Jerger and S. Jerger (1974, 1975) concluded that ipsilateral deficits are most commonly seen in extra-axial brainstem lesions, and contralateral ear effects are most commonly seen in intra-axial (i.e., above the cochlear nuclei) brainstem lesions.

Results Obtained from Children with CAPD

Dichotic listening tasks have been shown to differentiate normal children from children with learning disabilities (Hynd et al. 1979; Obrzut et al. 1981; Stubblefield and Young 1975). The expected right ear advantage is seen in children with auditory perceptual deficits and learning disabilities. However, left ear performance is typically depressed relative to normal controls (Baran and Musiek 1991; Musiek, Gollegly, and Baran 1984b; Pinheiro 1977; Willeford 1985) and is highly variable in subjects eight years and younger (Musiek and Pinheiro 1985).

Since dichotic digits appear moderately sensitive to brainstem, cortical, and interhemispheric dysfunction, they may serve as a useful screening tool for CAPD in children (Baran and Musiek 1991; Musiek 1983a; Sommers and Taylor

1972). Although normative data are available for children (Berlin, Hughes, et al. 1973; Berlin, Lowe-Bell, et al. 1973), the sensitivity of dichotic CV syllable tests for the assessment of central auditory processing function in children remains unclear (Dermody, Katsch, and Mackey 1983; Harris, Keith, and Novak 1983; Roeser, Millay, and Morrow 1983). In contrast, dichotic digits, SSW, and competing sentences were among the tests causing the greatest percentage of failures among children with CAPD (Musiek, Geurkink, and Keitel 1982). With the Pitch Patterns Sequence (PPS) test (described below in "Temporal Processing"), they exposed the auditory perceptual deficits of children with learning disabilities (Musiek, Gollegly, and Baran 1984b).

Several standardized dichotic word and sentence tests are available for use with school-aged children, including the SSW, the SCAN, the PSI contralateral competing message subtest, the SSI contralateral competing message subtest, and the Competing Sentence test.

Competing Sentence Test

The Competing Sentence (CS) test, developed by Willeford (1978), involves the dichotic presentation of natural sentences of similar length and semantic content. A right ear advantage is seen for the single ear response mode, and norms reveal improved performance between the ages of six and twelve years. Although comparative data are not available for children, Musiek (1983c) reported that the CS was the least sensitive of three dichotic speech tests administered to adult subjects with intracranial lesions. Moreover, only 48% of 150 children with learning disabilities obtained abnormal competing sentence scores (Willeford and Billger 1985).

Staggered Spondaic Word Test

The Staggered Spondaic Word (SSW) test involves the dichotic presentation of familiar spondees that are partially overlapped to deliver both noncompeting and competing syllables to each ear (Katz 1962). The leading ear is alternated on consecutive word pairs so that twenty word pairs are presented to the right ear first and the remaining twenty pairs are presented to the left ear first. The SSW is easily administered in ten to fifteen minutes and, with some practice, is relatively easy to score.

Depressed SSW recognition scores for competing syllables are typically observed for the ear contralateral to the cortical lesion involving the primary auditory reception area (Katz 1962; Katz, Basil, and Smith 1963; Lynn and Gilroy 1977). Results are less predictable in cases of brainstem lesion, although some investigators have reported depressed performance in such cases (Musiek 1983c; Musiek and Geurkink 1982; Pinheiro, Jacobson, and Boller 1982; Stephens and Thornton 1976).

Error patterns known as response biases are thought to localize cortical lesions in adults (Arnst and Katz 1982). These response biases include: ear effects, in which significantly greater numbers of errors are committed in response to words presented to the first or second ear receiving stimuli; order effects, in which significantly greater numbers of errors are committed for the first spondee or the second spondee; and reversals, in which a correct response is given but in improper sequence of syllables.

In addition to providing site of lesion information, the SSW has been used to evaluate children with suspected CAPD (Katz 1992). The SSW appears to differentiate children with CAPD from those without such difficulties (Johnson, Enfield, and Sherman 1981; Katz and Illmer 1972; Stubblefield and Young 1975). Musiek, Geurkink, and Keitel (1982) found the SSW to be among the more sensitive tests in confirming CAPD in children previously diagnosed.

Although SSW outcomes may reflect localized brain damage in some children, children's performance deficits on the SSW and other dichotic tests may also result from a developmental delay in the maturation of the auditory nervous system, a maturational delay correlated with learning problems (Keith 1983). Indeed, a maturational effect, including a strong right ear advantage, is seen when administering the SSW to normal children aged five to eleven years (Johnson et al. 1981; Keith 1983; Lukas and Guencher-Lucas 1985; Stubblefield and Young 1975; White 1977). Therefore, when administered to children, reduced scores in the competing conditions may be more appropriately interpreted as suggestive of auditory maturation or neurodevelopmental status, rather than brain lesions.

Invoking a maturational model, Keith (1983) suggested alternate interpretations for response biases in children, relating ear effects to directed attention deficits, order effects to memory deficits, and reversals to deficits in sequential memory. A functional deficits interpretation of SSW outcomes in children based on an auditory maturational model may not only offer a more accurate explanation but also provide a more explicit basis for management planning. In noting the large number of children with confirmed reading problems who do not display the expected response bias, Keith (1983) cautioned that the validity of the auditory maturational (i.e., functional deficits) interpretation of SSW outcomes must be substantiated.

Katz (1992) identified four categories of CAPD in children based on response biases that are commonly observed error patterns seen in learning disabled children who present with language deficits, memory deficits, reading comprehension difficulties, and general disorganization. Unlike the maturational model employed by Keith (1983), the taxonomy developed by Katz is derived from data generated by adults with brain lesions and implements a probable site of lesion model corroborated by similarities in symptoms shared by children and adults with brain lesions. Both approaches to interpreting SSW results, however, offer similar insights for management.

Competing Environmental Sounds

The Competing Environmental Sounds (CES) test is a nonlinguistic dichotic test for use along with the SSW (Arnst and Katz 1982; Johnson, Enfield, and Sherman 1981; Katz, Kushner, and Pack 1975). The listener is instructed to either verbalize or point to pictures depicting familiar everyday sounds. Limited data suggest that the CES may be less sensitive than is the SSW to CAPD.

Synthetic Sentence Identification

The Synthetic Sentence Identification (SSI) test, developed by Speaks and Jerger (1965), appears sensitive to brainstem and cortical lesions in adults (J. Jerger, Speaks, and Trammel 1968). Generally, patients with brainstem lesions demonstrate poorer sentence recognition on the SSI when the competing message is presented to the ear ipsilateral to the lesion (SSI-ICM). Patients with temporal lobe lesions perform more poorly when the competing message is presented to the ear contralateral to the lesion (SSI-CCM) (J. Jerger and S. Jerger 1975). J. Jerger and Hayes (1977) suggested comparing performance-intensity functions for monosyllabic words and sentences of the SSI to differentiate peripheral from central sites of lesion. Use of the SSI with younger children is limited because administration of the SSI requires that the subject read the list of ten possible sentences presented with either ipsilateral or contralateral competition.

OTHER BINAURAL INTERACTION TASKS

Masking Level Differences

THE difference between binaural masked thresholds obtained in a homophasic condition (masking noise and signal presented to both ears in-phase) and an antiphasic condition (i.e., one of the signals is presented 180° out-of-phase relative to the signal at the opposite ear) is known as binaural release from masking, masking level difference (MLD), or binaural unmasking. The binaural advantage seen in the MLD reveals the central auditory nervous system's sensitivity to binaural asymmetries and interaural phase differences (Durlach and Colburn 1978). Adult patients with low brainstem lesions do not show significant release from masking, whereas patients with lesions above the low brainstem show masking level differences comparable to normal subjects (Cullen and Thompson 1974; Lynn et al. 1981; Noffsinger 1982; Noffsinger, Martinez, and Schaèfer 1982; Olsen and Noffsinger 1976; Olsen, Noffsinger, and Carhart 1976).

Auditory processing of interaural cues underlying the MLD is mature at about age six years (Hall and Grose 1990); hence, reduced MLDs in children six years and older suggests difficulty interpreting binaural difference cues at the level of the brainstem. MLDs did not differentiate six- to twelve-year-old learning disabled children from normal children (Roush and Tait 1984) although

Sweetow and Reddell (1978) reported that some children with learning disabilities exhibit significantly reduced MLDs for tonal signals.

Binaural Fusion

Dichotic and diotic presentations of bandpass-filtered speech have been used to examine central auditory function. Although bandpass stimuli are not highly intelligible when presented monaurally, normal listeners generally achieve high recognition scores when stimuli are presented in tandem, either simultaneously to both ears (i.e., diotic) or to opposite ears (i.e., dichotic). Binaural fusion, thought to take place at the level of the brainstem (Matzker 1959), involves the integration of complementary information presented simultaneously to the two ears. Typically, the low- and high-pass bands comprising a word are presented to opposite ears, and the listener must summate binaurally. The task appears only moderately sensitive to brainstem lesions in adults (Linden 1964; Lynn and Gilroy 1975, 1977; Musiek 1983b; Musiek and Geurkink 1982; Ohta, Hayashi, and Morimoto 1967).

Although some investigators have reported the binaural fusion task capable of distinguishing children with learning disabilities from normal children (Ferre and Wilber 1986; Martin and Clark 1977; Willeford and Billger 1985), other investigators have reported binaural fusion to have only limited value in assessing CAPD in children (Harris 1963; Musiek, Geurkink, and Keitel 1982; Pinheiro 1977). Roush and Tait (1984) reported reduced word recognition scores under both diotic and dichotic conditions for children with learning disabilities between six and twelve years of age. Because these same subjects demonstrated normal MLDs and ABR, these results were interpreted as evidence of overall central auditory processing difficulty due to the distortion caused by the acoustic filtering rather than evidence of brainstem lesion or dysfunction.

Rapidly Alternating Speech Perception

Bocca and Calearo (1963) developed a "swinging speech test," in which the message alternates between ears. They reported the test to be sensitive to many cases of brainstem pathology but insensitive to diffuse cerebral pathology. Rapidly alternating speech perception (RASP) tests constructed in English have been shown sensitive only to grossly abnormal brainstem function in adults (Lynn and Gilroy 1977; Musiek 1983b; Musiek and Geurkink 1982), nor is RASP particularly sensitive to CAPD in children (Musiek et al. 1982; Pinheiro 1977; Willeford 1977; Willeford and Billger 1985).

TEMPORAL PROCESSING

TEMPORAL processing tasks (e.g., temporal sequencing, gap detection) have been used to examine the integrity and function of the central auditory nervous system. Temporal processing deficits have been reported fairly consistently in adult patients with cerebral lesions. Deficits in sequencing tonal patterns and ordering acoustic stimuli have also been reported in children with CAPD and learning disabilities (Musiek, Geurkink, and Keitel 1982; Musiek, Gollegly, and Baran 1984a, b; Pinheiro 1977; Tallal 1985; Tallal and Piercy 1973, 1974, 1975).

Pitch Patterns Sequence Test

The Pitch Patterns Sequence (PPS) Test is a monaural test that assesses several central auditory processes, including interhemispheric transfer, sequence analysis, and pattern perception (Musiek and Pinheiro 1987; Pinheiro 1977). A low (880 Hz) and a high (1430 Hz) frequency tone are presented in groups of three, with six possible sequences. The listener is required to hum, verbalize, or manually indicate the tonal pattern. Verbalizing or manually responding to the tone pattern requires coordinated processing in both hemispheres. Tonal patterns must be recognized in the right hemisphere and sequenced and encoded using a verbal or manual output in the left hemisphere, thereby requiring interhemispheric transfer across the corpus callosum (Musiek and Kibbe 1984; Musiek, Pinheiro, and Wilson 1980; Pinheiro 1977). Verbal responses reveal the integrity of the contralateral hemisphere and the corpus callosum. The PPS appears to be a sensitive measure (Musiek and Geurkink 1980) and is normed for children six to nine years old.

Patients with brainstem lesions may perform normally on the PPS (Musiek, Weider, and Mueller 1983); however, abnormal performance has also been reported (Musiek and Geurkink 1982; Pinheiro, Jacobson, and Boller 1982). Children with CAPD and learning disabilities present depressed tonal sequencing on the PPS. Demonstrating the benefits of a test battery including tasks requiring temporal processing as well as processing of monaural low-redundancy input, Musiek, Pinheiro, and Wilson (1980) suggested compromise of the auditory interhemispheric pathways based on findings of depressed pattern recognition scores on the PPS, coupled with normal filtered-speech scores.

Given the crucial role that temporal sequencing of acoustic and linguistic patterns serves for speech production and perception (Hirsh 1959, 1967; Lashley 1951; Neff 1964), the PPS offers a unique opportunity to assess central auditory processes underlying everyday function using a nonlanguage-based task (Musiek and Chermak 1995). Similar in task and processing demands, a duration pattern sequence test can be substituted for the PPS (Musiek, Baran, and Pinheiro 1990).

Willeford's Central Auditory Test Battery

Willeford (1977) normed a central auditory test battery developed for children. This battery consists of dichotic competing speech and dichotic binaural fusion subtests, a monotic filtered speech subtest, and a binaural rapidly alternating speech subtest. Maturation effects and large intersubject variability were documented for all subtests (except the rapidly alternating speech test) for children between five and ten years of age. Willeford reported performance deficits on at least one subtest for seven children with below expected academic performance or diagnosed learning disabilities. The rapidly alternating speech subtest appears least sensitive to CAPD (Willeford and Billger 1985).

SUMMARY

THE objectives of central auditory assessment with children are to determine the neuromaturational status and integrity of the central auditory nervous system and identify functional auditory processing deficits underlying communication and learning problems. Achieving these objectives requires a thorough evaluation, including a detailed case history and battery of tests of auditory perception and auditory-language or metalanguage. Basic audiologic testing must precede central testing because peripheral hearing impairment can influence central test outcomes. Although uncommon, some children with CAPD may have neurologic involvement or actual lesions of the central auditory nervous system (S. Jerger 1987; S. Jerger, Johnson, and Loiselle 1988; Musiek, Gollegly, and Ross 1985). Hence, children suspected of CAPD should get a medical examination to complement the audiologic assessment.

Given the heterogeneous nature of CAPD and the complexity of the central auditory nervous system, a test battery consisting of sensitive tests that assess a variety of auditory processes (e.g., binaural separation, binaural integration, and interhemispheric transfer) must be administered, appropriate for the patient's age, ability, and suspected dysfunction. Preliminary reports indicating the potential of late auditory event-related potentials to reveal CAPD in children suggest consideration of electrophysiologic measures for inclusion in the central test battery (Jirsa 1992; Jirsa and Clontz 1990; Stach, Loiselle, and Jerger 1988). Comprehensive test batteries employing distinct behavioral measures of auditory perception and auditory-language skills, as well as selected electrophysiologic measures, may assist in clarifying the relationships among CAPD, attention deficit disorders, and learning disabilities. Brain imaging may also offer new opportunities to reveal brain dysfunction (Duffy and McAnulty 1985; Finitzo and Pool 1987; Hynd, Semrud-Clikeman, and Lyytinen 1991; Kraus and McGee 1988).

The limited database pertaining to the relationship between central auditory test results and neurologic and functional deficits in children complicates interpretation of test results (Keith and Jerger 1991). Positive neurologic findings are uncommon in children with CAPD (Burd and Fisher 1986; Schain 1977; Willeford and Burleigh 1985; Wright et al. 1982). Typically, however, one is not able to establish whether diffuse neuromaturational disorder or maturational delay is the basis for observed functional deficits. Employing a comprehensive test battery, including audiologic tests and measures (e.g., Pitch Patterns Sequence test, dichotic speech) that reflect auditory maturational status and electrophysiologic measures (e.g., middle- and late-latency evoked potentials) that reveal neural synchrony may suggest the etiologic basis for the observed CAPD.

Identifying and assessing central auditory processing deficits in infants and toddlers are difficult given the task demands of behavioral tests and incomplete understanding and application of electrophysiologic and imaging techniques. Besides behavioral observation of their responses to sound, auditory evoked potentials (see chapter 7) and otoacoustic emissions (see chapter 8) provide insight into the capacity of the central auditory nervous system in infants (Northern and Downs 1991). Infants deemed at risk for central nervous system damage should be monitored closely for early signs of CAPD, focusing on speech and language developmental delays and other minimal signs of neurologic dysfunction or damage. Neurobehavioral assessment instruments, such as the Bayley Scales of Infant Development, may provide a window on the maturity and integrity of the central nervous system; however, such scales have limited predictive value and do not specifically implicate CAPD (Gibbs 1990).

Many tests and procedures are available for screening and assessing central auditory function in preschool-aged and older children. Given the common observation of selective attention deficits among children with CAPD, several commercially available instruments have been developed that incorporate a speech-in-noise or competing message task (Cherry 1980; S. Jerger and J. Jerger 1984; Keith 1986). Although some data are available, additional data must be collected documenting the efficiency of these tests and procedures (Chermak, O'Neill, and Seikel 1992; Stach 1992). Several checklists and performance inventories are also available to elucidate the impact of CAPD (Fisher 1980; Smoski et al. 1992).

Although norms for pediatric populations have not been published, a compact disc containing materials for central auditory assessment offers unprecedented acoustic-quality recordings of some experimental and many clinically known test materials (Musiek, Baran, and Pinheiro 1992). Included on the disc are speech masking level differences, dichotic digits, dichotic sentence identification, filtered words, frequency and duration pattern perception, time-compressed speech, and time-compressed speech with reverberation. These materials—and others designed specifically for children—may offer greater opportunity to explore functional deficits and resolve the etiologic basis for the heterogeneous manifestations of CAPD in children.

REFERENCES

Adams, J., E. Courchesne, R. Elmasian, and A. Lincoln. 1987. Increased amplitude of the auditory P2 and P3b components in adolescents with developmental dysphasia. In *Elec-*

troencephalography and clinical neurophysiology: Current trends in event-related potential research, ed. R. Johnson, J.W. Rohrbaugh, and R. Parasuraman. Amsterdam: Elsevier Science Publishers.

Allen, P., F. Wightman, D. Kistler, and T. Dolan. 1989. Frequency resolution in children. *Journal of Speech and Hearing Research* 32:317–322.

American Psychiatric Association. 1987. *Diagnostic and statistical manual of mental disorders*. 3d ed. Washington, D.C.: American Psychiatric Association.

American Speech-Language-Hearing Association. 1990. Guidelines for screening for hearing impairments and middle ear disorders. *Asha* (Suppl. 2) 32:17–30.

———. 1992. *Issues in central auditory processing disorders*. Rockville, MD: American Speech-Language-Hearing Association.

———. 1993. Guidelines for audiology services in the schools. *Asha* (Suppl. 10) 35:24–32.

Aoki, C., and P. Siekevitz. 1988. Plasticity in brain development. *Scientific American* 2596:56–64.

Arnst, D.J., and J. Katz. 1982. *Central auditory assessment: The SSW test—development and clinical use*. San Diego: College-Hill Press.

Baran, J.A., and F.E. Musiek. 1991. Behavioral assessment of the central auditory nervous system. In *Hearing assessment*, 2d ed., ed. by W.F. Rintelmann. Austin, TX: Pro-Ed.

Baran, J.A., F.E. Musiek, and A.G. Reeves. 1986. Central auditory function following anterior sectioning of the corpus callosum. *Ear and Hearing* 7:359–362.

Barr, D.F. 1976. *Auditory perceptual disorders*. 2d ed. Springfield, IL: Charles C. Thomas.

Bayley, N. 1969. *Bayley scales of infant development*. New York: Psychological Corporation.

Beasley, D.S., and B.A. Freeman. 1977. Time-altered speech as a measure of central auditory processing. In *Central auditory dysfunction*, ed. R.W. Keith, New York: Grune and Stratton.

Beasley, D.S., J.E. Maki, and D.J. Orchik. 1975. Children's perception of time-compressed speech using two measures of speech discrimination. *Journal of Speech and Hearing Disorders* 41:216–225.

Bench, J., Y. Collyer, L. Mentz, and I. Wilson. 1976. Studies in infant behavioral audiometry. I. Neonates. *Audiology* 15:85–105.

Bennett, M.J., and L.A. Weatherby. 1982. Newborn acoustic reflexes to noise and pure-tone signals. *Journal of Speech and Hearing Research* 25:383–387.

Bergman, M., H. Costeff, V. Koren, N. Koifman, and A. Reshef. 1984. Auditory perception in early lateralized brain damage. *Cortex* 20:233–242.

Berlin, C.I., J.K. Cullen, Jr., L.F. Hughes, H.L. Berlin, S.S. Lowe-Bell, and C.L. Thompson. 1975. Acoustic variables in dichotic listening. In *Proceedings of a symposium on central auditory processing disorders*, ed. M.D. Sullivan. Omaha: University of Nebraska Medical Center.

Berlin, C.I., L.J. Hood, R.P. Cecola, D.F. Jackson, and P. Szabo. 1993. Does type I afferent neuron dysfunction reveal itself through lack of efferent suppression? *Hearing Research* 65:40–50.

Berlin C.I., L.F. Hughes, S.S. Lowe-Bell, and H.L. Berlin. 1973. Dichotic right ear advantage in children 5 to 13. *Cortex* 9:394–402.

Berlin, C.I., S.S. Lowe-Bell, J.K. Cullen, Jr., S. Thompson, and C. Loovis. 1973. Dichotic speech perception: An interpretation of right-ear advantage and temporal offset effects. *Journal of the Acoustical Society of America* 53:699–709.

Berlin, C.I., S.S. Lowe-Bell, P.J. Jannetta, and D.G. Kline. 1972. Central auditory deficits of temporal lobectomy. *Archives of Otolaryngology* 96:4–10.

Berrick, J., G. Shubow, M. Schultz, H. Freed, S. Fournier, and J. Hughes. 1984. Auditory processing tests for children: Normative and clinical results on the SSW test. *Journal of Speech and Hearing Disorders* 49:318–325.

Blake, P.E., and J.W. Hall III. 1990. The status of statewide policies for neonatal hearing screening. *Journal of the American Academy of Audiology* 1:67–74.

Bocca, E. 1958. Clinical aspects of cortical deafness. *Laryngoscope* 68:301–309.

Bocca, E., and C. Calearo. 1963. Central hearing processes. In *Modern developments in audiology*, ed. J. Jerger. New York: Academic Press.

Bocca, E., C. Calearo, and V. Cassinari. 1954. A new method for testing hearing in temporal lobe tumors: Preliminary report. *Acta Oto-Laryngologica* 44:219–221.

Bocca, E., C. Calearo, V. Cassinari, and F. Migliavacca. 1955. Testing "cortical" hearing in temporal lobe tumors. *Acta Oto-Laryngologica* 42:289–304.

Boder, E. 1973. Developmental dyslexia: A diagnostic approach based on three atypical reading-spelling patterns. *Developmental Medicine and Child Neurology* 15:663–687.

Bornstein, M.H., and M.D. Sigman. 1986. Continuity in mental development from infancy. *Child Development* 57:251–274.

Bornstein, S.P., and F.E. Musiek. 1984. Implications of temporal processing for children with learning and language problems, In *Audition in childhood: Methods of study*, ed. D.S. Beasley and T.H. Shriner. San Diego: College-Hill Press.

———. 1992. Recognition of distorted speech in children with and without learning problems. *Journal of the American Academy of Audiology* 3:22–32.

Brazelton, T.B. 1984. *Neonatal behavioral assessment scale.* 2d ed. Philadelphia: J.B. Lippincott.

Brooks-Gunn, J., and M. Lewis. 1983. Screening and diagnosing handicapped infants. *Topics in Early Childhood Special Education* 3:14–28.

Burd, L., and W. Fisher. 1986. Central auditory processing disorder or attention deficit disorder? *Journal of Developmental and Behavioral Pediatrics* 7:215–216.

Calearo, C., and A.R. Antonelli. 1968. Audiometric findings in brainstem lesions. *Acta Oto-Laryngologica* 66:305–319.

Calearo, C., and A. Lazzaroni. 1957. Speech intelligibility in relation to the speed of the message. *Laryngoscope* 67:410–419.

Campbell, T.F., and M.R. McNeil. 1985. Effects of presentation rate and divided attention on auditory comprehension in children with an acquired language disorder. *Journal of Speech and Hearing Research* 28:513–520.

Chermak, G.D., and M.J. Montgomery. 1992. Form equivalence of the selective auditory attention test administered to 6-year-old children. *Journal of Speech and Hearing Research* 35:661–665.

Chermak, G.D., and F.E. Musiek. 1992. Managing central auditory processing disorders in children and youth. *American Journal of Audiology* 1:61–65.

Chermak, G.D., S.A. O'Neill, and J.A. Seikel. 1992. Criterion validity of the selective auditory attention test. Presented at annual convention of the American Speech-Language-Hearing Association.

Chermak, G.D., M. Vonhof, and R.B. Bendel. 1989. Word identification performance in the presence of competing speech and noise in learning disabled adults. *Ear and Hearing* 10:90–93.

Cherry, R.S. 1980. *Selective auditory attention test (SAAT).* St. Louis: Auditec.

Churchland, P.S., and T.J. Sejnowski. 1988. Perspectives on cognitive neuroscience. *Science* 242:741–746.

Cohen, M. and D. Prasher. 1988. The value of combining auditory brainstem responses and acoustic reflex threshold measurements in neuro-otological diagnosis. *Scandinavian Audiology* 17: 153–162.

Cohen, S.E., and A.H. Parmelee. 1983. Prediction of five-year Stanford-Binet scores in preterm infants. *Child Development* 54:1241–1253.

Cole, R., and J. Jakimik. 1980. A model of speech perception. In *Perception and production of fluent speech*, ed. R. Cole. Hillsdale, NJ: Lawrence Erlbaum Associates.

Collet, L., D.T. Kemp, E. Veuillet, R. Duclaux, A. Moulin, and A. Morgon. 1990. Effect of contralateral auditory stimuli on active cochlear micromechanical properties in human subjects. *Hearing Research* 43:251–262.

Cooper, F.S., P.C. Delattre, A.M. Liberman, J. Borst, and L. Gerstman. 1952. Some experiments on the perception of synthetic speech sounds. *Journal of the Acoustical Society of America* 24:597–606.

Cullen, J.K., and C.L. Thompson. 1974. Masking release for speech in subjects with temporal lobe resection. *Archives of Otolaryngology* 100:113–116.

Curati, W.L., M. Graif, D.P.E. Kingsley, T. King, C.L. Scholtz, and R.E. Steiner. 1986. MRI in acoustic neuroma: A review of 35 patients. *Neuroradiology* 28:208–214.

Cutler, A., and D. Norris. 1988. The role of strong syllables in segmentation for lexical access. *Journal of Experimental Psychology: Human Perception and Performance* 14:113–121.

D'Souza, S.W., E. McCartney, M. Nolan, and I.G. Taylor. 1981. Hearing, speech and language in survivors of severe perinatal asphyxia. *Archives of Diseases in Children* 56:245–252.

Dalebout, S., N. Nelson, P. Hletko, and B. Frentheway. 1991. Selective auditory attention and children with attention-deficit disorder: Effects of repeated measurement with and without methylphenidate. *Language, Speech, and Hearing Services in Schools* 22:219–228.

Dayal, V.S., L. Tarantino, and L.P. Swisher. 1966. Neurootologic studies in multiple sclerosis. *Laryngoscope* 76:1798–1809.

Dempsey, C. 1983. Selecting tests of auditory function in children. In *Central auditory processing disorders: Problems of speech, language and learning*, ed. E.Z. Lasky and J. Katz. Baltimore: University Park Press.

Dermody, P., R. Katsch, and K. Mackey. 1983. Auditory processing limitations in low verbal children: Evidence from a two-response dichotic listening task. *Ear and Hearing* 4:272–277.

Diefendorf, A.O. 1981. An investigation of one aspect of central auditory function in an infant population utilizing a binaural resynthesis fusion task. Ph.D. diss., University of Washington.

Duffy, F.H., J. Burchfield, and C. Lombroso. 1979. Brain electrical activity mapping. BEAM: A method for extending the clinical utility of EEG and evoked potential data. *Annals of Neurology* 5:309–321.

Duffy, F.H., M.B. Denckla, R.H. Bartell, and G. Sandini. 1980. Dyslexia: Regional differences in brain electrical activity by topographic mapping. *Annals of Neurology* 5:412–420.

Duffy, F.H., and G.B. McAnulty. 1985. Brain electrical activity in mapping. BEAM: The search for a physiology signature of dyslexia. In *Dyslexia: A neuroscientific approach to clinical evaluation*, ed. F.H. Duffy and N. Geschwind. Boston: Little, Brown and Co.

Durlach, N.I., and H.S. Colburn. 1978. Binaural phenomena. In *Handbook of perception*, vol. 4., ed. E.C. Carterette and M.F. Friedman. Orlando: Academic Press.

Eilers, R.E., W.R. Wilson, and J.M. Moore. 1977. Developmental changes in speech discrimination in infants. *Journal of Speech and Hearing Research* 20:766–780.

Elliott, L.L. 1979. Performance of children 9 to 17 years on a test of speech intelligibility in noise using sentence material with controlled word predictability. *Journal of the Acoustical Society of America* 66:651–653.

———. 1986. Discrimination and response bias for CV syllables differing in voice onset time among children and adults. *Journal of the Acoustical Society of America* 80:1250–1255.

Elliott, L.L., and M. Hammer. 1988. Longitudinal changes in auditory discrimination in normal children and children with language-learning problems. *Journal of Speech and Hearing Disorders* 53:467–474.

Elliot, L.L., and D. Katz. 1980. *Development of a new children's test of speech discrimination*. St. Louis: Auditec.

Farrer, S., and R. Keith. 1981. Filtered word testing in the assessment of children's central auditory abilities. *Ear and Hearing* 2:267–269.

Feagans, L.V., M. Sanyal, F. Henderson, A. Collier, and M. Applebaum. 1987. Relationship of middle ear disease in early childhood to later narrative and additional skills. *Journal of Pediatric Psychology* 12:581–594.

Ferre, J.M., and L.A. Wilber. 1986. Normal and learning disabled children's central auditory processing skills: An experimental test battery. *Ear and Hearing* 7:336–343.

Ferry, P.C. 1981. Neurological considerations in children with learning disabilities. In *Central auditory and learning disorders in children*, ed. R.W. Keith. Houston: College-Hill Press.

Fifer, R.C., J.F. Jerger, C.I. Berlin, E.A. Tobey, and J.C. Campbell. 1983. Development of a dichotic sentence identification test for hearing-impaired adults. *Ear and Hearing* 4:300–305.

Finitzo, T., and K.D. Pool. 1987. Brain electrical activity mapping. *Asha* 29:21–25.

Fisher, L. 1980. *Fisher's auditory problems checklist*. Cedar Rapids, IA: Grant Wood.

Freeman, B., and D. Beasley. 1978. Performance of reading-impaired and normal reading children on time-compressed monosyllabic and sentential stimuli. Paper presented at annual meeting of the American Speech and Hearing Association.

Frumkin, N.L., E.J. Potchen, A.S. Aniskiewicz, J.B. Moore, and P.A. Cooke. 1989. Potential impact of magnetic resonance imaging on the field of communication disorders. *Asha* 31:95–99.

Fujisaki, H., K. Nakamura, and T. Imoto. 1975. Auditory perception of duration of speech and nonspeech stimuli. In *Auditory analysis and perception of speech*, ed. G. Fant and M. Tatham. New York: Academic Press.

Galaburda, A., G. Sherman, G. Rosen, F. Aboitiz, and N. Geschwind. 1985. Developmental dyslexia: Four consecutive patients with cortical anomalies. *Annals of Neurology* 18:222–233.

Garstecki, D., C.L. Hutton, M.A. Nerbonne, C.W. Newman, and W.J. Smoski. 1990. Case study examples using self-assessment. *Ear and Hearing* (Suppl.) 11:48S–56S.

Gascon, G.G., R. Johnson, and L. Burd. 1986. Central auditory processing and attention deficit disorders. *Journal of Child Neurology* 1:27–33.

Gerber, S.E., E. Wile, and N.T. Hamai. 1985. Central auditory dysfunction in deaf children. *Human Communication* 9:39–44.

Gibbs, E.D. 1990. Assessment of infant mental ability: Conventional tests and issues of prediction. In *Interdisciplinary assessment of infants: A guide for early intervention professionals*, ed. E.D. Gibbs and D.M. Teti. Baltimore: Paul H. Brookes Publishing Co.

Gillberg, C., U. Rosenhall, and E. Johansson. 1983. Auditory brainstem responses in children. *Journal of Autism and Developmental Disorders* 13:181–195.

Goodglass, H. 1967. Binaural digit presentation and early lateral brain damage. *Cortex* 3:295–306.

Grandori, F. 1986. Field analysis of auditory evoked brain-stem potentials. *Hearing Research* 21:51–58.

Gravel, J.S., and I.F. Wallace. 1992. Listening and language at four years of age: Effects of early otitis media. *Journal of Speech and Hearing Research* 35:588–595.

Greisen, D., and P. Rasmussen. 1970. Stapedius muscle reflexes and otoneurological examinations in brain stem tumors. *Acta Oto-Laryngologica* 70:366–370.

Gunnarson, A.D., and T. Finitzo. 1991. Conductive hearing loss in infancy: Effects on later auditory brain stem electrophysiology. *Journal of Speech and Hearing Research* 34:1207–1215.

Hall, J.W., III. 1992. *Handbook of auditory evoked responses*. Boston: Allyn and Bacon.

Hall, J.W., III, and J.H. Grose. 1990. The masking-level difference in children. *Journal of the American Academy of Audiology* 1:81–88.

———. 1991. Notched-noise measures of frequency selectivity in adults and children using fixed-masker-level and fixed-signal-level presentation. *Journal of Speech and Hearing Research* 34:651–660.

Harris, R. 1963. Central auditory functions in children. *Perceptual and Motor Skills* 16:207–214.

Harris, V., R. Keith, and K. Novak. 1983. Relationship between two dichotic listening tests and the token test for children. *Ear and Hearing* 4:278–282.

Hassmannova, J., J. Myslivecek, and V. Novakova. 1981. Effects of early auditory stimulation on cortical areas. In *Neuronal mechanisms of hearing*, ed. J. Syka and L. Aitkin. New York: Plenum Press.

Hedrick, D., E. Prather, and A. Tobin. 1984. Sequenced inventory of communication development. Seattle: University of Washington Press.

Heilman, K.M., L.C. Hammer, and B.J. Wilder. 1973. An audiometric defect in temporal lobe dysfunction. *Neurology* 23:384–386.

Hier, D.B., M. LeMay, P.B. Rosenberger, and V.P. Perlo. 1978. Developmental dyslexia: Evidence for a subgroup with a reversal of cerebral asymmetry. *Archives of Neurology* 35:90–92.

Hirsh, I.J. 1959. Auditory perception of temporal order. *Journal of the Acoustical Society of America* 31:759–767.

———. 1967. Information processing in input channels for speech and language: The significance of serial order of stimuli. In *Brain mechanisms underlying speech and language*, ed. C.H. Millikan and F.L. Darley. New York: Grune and Stratton.

Honzik, M.P. 1976. Value and limitations of infant tests: An overview. In *Origins of intelligence*, ed. M. Lewis. New York: Plenum Press.

Hubatch, L.M., C.J. Johnson, D.J. Kistler, W.J. Burns, and W. Moneka. 1985. Early language abilities of high-risk infants. *Journal of Speech and Hearing Disorders* 50:195–207.

Hynd, G.W., J. Obrzut, W. Weed, and C. Hynd. 1979. Development of cerebral dominance: Dichotic listening asymmetry in normal and learning-disabled children. *Journal of Experimental Child Psychology* 28:445–454.

Hynd, G.W., and M. Semrud-Clikeman. 1989. Dyslexia and brain morphology. *Psychological Bulletin* 106:447–482.

Hynd, G.W., M. Semrud-Clikeman, A.R. Lorys, E.S. Novey, and D. Eliopulos. 1990. Brain morphology in developmental dyslexia, attention deficit disorder/hyperactivity. *Archives of Neurology* 47:919–926.

Hynd, G.W., M. Semrud-Clikeman, and H. Lyytinen. 1991. Brain imaging in learning disabilities. In *Neuropsychological foundations of learning disabilities*, ed. J.E. Obrzut and G.W. Hynd. San Diego: Academic Press.

Jerger, J. 1960a. Audiological manifestations of lesions in the auditory nervous system. *Laryngoscope* 70:417–425.

———. 1960b. Observations on auditory behavior in lesions of the central auditory pathways. *Archives of Otolaryngology* 71:797–806.

———. 1975. Diagnostic use of impedance measures. In *Handbook of clinical impedance audiometry*, ed. J. Jerger. Dobbs Ferry, NY: American Electromedics Corp.

Jerger, J., L. Anthony, S. Jerger, and L. Mauldin. 1974. Studies in impedance audiometry: Middle ear disorders. *Archives of Otolaryngology* 99:165–171.

Jerger, J., P. Burney, L. Mauldin, and B. Crump. 1974. Predicting hearing loss from the acoustic reflex. *Journal of Speech and Hearing Disorders* 39:11–22.

Jerger, J., and D. Hayes. 1977. Diagnostic speech audiometry. *Archives of Otolaryngology* 103:216–222.

Jerger, J., and S. Jerger. 1971. Diagnostic significance of PB word function. *Archives of Otolaryngology* 93:573–580.

———. 1974. Auditory findings in brain stem disorders. *Archives of Otolaryngology* 99:342–350.

———. 1975. Clinical validity of central auditory tests. *Scandinavian Audiology* 4:147–163.

———. 1977. Diagnostic value of crossed versus uncrossed acoustic reflexes: Eighth nerve and brainstem disorders. *Archives of Otolaryngology* 103:445–450.

Jerger, J., K. Johnson, S. Jerger, N. Coker, F. Pirozzolo, and L. Gray. 1991. Central auditory processing disorder: A case study. *Journal of the American Academy of Audiology* 2:36–54.

Jerger, J., and J.L. Northern. 1980. *Clinical impedance audiometry*. Acton, MA: American Electromedics Corp.

Jerger, J., C. Speaks, and J. Trammel. 1968. A new approach to speech audiometry. *Journal of Speech and Hearing Disorders* 33:318–328.

Jerger, J., N. Weikers, F. Sharbrough, and S. Jerger. 1969. Bilateral lesions of the temporal lobe: A case study. *Acta Oto-Laryngologica* (Suppl.) 258:1–51.

Jerger, S. 1980. Evaluation of central auditory function in children. In *Central auditory and language disorders in children*, ed. R.W. Keith. Houston: College-Hill Press.

———. 1983. Decision matrix and information theory analyses in the evaluation of neuroaudiological tests. *Seminars in Hearing* 4:121–132.

———. 1987. Validation of the pediatric speech intelligibility test in children with central nervous system lesions. *Audiology* 26:298–311.

Jerger, S., and J. Jerger. 1983. Evaluation of diagnostic audiometric tests. *Audiology* 22:144–161.

———. 1984. *Pediatric speech intelligibility test: Manual for administration*. St. Louis: Auditec.

Jerger, S., J. Jerger, and S. Abrams. 1983. Speech audiometry in the young child. *Ear and Hearing* 4:56–66.

Jerger, S., J. Jerger, B.R. Alford, and S. Abrams. 1983. Development of speech intelligibility in children with recurrent otitis media. *Ear and Hearing* 4:138–145.

Jerger, S., K. Johnson, and L. Loiselle. 1988. Pediatric central auditory dysfunction: Comparison of children with confirmed lesions versus suspected processing disorders. *American Journal of Otology* 9:63–71.

Jerger, S., R. Martin, and J. Jerger. 1987. Specific auditory perceptual dysfunction in a learning disabled child. *Ear and Hearing* 8:78–86.

Jerger, S., and R. Zeller. 1989. Dichotic listening in a child with a cerebral lesion: The "paradoxical" ipsilateral ear deficit. *Ear and Hearing* 10:167–172.

Jirsa, R.E. 1992. The clinical utility of the P3 AERP in children with auditory processing disorders. *Journal of Speech and Hearing Research* 35:903–912.

Jirsa, R.E., and K.B. Clontz. 1990. Long latency auditory event-related potentials from children with auditory processing disorders. *Ear and Hearing* 11:222–232.

Johnson, D., M. Enfield, and R. Sherman. 1981. The use of the staggered spondaic word test and the competing environmental sounds test in the evaluation of central auditory function in hearing disabled children. *Ear and Hearing* 2:70–77.

Kalil, R.E. 1989. Synapse formation in the developing brain. *Scientific American* 2616:76–85.

Katz, J. 1962. The use of staggered spondaic words for assessing the integrity of the central auditory system. *Journal of Auditory Research* 2:327–337.

———. 1970. Audiologic diagnosis: Cochlea to cortex. *Menorah Medical Journal* 1:25–38.

———. 1983. Phonemic synthesis. In *Central auditory processing disorders: Problems of speech, language, and learning*, ed. E.Z. Lasky and J. Katz. Baltimore: University Park Press.

———. 1992. Classification of auditory processing disorders. In *Central auditory processing: A transdisciplinary view*, ed. J. Katz, N.A. Stecker, and D. Henderson. St. Louis: Mosby Year Book.

———. 1994. *Handbook of clinical audiology.* 4th ed. Baltimore: Williams and Wilkins.

Katz, J., R.A. Basil, and J.M. Smith. 1963. A staggered spondaic word test for detecting central auditory lesions. *Annals of Otology, Rhinology, and Laryngology* 72:906–917.

Katz, J., and R. Illmer. 1972. Auditory perception in children with learning disabilities. In *Handbook of clinical audiology*, ed. J. Katz. Baltimore: Williams and Wilkins.

Katz, J., D. Kushner, and G. Pack. 1975. The use of competing speech SSW and environmental sounds: CES tests for localizing brain lesions. Presented at annual convention of the American Speech and Hearing Association.

Katz, J., and L. Wilde. 1985. Auditory perceptual disorders in children. In *Handbook of clinical audiology*, 3d ed., ed. J. Katz. Baltimore: Williams and Wilkins.

Kaufman, N.L. 1980. Review of research on reversal errors. *Perceptual and Motor Skills* 51:55–79.

Keith, R.W. 1981a. Audiological and auditory-language tests of central auditory function. In *Central auditory and language disorders in children*, ed. R.W. Keith. Houston: College-Hill Press.

———. 1981b. Tests of central auditory function. In *Auditory disorders in school children*, ed. R.J. Roeser and M.P. Downs. New York: Thieme-Stratton, Inc.

————. 1983. Interpretation of the staggered spondee word (SSW) test. *Ear and Hearing* 4:287–292.

————. 1986. *SCAN: A screening test for auditory processing disorders.* San Antonio: Psychological Corp.

————. 1988. Central auditory tests. In *Handbook of speech, language pathology, and audiology,* ed. N.J. Lass, L.V. McReynolds, and J.L. Northern. Philadelphia: B.C. Decker.

Keith, R.W., ed. 1977. *Central auditory dysfunction.* New York: Grune and Stratton.

Keith, R.W., and P. Engineer. 1991. Effects of methylphenidate on the auditory processing abilities of children with attention deficit-hyperactivity disorder. *Journal of Learning Disabilities* 24:630–363.

Keith, R.W., and S. Jerger. 1991. Central auditory disorders. In *Diagnostic audiology,* ed. J.T. Jacobson and J.L. Northern. Austin, TX: Pro-Ed.

Keith, R.W., J. Rudy, P.A. Donahue, and B. Katbamna. 1989. Comparison of SCAN results with other auditory and language measures in a clinical population. *Ear and Hearing* 10:382–386.

Keller, W.D. 1992. Auditory processing disorder or attention-deficit disorder? In *Central auditory processing: A transdisciplinary view,* ed. J. Katz, N.A. Stecker, and D. Henderson. St. Louis: Mosby Year Book.

Kemp, D.T., P. Bray, L. Alexander, and A.M. Brown. 1986. Acoustic emission cochleography: Practical aspects. *Scandinavian Audiology Supplementum* 25:71–96.

Kimura, D. 1961a. Cerebral dominance and the perception of verbal stimuli. *Canadian Journal of Psychology* 15:166–171.

————. 1961b. Some effects of temporal lobe damage on auditory perception. *Canadian Journal of Psychology* 15:157–165.

————. 1964. Left-right differences in the perception of melodies. *Quarterly Journal of Experimental Psychology* 14:355–358.

Kinsbourne, M. 1973. Minimal brain dysfunction as a neurodevelopmental lag. *Annals of the New York Academy of Sciences* 205:268–273.

Kraus, N., and T. McGee. 1988. Color imaging of the human middle latency response. *Ear and Hearing* 9:159–167.

Kraus, N., O. Ozdamar, L. Stein, and N. Reed. 1984. Absent auditory brain stem response: Peripheral hearing loss or brain stem dysfunction? *Laryngoscope* 94:400–406.

Kreul, J., J. Nixon, K. Kryter, D. Bell, S. Lang, and E. Schubert. 1968. A proposed clinical test of speech discrimination. *Journal of Speech and Hearing Research* 11:536–552.

Kurdziel, S., D. Noffsinger, and W. Olsen. 1976. Performance by cortical lesion patients on 40% and 60% time-compressed materials. *Journal of the American Audiological Society* 2:3–7.

Lashley, K.S. 1951. The problem of serial order in behavior. In *Cerebral mechanisms in behavior,* ed. L.A. Jeffress. New York: Wiley.

Lasky, E.Z., and J. Katz, eds. 1983. *Central auditory processing disorders.* Baltimore: University Park Press.

Lasky, E.Z., and H. Tobin. 1973. Linguistic and nonlinguistic competing message effects. *Journal of Learning Disabilities* 6:243–250.

Liberman, A. 1970. The grammars of speech and language. *Cognitive Psychology* 1:301.

Linden, A. 1964. Distorted speech and binaural speech resynthesis tests. *Acta Oto-Laryngologica* 58:32–48.

Lubert, N. 1981. Auditory perceptual impairments in children with specific language disorders. *Journal of Speech and Hearing Disorders* 46:3–9.

Luce, P. 1986. Neighborhoods of words in the mental lexicon: Research on speech perception. Technical Report no. 6. Bloomington: Indiana University Department of Psychology, Speech Research Laboratory.

Lukas, R.A., and J. Guenchur-Lukas. 1985. Spondaic word tests. In *Handbook of clinical audiology*, 3d ed., ed. J. Katz. Baltimore: Williams and Wilkins.

Lynn, G.E., and J. Gilroy. 1972. Neuroaudiological abnormalities in patients with temporal lobe tumors. *Journal of Neurological Sciences* 17:167–184.

———. 1975. Effects of brain lesions on the perception of monotic and dichotic speech stimuli. In *Proceedings of symposium on central auditory processing disorders*, ed. H. Sullivan. Omaha: University of Nebraska Medical Center.

———. 1977. Evaluation of central auditory dysfunction in patients with neurological disorders. In *Central auditory dysfunction*, ed. R.W. Keith. New York: Grune and Stratton.

Lynn, G.E., J. Gilroy, P.C. Taylor, and R.P. Leiser. 1981. Binaural masking-level differences in neurological disorders. *Archives of Otolaryngology* 107:357–362.

Manning, W., K. Johnston, and D. Beasley. 1977. The performance of children with auditory perceptual disorders on a time-compressed speech discrimination measure. *Journal of Speech and Hearing Disorders* 42:77–84.

Marslen-Wilson, W.D. 1987. Functional parallelism in spoken word-recognition. *Cognition* 25:71–102.

Martin, F.N., and J.G. Clark. 1977. Audiologic detection of auditory processing disorders in children. *Journal of the American Audiology Society* 3:140–146.

Massaro, D.W. 1987. *Speech perception by ear and eye: A paradigm for psychological inquiry*. Hillsdale, NJ: Lawrence Erlbaum.

Matkin, N.D., and P.E. Hook. 1983. A multidisciplinary approach to central auditory evaluations. In *Central auditory processing disorders: Problems of speech, language, and learning*, ed. E.Z. Lasky and J. Katz. Baltimore: University Park Press.

Matzker, J. 1959. Two methods for the assessment of central auditory functions in cases of brain disease. *Annals of Otology, Rhinology, and Laryngology* 68:1155–1197.

———. 1962. The binaural test. *International Audiology* 1:209–211.

Maxon, A.B., and I. Hochberg. 1982. Development of psychoacoustic behavior: Sensitivity and discrimination. *Ear and Hearing* 3:301–308.

McCall, R.B. 1983. A conceptual approach to early mental development. In *Origins of intelligence*, ed. M. Lewis. New York: Plenum Press.

McClelland, J.L., and J.L. Elman. 1986. The TRACE model of speech perception. *Cognitive Psychology* 18:1–86.

McMillan, P.M., M.J. Bennett, C.D. Marchant, and P. Shurin. 1985. Ipsilateral and contralateral acoustic reflexes in neonates. *Ear and Hearing* 6:320–324.

Mencher, G.T. 1985. Hearing screening programs and identification of central auditory disorders. *Human Communication* 9:45–49.

Mikhael, M.A., I.S. Ciric, and A.P. Wolff. 1987. MR diagnosis of acoustic neuromas. *Journal of Computer Assisted Tomography* 11:232–235.

Milner, B., S. Taylor, and R. Sperry. 1968. Lateralized suppression of dichotically presented digits after commissural section in man. *Science* 161:184–185.

Morales-García, C., and J.O. Poole. 1972. Masked speech audiometry in central deafness. *Acta Oto-Laryngologica* 74:307–316.

Morest, D.K. 1983. Degeneration in the brain following noise exposure. In *New perspectives in noise induced hearing loss*, ed. R.P. Hammernik, D. Henderson, and R.J. Salvi. New York: Raven Press.

Mott, J.B., S.T. Norton, S.T. Neely, and B. Warr. 1989. Changes in spontaneous otoacoustic emissions produced by acoustic stimulation of the contralateral ear. *Hearing Research* 38:229–242.

Mueller, H.G., W.G. Beck, and R.K. Sedge. 1987. Comparison of the efficiency of cortical level speech tests. *Seminars in Hearing* 8:279–298.

Musiek, F.E. 1983a. Assessment of central auditory dysfunction: The dichotic digit test revisited. *Ear and Hearing* 4:79–83.

———. 1983b. The evaluation of brainstem disorders using ABR and central auditory tests. *Monographs in Contemporary Audiology* 4:1–24.

———. 1983c. The results of three dichotic speech tests on subjects with intracranial lesions. *Ear and Hearing* 4:318–323.

———. 1989. Probing brain function with acoustic stimuli. *Asha* 31:100–108.

Musiek, F.E., and J.A. Baran. 1987. Central auditory assessment: Thirty years of challenge and change. *Ear and Hearing* 8:22S–35S.

Musiek, F.E., J.A. Baran, and M.L. Pinheiro. 1990. Duration pattern recognition in normal subjects and patients with cerebral and cochlear lesions. *Audiology* 29:304–313.

———. 1992. P300 results in patients with lesions of the auditory areas of the cerebrum. *Journal of the American Academy of Audiology* 3:5–15.

Musiek, F.E., and G.D. Chermak. 1994. Three commonly asked questions about central auditory processing disorders: Assessment. *American Journal of Audiology* 3:23–27.

Musiek, F.E., and G.D. Chermak. 1995. Three commonly asked questions about central auditory processing disorders: Management. *American Journal of Audiology* 4:15–18.

Musiek, F.E., and N.A. Geurkink. 1980. Auditory perceptual problems in children: Considerations for the otolaryngologist and audiologist. *Laryngoscope* 90:962–971.

———. 1982. Auditory brainstem response (ABR) and central auditory test (CAT) findings for patients with brainstem lesions: A preliminary report. *Laryngoscope* 92:891–900.

Musiek, F.E., N.A. Geurkink, and S. Keitel. 1982. Test battery assessment of auditory perceptual dysfunction in children. *Laryngoscope* 92:251–257.

Musiek, F.E., and K.M. Gollegly. 1988. Maturational considerations in the neuroauditory evaluation of children. In *Hearing impairment in children*, ed. F.H. Bess. Parkton, MD: York Press.

Musiek, F.E., K.M. Gollegly, and J.A. Baran. 1984a. Myelination of the corpus callosum and auditory processing problems in learning disabled children: Theoretical and clinical correlates. *Seminars in Hearing* 5:219–242.

———. 1984b. Myelination of the corpus callosum in learning disabled children: Theoretical and clinical correlates. *Seminars in Hearing* 5:219–229.

Musiek, F.E., K.M. Gollegly, and M.K. Ross. 1985. Profiles of types of central auditory processing disorders in children with learning disabilities. *Journal of Childhood Communication Disorders* 9:43–61.

Musiek, F.E., and K. Kibbe. 1984. Audiologic test results in patients with commissurotomy. In *Epilepsy and the corpus callosum*, ed. A.G. Reeves. New York: Plenum Press.

Musiek, F.E., S. Lenz, and K. Gollegly. 1991. Neuroaudiologic correlates to anatomical changes of the brain. *American Journal of Audiology* 1:19–24.

Musiek, F.E., D. Noffsinger, R. Wilson, S. Bornstein, and C. Martinez. 1992. Tonal and speech materials for central auditory assessment. Presented at annual convention of the American Speech-Language-Hearing Association. San Antonio, Texas.

Musiek, F.E., and M.L. Pinheiro. 1985. Dichotic speech tests in the detection of central auditory dysfunction. In *Assessment of central auditory dysfunction: Foundations and clinical correlates*, ed. M.L. Pinheiro and F.E. Musiek. Baltimore: Williams and Wilkins.

———. 1987. Frequency patterns in cochlear, brainstem and cerebral lesions. *Audiology* 26:79–88.

Musiek, F.E., M.L. Pinheiro, and D.H. Wilson. 1980. Auditory pattern perception in "split brain" patients. *Archives of Otolaryngology* 106:610–612.

Musiek, F.E., S.B. Verkest, and K.M. Gollegly. 1988. Effects of neuromaturation on auditory-evoked potentials. In *Seminars in hearing*, ed. D.W. Worthington. New York: Thieme Medical Publishers, Inc.

Musiek, F.E., D.J. Weider, and R.J. Mueller. 1983. Reversible audiologic results in a patient with an extra-axial brain stem tumor. *Ear and Hearing* 4:169–172.

Musiek, F.E., and D.H. Wilson. 1979. SSW and dichotic digit results pre- and postcommissurotomy: A case report. *Journal of Speech and Hearing Disorders* 44:528–533.

Musiek, F.E., D.H. Wilson, and M.L. Pinheiro. 1979. Audiological manifestations in split-brain patients. *Journal of the American Auditory Society* 5:25–29.

Nass, R. 1984. Case report: Recovery and reorganization after congenital unilateral brain damage. *Perceptual and Motor Skills* 59:867–874.

National Institutes of Health. 1993. Early identification of hearing impairment in infants and young children. *NIH Consensus Statement* 11:1–24. Washington, D.C.: National Institutes of Health.

Neff, W.D. 1964. Temporal pattern discrimination in lower animals and its relation to language perception in man. In *Disorders of language*, ed. A.V.S. deRueck and M. O'Connor. Boston: Little, Brown.

Newhoff, M., M.J. Cohen, G.W. Hynd, J.J. Gonzalez, and C.A. Riccio. 1992. Etiological, educational and behavioral correlates of ADHD and language disabilities. Presented at annual convention of the American Speech-Language-Hearing Association, San Antonio, Texas.

Niccum, N., A. Rubens, and C. Speaks. 1981. Effects of stimulus material on the dichotic listening performance of aphasic patients. *Journal of Speech and Hearing Research* 24:526–534.

Nodar, R.H., J. Hahn, and H.L. Levine. 1980. Brain stem auditory evoked potentials in determining site of lesion of brain stem gliomas in children. *Laryngoscope* 90:258–266.

Noffsinger, D. 1982. Clinical application of selected binaural effects. *Scandinavian Audiology Supplement* 15:157–165.

Noffsinger, D., C.D. Martinez, and A.B. Schaefer. 1982. Auditory brainstem responses and masking level differences from persons with brainstem lesions. *Scandinavian Audiology Supplement* 15:81–93.

Noffsinger, D., W.O. Olsen, R. Carhart, C.W. Hart, and V. Sahgal. 1972. Auditory and vestibular aberrations in multiple sclerosis. *Acta Oto-Laryngologica* (Suppl.) 303:1–63.

Northern, J.L. 1981. Impedance measurement in infants. In *Early management of hearing loss*, ed. G.T. Mencher and S.E. Gerber. New York: Grune and Stratton.

Northern, J.L., and M.P. Downs. 1991. *Hearing in children*. 4th ed. Baltimore: Williams and Wilkins.

Norton, S.J. 1993. Application of transient evoked otoacoustic emissions to pediatric populations. *Ear and Hearing* 14:64–73.

Obrzut, J., G. Hynd, A. Obrzut, and F. Pirozzolo. 1981. Effects of directed attention on cerebral asymmetries in normal and learning-disabled children. *Developmental Psychology* 17:118–125.

Obrzut, J., W. Weed, and C. Hynd. 1979. Development of cerebral dominance: Dichotic listening asymmetry in normal and learning-disabled children. *Journal of Experimental Child Psychology* 28:445–454.

Ohta, F., R. Hayashi, and M. Morimoto. 1967. Differential diagnosis of retrocochlear deafness: Binaural fusion test and binaural separation test. *International Audiology* 6:58–62.

Olsen, W.O., and D. Noffsinger. 1976. Masking level differences for cochlear and brain stem lesions. *Annals of Otology, Rhinology, and Laryngology* 85:820–825.

Olsen, W.O., D. Noffsinger, and R. Carhart. 1976. Masking level differences encountered in clinical populations. *Audiology* 15:287–301.

Olsen, W.O., D. Noffsinger, and S. Kurdziel. 1975. Speech discrimination in quiet and in white noise by patients with peripheral and central lesions. *Acta Oto-Laryngologica* 80:375–382.

Pickles, J.O. 1982. *An introduction to the physiology of hearing*. New York: Academic Press.

Picton, T.W., D.L. Woods, J. Baribeau-Braun, and T.L. Healey. 1977. Evoked potential audiometry. *Journal of Otolaryngology* 6:90–119.

Pinheiro, M.L. 1977. Tests of central auditory function in children with learning disabilities. In *Central auditory dysfunction*, ed. R.W. Keith. New York: Grune and Stratton.

Pinheiro, M.L., G.P. Jacobson, and F. Boller. 1982. Auditory dysfunction following a gunshot wound of the pons. *Journal of Speech and Hearing Disorders* 47:296–300.

Pinheiro, M.L., and F.E. Musiek. 1985. Sequencing and temporal ordering in the auditory system. In *Assessment of central auditory dysfunction: Foundations and clinical correlates*, ed. M. Pinheiro and F. Musiek. Baltimore: Williams and Wilkins.

Pinheiro, M.L., and F.E. Musiek, eds. 1985. *Assessment of central auditory dysfunction*. Baltimore: Williams and Wilkins.

Pohl, P. 1979. Dichotic listening in a child recovering from acquired aphasia. *Brain and Language* 8:372–379.

Protti, E. 1983. Brainstem auditory pathways and auditory processing disorders: Diagnostic implications of subjective and objective tests. In *Central auditory processing disorders*, ed. E. Lasky and J. Katz. Baltimore: University Park Press.

Rauschecker, J.P., and P. Marler. 1987. Cortical plasticity and imprinting: Behavioral and physiological contrasts and parallels. In *Imprinting and cortical plasticity*, ed. J.P. Rauschecker and P. Marler. New York: John Wiley.

Rintelmann, W.F., and G.E. Lynn. 1983. Speech stimuli for assessment of central auditory disorders. In *Principles of speech audiometry*, ed. D.F. Konkle and W.F. Rintelmann. Baltimore: University Park Press.

Roberts, J.E., M.R. Burchinal, B.P. Davis, A.M. Collier, and F.W. Henderson. 1991. Otitis media in early childhood and later language. *Journal of Speech and Hearing Research* 34:1158–1168.

Robertson, D., and D.R.F. Irvine. 1989. Plasticity of frequency organization in auditory cortex of guinea pigs with partial unilateral deafness. *Journal of Comparative Neurology* 282:456–471.

Roeser, R., K. Millay, and J. Morrow. 1983. Dichotic consonant-vowel (cv) perception in normal and learning-impaired children. *Ear and Hearing* 4:293–299.

Rosenberger, P., and D. Hier. 1980. Cerebral asymmetry and verbal intellectual deficits. *Annals of Neurology* 8:300–304.

Ross, M. and J. Lerman. 1971. *Word intelligibility by picture identification.* Pittsburgh: Stanwix House.

Roush, J., and C.A. Tait. 1984. Binaural fusion, masking level differences, and auditory brain stem responses in children with language-learning disabilities. *Ear and Hearing* 5: 37–41.

Salvia, J., and J.E. Ysseldyke. 1981. *Assessment in special and remedial education.* 2d ed. Boston: Houghton Mifflin Co.

Sanderson-Leepa, M.E., and W.F. Rintelmann. 1976. Articulation function and test-retest performance of normal-hearing children on three speech discrimination tests: WIPI, PBK 50, and NU auditory test no. 6. *Journal of Speech and Hearing Disorders* 41: 503–519.

Schain, R. 1977. *Neurology of childhood learning disorders.* 2d ed. Baltimore: Williams and Wilkins.

Schlaggar, B.L., and D.D.M. O'Leary. 1991. Potential of visual cortex to develop an array of functional units unique to somatosensory cortex. *Science* 252:1556–1560.

Schmitt, B.D. 1975. The minimal brain dysfunction myth. *American Journal of Diseases of Children* 129:1313–1318.

Shimizu, H., and F. Brown. 1981. ABR in children with MBD. Presented at annual convention of the American Speech-Language-Hearing Association, Los Angeles.

Silman, S., and C.A. Silverman. 1991. *Auditory diagnosis: Principles and applications.* San Diego: Academic Press.

Sloan, C. 1980. Auditory processing disorders and language development. In *Auditory processing and language: Clinical and research perspectives*, ed. P.J. Levinson and C. Sloan, 101–115. New York: Grune and Stratton.

Smoski, W.J. 1990. Use of CHAPPS in a children's audiology clinic. *Ear and Hearing* (Suppl.) 11:53–56.

Smoski, W.J., M.A. Brunt, and C. Tannahill. 1992. Listening characteristics of children with central auditory processing disorders. *Language, Speech, and Hearing Services in Schools* 23:145–152.

Sohmer, H., and M. Student. 1978. Auditory nerve and brainstem evoked responses in normal, autistic, minimal brain dysfunction and psychomotor retarded children. *Electroencephalography and clinical neurophysiology* 44:380–388.

Sommers, R.K., and M.L. Taylor. 1972. Cerebral speech dominance in language-disorderd and normal children. *Cortex* 8:224–232.

Sparks, R., and N. Geschwind. 1968. Dichotic listening in man after section of neocortical commissures. *Cortex* 4:3–16.

Speaks, C., T. Gray, J. Miller, and A. Rubens. 1975. Central auditory deficits and temporal-lobe lesions. *Journal of Speech and Hearing Disorders* 40:192–205.

Speaks, C., and J. Jerger. 1965. Method for measurement of speech identification. *Journal of Speech and Hearing Research* 8:185–194.

Speaks, C., N. Niccum, and D. van Tassel. 1985. Effects of stimulus material on the dichotic listening performance of patients with sensorineural hearing loss. *Journal of Speech and Hearing Research* 18:16–25.

Sprague, B.H., T.L. Wiley, and R. Goldstein. 1985. Tympanometric and acoustic reflex studies in neonates. *Journal of Speech and Hearing Research* 28:265–272.

Squires, K., and K. Hecox. 1983. Electrophysiological evaluation of higher level auditory processing. *Seminars in Hearing* 4:415–432.

Stach, B.A. 1992. Controversies in the screening of central auditory processing disorders. In *Screening children for auditory function*, ed. F.H. Bess and J.W. Hall III. Nashville: Bill Wilkerson Center Press.

Stach, B.A., L.H. Loiselle, and J.F. Jerger. 1988. Auditory evoked potential abnormalities in children with central auditory disorder. *Asha* 30:133 (abstract).

Stephens, S., and A. Thornton. 1976. Subjective and electrophysiologic tests in brainstem lesions. *Archives of Otolaryngology* 102:608–613.

Stubblefield, J., and C. Young. 1975. Central auditory dysfunction in learning-disabled children. *Journal of Learning Disabilities* 8:32–37.

Sussman, J.E. 1991. Stimulus ratio effects on speech discrimination by children and adults. *Journal of Speech and Hearing Research* 34:671–678.

Sweetow, R., and R. Reddell. 1978. The use of masking level differences in the identification of children with perceptual problems. *Journal of the American Auditory Society* 4: 52–56.

Swisher, L., and I. Hirsh. 1972. Brain damage and the ordering of two temporally successive stimuli. *Neuropsychologia* 10:137–152.

Tallal, P. 1985. Neuropsychological research approaches to the study of central auditory processing. *Human Communication* 9 (Part 1):17–22.

Tallal, P., and M. Piercy. 1973. Developmental aphasia: Impaired rate of nonverbal processing as a function of sensory modality. *Neuropsychologia* 11:389–398.

———. 1974. Developmental aphasia: Rate of auditory processing and selective impairment of consonant perception. *Neuropsychologia* 12:83–94.

———. 1975. Developmental aphasia: The perception of brief vowels and extended consonants. *Neuropsychologia* 13:69–74.

Teatini, G.P. 1970. Sensitized speech tests: Results in normal subjects. In *Speech audiometry*, ed. C. Rojskjaer. Odense: Danavox.

Thoman, E.B., and P.T. Becker. 1979. Issues in assessment and prediction for the infant born at risk. In *Infants born at risk*, ed. T. Field. Jamaica, NY: Spectrum.

Tobey, E.A., and J.K. Cullen, Jr. 1984. Temporal integration of tone glides by children with auditory-memory and reading problems. *Journal of Speech and Hearing Research* 27: 527–533.

Tokioka, A.B., D.H. Crowell, and J.W. Pierce. 1987. Electrophysiological investigation of cognition in infants. In *Thinking across cultures: The third international conference on thinking*, ed. D.M. Topping, D.C. Crowell, and V.N. Kobayashi. Hillsdale, NJ: Lawrence Erlbaum Associates.

Turner, R.G., and D.W. Nielsen. 1984. Application of clinical decision analysis to audiological tests. *Ear and Hearing* 5:125–133.

Warren, R.M. 1983. Multiple meanings of "phoneme": Articulatory, acoustic, perceptual, graphemic, and their confusions. In *Speech and language: Advances in basic research and practice*, vol. 9., ed. N.J. Lass. New York: Academic Press.

Webster, D.B., and M. Webster. 1977. Neonatal sound deprivation affects brainstem auditory nuclei. *Archives of Otolaryngology* 103:392–396.

Werner, L.A. 1992. Interpreting developmental psychoacoustics. In *Developmental psychoacoustics*, ed. L.A. Werner and E.W. Rubel. Washington, D.C.: American Psychological Association.

White, E.J. 1977. Children's performance on the SSW test and Willeford battery: Interim clinical data. In *Central auditory dysfunction*, ed. R.W. Keith. New York: Grune and Stratton.

Willeford, J.A. 1976. Differential diagnosis of central auditory dysfunction. In *Audiology: An audio journal for continuing education*, vol. 2, ed. L. Bradford. New York: Grune and Stratton.

———. 1977. Assessing central auditory behavior in children: A test battery approach. In *Central auditory dysfunction*, ed. R.W. Keith. New York: Grune and Stratton.

———. 1978. Sentence tests of central auditory function. In *Handbook of clinical audiology*, 2d ed., ed. J. Katz. Baltimore: Williams and Wilkins.

———. 1980. Central auditory behaviors in learning disabled children. *Seminars in Speech Language and Hearing* 1:127–140.

———. 1985. Assessment of central auditory disorders in children. In *Assessment of central auditory dysfunction: Foundations and clinical correlates*, ed. M.L. Pinheiro and F.E. Musiek. Baltimore: Williams and Wilkins.

Willeford, J.A., and J.M. Billger. 1985. Auditory perception in children with learning disabilities. In *Handbook of clinical audiology*, 3d ed., ed. J. Katz. Baltimore: Williams and Wilkins.

Willeford, J.A., and J.M. Burleigh. 1985. *Handbook of central auditory processing disorders in children*. Orlando: Grune and Stratton.

Willott, J.F., R.M. Demuth, and S.M. Lu. 1984. Excitability of auditory neurons in the dorsal and ventral cochlear nuclei of DBA/2 and C57BL/6 mice. *Experimental Neurology* 83:495–506.

Willows, D.M., J.R. Kershner, and E. Corcos. 1986. Visual processing and visual memory in reading and writing disabilities: A rationale for reopening a "closed case." Paper presented at symposium, The Role of Visual Processing and Visual Memory in Reading and Writing. Annual meeting of the American Educational Research Association, April, San Francisco.

Wilson, W.R., and G. Thompson. 1984. Behavioral audiometry. In *Pediatric audiology: Current trends*, ed. J. Jerger. San Diego: College-Hill Press.

Witkin, B.R. 1971. Auditory perception: Implications for language development. *Language, Speech, and Hearing Services in Schools* 4:31–52.

World Health Organization. 1971. *Mass health examinations*. Public Health Papers no. 45: 81–82. Geneva: World Health Organization.

Worthington, D. 1981. ABR in special populations. Paper presented at ABR workshop, Cleveland, Ohio.

Wright, F., R. Schain, W. Weinberg, and R. Ischelle. 1982. Learning disabilities and associated conditions. In *The practice of pediatric neurology*, ed. K. Swaiman and F. Wright. St. Louis: C.V. Mosby.

Yellin, M.W., J.F. Jerger, and R.C. Fifer. 1983. Norms for disproportionate loss in speech intelligibility. Presented at American Speech-Language-Hearing Association convention, Cincinnati.

10

Amplification

Dale O. Robinson and Frances Eldis

THE goal of this chapter is to present the reader with practical information concerning the provision for and management of amplification with
real children encountered in real clinical settings. We are interested in
sharing our experiences in a way that is helpful to the working clinician by
bringing together the theoretical selection and fitting procedures taught in the
classroom or workshop with the reality of clinical application. This is not an attempt to present a technical or academic review of the many fine hearing aid
selection procedures detailed in the literature. Those are best presented by the
original authors. Several excellent overviews of selection procedures can be
found in texts such as those by Hodgson (1986), Mueller, Hawkins, and Northern (1992), Pollack (1988), and Skinner (1988), and in professional journals.

THE HEARING AID SELECTION

ONCE a child is identified as hearing impaired, it is critical that an intervention program be initiated. A key component of this is the selection of appropriate amplification. Through amplification the child will have an opportunity
to hear spoken language and speech and have contact with the world of sound.
Even profoundly hearing-impaired children, who may never receive speech, may
benefit from amplification to help them make contact with the acoustic environment. Therefore, the hearing aid selection process is a critical step in habilitation.

Accurate measurement of hearing in children requires extensive experience
with the pediatric population. Often, the audiologist must make clinical decisions that may not be based on documented responses. In the hands of an inex-
perienced individual, this could be a catastrophe. The same is true for hearing
aid selection procedures. A large percentage of children in the clinical setting
will not be able to tolerate the probe tube for real ear measurements, for example. There is no substitute for competent clinical judgment in the hands of an
audiologist experienced in working with children.

We believe that the hearing aid selection process for children consists of three elements: (1) choosing the most appropriate type of earmolds; (2) selecting the instrument that best meets the hearing-impaired child's needs; and (3) involving the parent or caregiver in the process from the beginning. It is our opinion that parental involvement is critical to the successful use of hearing aids and to a successful habilitation program.

This introduction is presented to help lay the groundwork for the discussion of hearing aid selection procedures. The primary purpose of fitting any type of amplification is to improve the child's communication ability; in fact, the hearing aid has become the central point around which all other aspects of auditory habilitation are planned. Traditionally, hearing aid selection and fitting procedures have relied on clinical measures of communicative ability that involved the application of some type of speech material that requires a voluntary response from the patient. The results of these measures provide data that help the audiologist in making the final recommendation of amplification devices.

The major challenge in selecting and fitting hearing aids for hearing-impaired children is the children's ability to cooperate in the process. Frequently, that ability is significantly limited for reasons of age, maturation, development, multiplicity of impairments, or the degree of hearing loss. Although reasons may be age related, this is not always the case. For example, a child may be fifteen years of age chronologically but unable to participate in customary hearing aid selection procedures because of cognitive difficulties, severity of the hearing loss, age of onset, quality and quantity of educational intervention, or other factors. Nevertheless, a child of fifteen years cannot and should not be managed in the same manner as a six-year-old child with similar problems affecting the ability to cooperate.

Some generalizations can be made based on age, and we attempt to do so in this chapter. Deviations from the usual, however, are many and significant. In addition, those features deemed important in hearing aid selection and fitting procedures are normally not tied to a specific age group.

The first challenge for the audiologist is to realize that each child is an individual, one who is very likely to need an approach or procedure different from the last child or the next. Flexibility, extensive technical knowledge, and a high level of expertise with children are therefore critical requirements for the audiologist. As audiologists we must be equipped and able to apply both objective and functional measures, often in nonstandard ways, to select and fit hearing aids for children successfully.

Functioning within one's clinical "means" is an important but often overlooked pragmatic of the real world. Audiology services are offered to children in a variety of settings with varied and, almost always, limited instrumentation. The minimum equipment needed for hearing aid selections must allow for testing in a soundfield environment for presentation of speech material and frequency-modulated pure tones as well as equipment for immittance measurements, electroacoustic analysis of hearing aids, and real ear measurements.

It is unlikely that all clinical settings will have a full complement of contemporary evaluation instruments. It is also unlikely that all audiologists are fully aware of, and skilled in, the entire range of procedures described in the literature. Operating from a base of ethical principles and realistic goals, therefore, might be more important than the specific practices utilized. It is simply impossible to offer every client all the newest applications; it is also unnecessary.

The goal of improving the hearing-impaired child's ability to develop and use communication should be the audiologist's primary consideration. It is critical to approach this goal from the basis of principles that address it. This may mean that the audiologist will make good use of the practices learned in the classroom or written about in texts. Or the audiologist may disregard those practices completely, maintain the principles behind them, and use creative nonstandard techniques never before used but effective and in the best interest of the child. This is where the audiologist's knowledge must be fully supported by flexibility and pediatric experience. We believe very strongly that the audiologist who cannot be flexible or who lacks experience with children should reconsider working with these young patients, at least until supervised experience is gained.

As audiologists, we must recognize that, although both age of onset of the hearing loss and its degree will help determine impact on the linguistic development of the hearing-impaired child, neither the audiogram nor real ear measures will be able to predict the effectiveness of amplification for spoken language acquisition or other areas of development. Therefore, selecting amplification based on the audiogram or real ear measurements, alone or together, is acceptable neither in principle nor in practice.

Finally, given the importance of early spoken language stimulation in the developmental process, we believe that it is imperative to stress the need for providing amplification as soon as possible after a hearing loss is identified.

PRESELECTION CONSIDERATIONS

SEVERAL decisions can be made before initiating the formal hearing aid selection procedure. Among these are: (1) type of hearing aid, instrument style, microphone directionality (if there is a choice); (2) type of fitting to be done (e.g., BTE); (3) auditory input alternative or telecoil options such as earmold style, acoustics, material, and color. These decisions are not mutually exclusive, but the audiologist must prioritize choices based on attitudes of the child and parent or caregiver, economic circumstances of the family, and the audiologist's knowledge, experience, and biases.

Electroacoustic characteristics of hearing aids are frequently the primary focus both in the professional literature and in the minds of some audiologists. Allowing frequency, gain, and output characteristics to become primary determining factors for making a recommendation for hearing aids can result in a real world disaster. Although these factors are important and must be considered seriously, it is critical to remember that hearing-impaired children must first wear the hearing aids if they are to receive benefit from amplification. Therefore, factors such as style, size, brand, controls, and so forth must be considered for many children.

Binaural vs. Monaural Fitting

Fitting children binaurally seems to be the common wisdom (Bentler 1993; Langford and Faires 1973; Lidén and Hartford 1985; Maxon 1981; Mueller 1986; Northern, Gabbard, and Kinder 1990). We prefer binaural hearing aid fittings whenever possible and believe that Mueller and Hawkins (1990) offered sufficient support for this position in their description of the primary advantages of binaural amplification. These advantages were identified as binaural summation (6–10 dB), elimination of head shadow, and binaural squelch (more effective reduction of noise and reverberation with binaural input).

The long-time concern over whether a binaural fitting improves speech recognition in quiet continues. However, there is now apparently some agreement that there is improved speech recognition in noise (perhaps as a result of the advantages described by Mueller, Hawkins, and Northern 1992) as well as improved localization. In addition, our experience is consistent with many previous accounts such as those of Northern and Downs (1991) that users of binaural amplification report improved sound quality, better fidelity, and easier listening.

Occasionally there will be a child who has significant difficulty tolerating binaural hearing aids. The child may be able to do well with a monaural fitting when the second aid simply causes a disruption in the processing of incoming information. In very young children, this may be evident by the tolerance of one aid but the rejection of both when the second aid is placed. Children who are able to communicate will inform the audiologist of the problem. We must be alert and sensitive to those who communicate poorly.

Obviously, fitting binaurally is easiest when there is a symmetrical, bilateral, sensorineural hearing loss. However, there is no reason that asymmetrical hearing loss could not be fit binaurally if there is flexibility with regard to internal adjustments or hearing aid makes and models. Similarly, if a child has a bilateral conductive hearing loss and there are no contraindications for personal amplification, we recommend a binaural hearing aid selection.

The CROS type fitting was developed by Harford and Barry (1965) to be used for patients with unilateral hearing loss. Since then, many variations on the idea have been published. One of these is the BICROS, developed for use with asymmetrical hearing loss. These fittings are recommended for specific losses (Bess and Tharpe 1984; Hodgson 1986; Matkin and Thomas 1972). Both theoretical and experimental benefits are quite real. In our experience, however, the practical management of CROS and BICROS fittings has been very difficult. As a result, we recommend these fittings only when there is no alternative. We have never experienced either a wired or radio version that performed up to manufacturer's specification for an entire school year; and the younger the child, the more frequent the problems seem to be. Moreover, the management of CROS and BICROS seems to intimidate both parents and teachers.

Type of Hearing Aid

Digitally programmed hearing aids have the advantage of greater precision. The multichannel type has the additional benefit of greater electroacoustic flexibility and performance in noisy environments, but the cost can be as much as 100% more than for a conventional aid. Nevertheless, we believe that the precision and flexibility offered by the multichannel automatic signal processing units are well worth the investment for the child who can participate to the necessary degree in the selection process and, of course, if the units are available through the child's audiologist.

Educational type FM amplification units might also be considered as the initial or primary fitting for neonates and infants in the critical language development period. Madell (1992) presents several convincing reasons for the use of FM amplification on preschool-age children. Among them are improved communication between child and parent, improved signal-to-noise ratio, somewhat better frequency gain characteristics (as shown by audiological testing), and improved speech perception.

Instrument Style

In our experience, body hearing aids are seldom, if ever, used. There is little reason to prescribe this type of instrument unless there is a compelling need. Such a need might occur when a hearing-impaired child has a neuromotor disorder such as cerebral palsy that interferes with the ability to handle the smaller, postauricular instruments. The child might be capable of managing a hearing aid if it were in front. At times, we have encountered a parent who was unable to handle the smaller devices but could manage the larger, body-type instrument. For the most part, children of any age can be fitted with behind-the-ear instruments. This is true also for children who are multiply-impaired because they do not usually manipulate their own hearing aids.

It is obvious that behind-the-ear aids (BTEs) have become used most widely with children. BTEs have many advantages over the body-style aids, including reasonably good binaural qualities, flexible electroacoustics, a variety of sizes, and a wide range of powers so that even a profound loss can be fitted. In addition, some manufacturers offer a variety of bright colors or even see-through models, which can help capture the interest of children and encourage in them a positive attitude toward hearing aids. It should be noted here, however, that the parents must have completed the grieving process to the point of accepting the hearing loss before they can accept the child's choice of either hearing aids or earmolds in nonstandard colors or styles (see chapter 13).

In-the-ear (ITE) hearing aids provide better binaural qualities than do BTEs, and binaural qualities are thought to improve speech recognition in the classroom. Nevertheless, ITEs are not often recommended for children under the age of ten years because they are still growing, and the instruments would have to be recased too often to keep up with growth. Bentler (1993) suggested two other limitations: poor telecoil response and no provision for direct audio input. Of these two, we consider the lack of audio input to be the more detrimental. However, we agree with Northern and Downs (1991), who suggest that ITEs or in-the-canal (ITC) hearing aids should be fitted as often as possible. They report successful fitting of ITEs for children as young as two years, and we encourage this. ITEs can be fitted to provide enough power to all but the most severe hearing losses. They have adequate frequency-gain flexibility; output-limiting microphone directionality is natural; and recasing is only a matter of days if a reputable company is notified of the need to rush an order.

Although telecoil and direct audio input limitations need to be considered, we find that many of our children do not use the telecoils for telephone use even when they have the option. If booting to an FM system is a requirement, then BTE instruments are the answer. Of course, not all BTEs have equally good telecoils. If this is of real concern to the audiologist, then choice of instruments will be limited to only a handful of companies who produce top quality telecoil response characteristics and who actually check the instrument's function to ensure that it meets ANSI specifications before delivery.

Finally, it is easy to assume that children as young as five or six years of age are not vain. Our observations indicate that they are indeed conscious of their appearance, which makes the cosmetic effect of a hearing aid an important ingredient in the child's decision to accept and wear the instrument.

Insurance

Although we prefer not to be concerned about the cost of amplification, in reality it is an issue of great concern. Many insurance carriers provide no hearing benefits. Others place restrictions on the use of hearing benefits, such as stipulating which hearing aid dealers may dispense the instruments or which brand of hearing aids must be used. Often earmolds are provided only once per year and sometimes only one earmold per year may be allowed. Further, some carriers will cover only one hearing aid every three years. In the United States, all fifty states have some state or federally mandated insurance program for children with chronic illnesses or disabilities. Although the program goes by different names in different locations, hearing-impaired children are typically covered. This insurance usually provides hearing aids, earmolds, and sometimes even batteries at no cost to the families. However, to qualify for coverage by such programs, families must meet financial eligibility guidelines. The result is that payment for assessments, hearing aids, earmolds and batteries must be made directly by the parents. This can, and often does, place a heavy financial burden on many families of hearing-impaired children. A factor such as economics of necessity may influence whether the audiologist will prescribe monaural or binaural fittings or whether the instrument that would best meet the child's needs electroacoustically will be prescribed at all.

EARMOLDS

THE earmold is a critical part of the amplification system because it connects the hearing aid to the child and significantly affects the acoustics delivered to the tympanic membrane. The earmold is often the most problematic component in the system. Feedback occurs frequently due to an inadequate fit, broken or hard tubing, a vent that is too large, and so on.

Discomfort is also a frequent complaint. The better the earmold is at the beginning, the fewer the problems later. Our experience is that many clinical audiologists seldom, if ever, see the earmold problems once the child has been fitted with hearing aids because they often do not follow up beyond the hearing aid pick-up or orientation appointments. Subsequent earmolds might best be made by the educational audiologist, if available, as this individual has the opportunity to see the child and communicate with teachers regularly. Badly made, poorly fitting earmolds are a significant management problem that must be addressed if successful use of amplification is to be achieved.

Earmold Impression

When making an impression, children to two years of age are usually held by their parents or caregivers, positioned on the lap with the adult's arms wrapped around the infant. If necessary, the child's legs can be caught between the adult's legs. Some children from 18 to 24 months are able to sit quietly enough to cooperate in the process of obtaining earmold impressions. A highchair is ideal for those who can sit independently as the tray serves to hold a mirror and something with which to play. If the child is too large for a highchair, a standard, comfortable chair can be used.

One effective technique is to place a mirror in front of the child who can then watch what you are doing. The ability to see themselves in the mirror while you work serves to reduce anxiety. For children who are able to comprehend, showing them the tools and materials you will be using also helps them to relax.

It is necessary, of course, to ensure that the ear canal is reasonably clean and free of debris before proceeding. It is best to do so at the time of the otologic visit so that the physician can clean the ears if necessary. However, the audiologist should be trained and prepared to do the cleaning if the canals are not clear and ENT services are not readily available.

Because children do not stop talking or moving their mouths when they are wearing their earmolds, no attempt is made to keep them from talking or moving their mouths while the impression material is setting. This will lead to a better earmold fit. It is imperative that the audiologist not attempt to pack or push the material into the ear. Children's ears are so pliable that the slightest pressure will push them out of a natural shape, adversely affecting the impression.

The length of the canal piece is a critical factor in obtaining a good earmold fit for children with severe or profound hearing impairments. Be certain that the impression material gets into the canal deeply enough to obtain an appropriate canal fit. A good helix is important in maintaining a lock on the fit of the earmold, especially for younger children.

For children who will be fitted with postauricular hearing aids (most of our patients), impressions should be obtained only with the hearing aid in place over the pinna and with the battery in the hearing aid. This is crucial for children who are still growing. Actually, it is good practice to do this with all clients. Some people have pinnae that are very pliable or abnormal in shape or position (e.g., too close to the skull, rotated backward, low set, or malformed in another manner). As a result, we have found poor earmold fit when impressions were obtained without the hearing aids in place. If the children wear glasses, we recommend that the glasses be in place with the hearing aids because it is likely that they will be utilizing their amplification while they also will be wearing their glasses.

Showing video cartoons during the time it takes the impression material to set has been successful in containing children of all ages. The child may prefer to play with toys at a table, and this too is acceptable as long as playing does not require standing up and moving around the room. Often, children three years of age or older enjoy playing with the unused impression material while they wait. This should be permitted only under supervision. The excess material should ordinarily be taken from the child after the process because some children will attempt to mimic the procedure by putting the leftover material in their ear canals when alone.

Style and Material for Earmolds

We prefer a soft material such as silicone or vinyl. Although silicone is more difficult to modify, it has two advantages over vinyl. First, it is an inert material (hypoallergenic) and is softer, thus permitting a tighter fit and reduced probability of feedback. Soft earmolds are best accepted by parents, teachers, and children alike. Also, they do not work their way out of the ear as easily as those made from hard material. The type of material is essential to the fit, comfort, and performance, and should be specified by the audiologist.

In our practice, we have found the Select-A-Vent to be the least useful modification to earmolds, even for those children who need less low frequency gain. However, it is necessary to have a pressure vent for some of these children because they will otherwise complain about the quality of the sound. Our most frequently used modification is the continuous flow adapter (C.F.A.), which is ordered for virtually all our infants and young children who have hearing losses ranging from mild to severe and sometimes profound. Our clinical experience has demonstrated that high frequency enhancement is often better with C.F.A. than that produced by a horn modification. In addition, the fit is better because the connector makes the tubing adjustable to some degree. Finally, the size of the ear canal is not a problem as it is with the horn-type bore. The C.F.A. is not without problems, however. The elbow fit may loosen, causing feedback, and the connection breaks down faster. We advise parents to have spare elbows available, and we teach them how to replace elbows and tubing.

A horn modification can be utilized when the child is older and the ears have stopped growing. To benefit from the horn, one needs the correct length and cross-sectional dimensions, but many children do not have large enough canals to accommodate even a three-millimeter horn.

Of course, the more severe the hearing loss, the thicker the tubing needed for the earmold. We order the thicker tubing routinely, except for those children with mild hearing losses, because it also adds stability to the hearing aid placement and is more durable. It is also helpful to know that a product known as "dry tube" is available for children who collect excessive moisture in the tubing. Dry tube is earmold tubing that prevents condensation from forming within the tubing.

In general, we order a full shell earmold for most of our hearing-impaired children. Whenever appropriate, and with parent or caregiver permission, we let children select the color of earmold they prefer. The neon colors, while a little more expensive, are very popular, and we believe this helps reduce the perceived stigma of hearing aids.

Finally, keep handy a plentiful supply of a lubricating cream such as Oto-ferm. It not only eases insertion of the earmold, especially when the mold has a long canal piece, but it also improves the seal that aids in preventing feedback.

Real Ear Measurements

Real ear or probe tube measurement is the preferred method for beginning the hearing aid selection; unfortunately, it is not always feasible. Infants and toddlers, as a rule, are unable to cooperate. We choose not to sedate children to obtain real ear data. Furthermore, we strongly recommend that, in the selection procedure, behavioral measurements be used to corroborate data from real ear measurements before a final recommendation of instrument is made. Of course, behavioral measurements may also be difficult to obtain.

Using real ear or probe tube measurements requires a fairly quiet location. The ear canals should be free of debris, and the child's personal earmolds should be utilized. Therefore, the child must be tolerant of the earmolds in the ears. To do this, it may be necessary for some children to become accustomed to wearing their earmolds before the hearing aid selection procedure. We prefer to do this with amplification attached. Unfortunately, the child must be able to leave the earmolds in place if further progress is to be made. Tolerance for the earmolds becomes essential for those children who are tactilely defensive.

When making real ear measurements, we routinely use the NAL-R formula for mild to moderate hearing losses, and POGO is used for severe and profound losses. Other procedures such as the CID: Phase IV or the DSL may be useful also. (See Mueller et al. [1992] for an overview of these methods.) Each audiologist will need to make an individual choice regarding a formula and must take into account the child's needs.

As in obtaining earmold impressions, it is helpful to place a mirror in front of children during real ear measurements so that they can watch what is happening and not be fearful. The equipment that will be used should be shown to the children. Use of video cartoons with the sound off has been found to be helpful in entertaining many children during this procedure.

If two different hearing aids appear to meet your target for the child, then it is important to make your choice based on another factor. The choice may be based on the size of the hearing aids, if desired, but only after behavioral measurements are done in the soundfield and an aided audiogram is obtained. Again, if two or more aids perform equally well, the decision may need to be based on how the child does at speech awareness with the Ling five-sound test (see chapter 5) or speech recognition at a distance, or perhaps in noise. Children who are experienced hearing aid users or who are old enough and have adequate language will be able to tell the audiologist if they prefer one instrument to another. Finally, the choice of instruments may be based on economics or on the preference of the parent or audiologist.

Whenever possible, MCL and UCL levels (both with real ear measurements) should be obtained while you are obtaining the aided audiogram.

Setting Targets

When determining how much amplification is appropriate for the hearing-impaired child, the target should be as close to the speech range as it is possible to get without distortion or discomfort; an additional pitfall to avoid is exceeding what we consider the safe limit.

What is the safe limit? Although there is no general agreement, temporary and permanent threshold shifts due to overamplification have been documented and reported in the literature (Hawkins, 1982; Heffernan and Simons 1979; Rintelmann and Bess 1988). Clinically, we have seen incidents of temporary (fortunately) threshold shift in children using high levels of maximum power output. These have occurred when hearing aids have been repaired and placed on the child without readjustment of internal settings. Our rule of thumb is never to exceed 124 to 128 dB SPL as a protection against possible deterioration of hearing levels. This can best be measured by real ear procedures.

Besides the safety issue, it appears that high levels of maximum power output contribute nothing to improved speech awareness or recognition when compared to lower levels. A pilot study done at Children's Hospital of Michigan (Schneider, Rich, and Bazell 1989) evaluated a group of hearing-impaired children with severe to profound degrees of loss. They were tested under two conditions: With their hearing aids set at full on (130 dB SSPL or greater) and the SSPL levels as close to 125 dB as it was possible to set the instruments. Measures obtained included aided thresholds, correct perception of the Ling Five Sound Test with sounds presented directly behind the child, and at three, five, and ten feet from the child. Where possible, speech recognition scores were obtained using standard lists.

The results of the pilot study indicated that aided audiograms were not substantially different between the two conditions. When high SSPL settings resulted in better thresholds for frequency modulated pure tones, the difference was five to ten dB at two or three frequencies. However, even when the higher settings elicited better thresholds for tones, discrimination or detection of the Ling sounds was poorer than at the lower power setting. Speech recognition scores, where obtained, were also poorer at the higher power settings.

Our preferred target for setting internal controls on hearing aids is a volume use of three (3) when the dial ranges from one (1) to four (4) for severe and profound hearing loss, or one-half to two-thirds of the maximum on the volume control. This affords some leeway for adjusting volume up or down as suggested by Mueller, Hawkins, and Northern (1992). Whatever volume setting is chosen, it should provide the child with the targeted frequency gain characteristics.

The reader is referred to Mueller, Hawkins, and Northern (1992) for a complete discussion of real ear measurements in the hearing aid evaluation process.

Alternatives to Real Ear Measurements

There are alternatives to the use of real ear measurements for hearing aid selection if equipment is not available. We stress, however, that extensive pediatric experience is required to utilize behavioral procedures well. The major problem in using the calibrated soundfield is the lack of cooperation or ability to respond by the child. Visual reinforcement procedures may or may not be usable. VRA is not usable with infants below six months of age. In addition, ability to respond to this technique relies on cognitive level and neuromotor control.

When using behavioral measures to select amplification, the targets remain the same. That is, maximum power is limited to 125 to 128 dB SPL. Internal settings are made with the goal of using a volume level that will yield the preferred power output; another aim is to select hearing aids that will provide amplification as close to the speech range as it is possible to get without distortion, discomfort, or exceeding the safe limit.

Sometimes the hearing aid selection is done using the "by guess and by gosh" procedure because all other attempts have failed, and it is imperative that amplification be provided. In this instance, the ideal situation would be to have a large stock of loaner hearing aids from which various instruments can be tried on the child for a week or two. This permits the audiologist to follow the child closely and receive feedback from the parent or caregiver regarding behavior while wearing the hearing aids. Often, once the child has worn some type of amplification for a week or two, responses begin to emerge and further testing can be undertaken.

General Procedures

Regardless of whether the audiologist uses real ear measurements, a minimum of three hearing aids should be tried out in the selection process. At times more will be used. With very young children, it may be necessary to conduct the hearing aid selection in two appointments to complete all the assessments or measurements.

The size of the hearing aid may be a consideration, especially for very young children or those with small, malformed, or close-set ears. However, the size of the instrument should never be the critical feature in the choice of a hearing aid.

In a pediatric practice, it is necessary to have an ample supply of "baby" ear hooks. One must be aware, of course, that these change the frequency response of the hearing aids. If a pediatric-size hook is utilized, the selection process must be done with that hook on the hearing aid. If not, real ear measurements will have to be repeated at the conformity to determine exactly what the ear is receiving. We also mention here the often overlooked availability of the Etymotic hooks. Although they are not particularly attractive, we have found them to be effective in achieving certain response characteristics.

All hearing aids selected through real ear measurements should be evaluated in the soundfield also. In addition to obtaining responses to aided frequency-modulated pure tones, speech recognition should be tested if possible. At the very least, speech detection thresholds must be obtained, and the Ling Five Sound Test should be utilized. The Ling sounds should be presented both in the soundfield and at distances of five and ten feet. We believe it is critical to fit hearing aids for distance as well as for near settings. Other speech material may be utilized. For example, numbers are frequently recognized even by children with the severest of hearing impairments.

Our target for aided responses to the Ling sounds is 46 dB HL. If the child is unable to respond at that intensity level, increase gain until all five sounds elicit responses or until best performance is obtained. Then adjust the aid accordingly.

Finally, we caution that the shape of the aided audiogram should never be precipitous. That is, do not permit amplification to produce an aided audiogram that results in responses of 10 dB at 250 Hz, 20 dB at 500 Hz, and 50 dB or more at 1000 Hz and above. In this condition, the low frequency amplification masks information at the other frequencies.

Fitting the Hearing Aid

Before delivering the hearing aids to the child, an electroacoustic analysis should be completed for each instrument. It is important to run the instruments according to ANSI specifications in order to compare them to the manufacturer's specifications. However, we believe it is equally important to run the hearing aids at the "to be worn" setting based on the results of the hearing aid selection procedure. This includes the correct internal control settings and the target volume selected for the child.

A conformity test, which should include the same measures that were done when the hearing aids were selected, is performed when the hearing aids are delivered. If the child's aided performance does not match that obtained at the time of the selection, one must consider doing real ear measurements to identify the reason for the poorer performance. We recommend that real ear measures be made routinely at the time of the conformity to fine-tune targets. It will be necessary at times for first-time hearing aid users to be fitted with gain below the target so that they can become used to amplified sound gradually. If the audiologist is unsure about the exact internal settings for the hearing aids (and this does happen), the gain should be estimated on the low side and increased as needed.

Caregiver Training

At the time the hearing aids are delivered, the parent or caregiver is trained to manage the instruments. Of course, the audiologist demonstrates battery insertion, attachment of the earmold to the ear-hook, and the on-off switch and volume settings. The adult should then repeat the process. Inserting the earmold in the ear is then demonstrated. Many children will be able to learn how to handle the hearing aids at the time of fitting. We have had children as young as two years of age be able to put on their own instruments. If the audiologist has concerns about the ability of the adult (or child) to manage the hearing aids, weekly appointments should be scheduled until management is mastered. The initial orientation should include some techniques parents can use to initiate auditory training for the child. Some of these are discussed in the last section of this chapter.

Keeping the Hearing Aids on the Ears

It is often difficult to keep hearing aids in place on a young child's ears. This problem results in failure to receive full benefit from amplification and may also result in lost or broken devices. Several products have been used—with various degrees of success—to alleviate this problem. Two-sided tape that is reported not to irritate skin will sometimes work. In our experience, even this tape irritates the skin in young children. A device such as the Huggie Aid assists in keeping the hearing aid in place and may help prevent tampering with the battery drawer or volume control. However, we find that some children use this device as a faster way to pull their hearing aids out because it is easy to grab and pull.

We have found that an eyeglass cord used to suspend glasses from the neck when not being worn works very well in helping avoid lost hearing aids. The cord is attached to the hearing aids, and the center is pinned to the inside of a shirt, dress, or sweater. If an aid should fall out, the cord keeps it from falling to the ground or being lost. Parents have also reported some success with an elastic sports band that holds glasses in place for the physically active. On occasion, we have had to resort to sweat bands or ski bands to keep the aids in place and stop the child from pulling them off. One must exercise care that the hearing aid microphones are not covered by the fabric.

Continuing Follow-up

Following the initial hearing aid fitting—and assuming the audiologist is comfortable with the parent's or caregiver's ability to manage the hearing aids—our experience is that a follow-up visit should be scheduled in three months. At the first follow-up visit, a hearing aid conformity examination should be conducted. It is recommended that the same test materials utilized during the selection and the fitting be used again at this time. The parent or caregiver is asked to demonstrate the management of the hearing aids. Any questions that have occurred since the child was last seen can be answered. The follow-up visit also provides an opportunity to ensure that the recommendations for educational placement are being followed.

The second follow-up visit should occur six months after the first, and the procedures should be the same. Now the child may be capable of further testing. The audiologist should keep in mind the need to conduct formal testing as soon as possible. Any standardized test with which the audiologist is comfortable and that is consistent with the age of the child can be used.

Attitudes

It is imperative that the use of hearing aids be presented to the child, regardless of age, in the most positive light possible. Parents must understand that their attitude about amplification will influence how their child adapts to the use of hearing aids. Therefore, the aids need to be viewed by all concerned as absolutely wonderful. The experienced audiologist will understand the need to provide skills and techniques to the parents to help them initiate habilitation. The parents need to have some positive feedback as soon as possible so that the child can be positively reinforced. This is best achieved when the adults are able to see the effects of amplification by obtaining responses from the child. This creates a positive reinforcement for both parent and child.

THE SCHOOL PROGRAM

THE presence of an educational audiologist within a school program makes life easier because that person serves as the contact for the clinical audiologist. Only through the educational audiologist can we be assured that the child's hearing aids will be monitored periodically, earmold fit will be checked routinely, and any internal settings for the hearing aid are reset following repairs. It is imperative that the school program know the correct hearing aid settings for any hearing-impaired child. If the child is not receiving school services for the hearing loss, parents must be made aware that hearing aids are never to be put back on the child's ears following repair unless first seen by an audiologist. We have had some parents who were perfectly capable of resetting hearing aids following repair. However, only the audiologist in a clinical or educational setting will be able to evaluate the devices electroacoustically.

FM Amplification

The audiologist who has done the hearing aid selection for the child and the educational audiologist, if available, should work together to determine the most appropriate settings for any FM amplification system that will be used in school. We recommend that these devices be set as close as possible to the chosen settings for the hearing aids. This may be done most precisely by use of real ear measurements to ensure that the children are not overamplified and, possibly, provide some consistency in input between the hearing aid and FM unit.

This is not always possible, however, particularly with neonates and infants. Moreover, the instrumentation for real ear measurements may not be available. A clear description of the procedures for this as well as other aspects of FM amplification system selection and use can be found in Ross (1992).

PARENTS, CAREGIVERS, AND THE HEARING AID SELECTION PROCESS

Parents As Partners

PARENTS are the critical link between the hearing aid fitting and successful adaptation and use of amplification by the child. Adult attitudes about amplification will influence the child's response. When aids are considered to be a wonderful invention, that feeling is transmitted to the youngster. The audiologist must spend sufficient time counseling the adult regarding the need for a positive attitude, both at the beginning of the hearing aid selection process and during fitting and follow-up visits. However, this is to be done only when the caregivers are ready (see chapter 13).

Care and Maintenance of the Hearing Aids

Training in the care and maintenance of hearing aids is, of course, very important. An excellent discussion of all the features of a maintenance program is presented by Musket (1988). Clinically, we have found that parents function best when provided with tangible material to which they can refer as necessary. The addendum to this chapter is a sample of the material we provide to parents of hearing-impaired children.

Grief and Grieving

Audiologists must recognize the grieving process and all its stages in order to work effectively with the parents of hearing-impaired children (see chapter 13). It is important to recognize in what stage parents may be and to know what type of responses to expect from them. Often the audiologist who first identifies a child's hearing loss becomes the villain in the scene. When this occurs, parents may seek out second and even third opinions. In our experience, parents invariably make a full circle back to the original professional.

Audiologists must also recognize their own limitations in counseling parents through the grieving process. At times it may be necessary only to sit and listen, whereas at other times it may be essential to make comments and suggestions. Appropriate referrals should be made when needed for available support services. Although it is often difficult to find counseling professionals who have an understanding of hearing impairment and its effects on families, it may be vital to have access to such individuals. We have found that deaf parents of deaf children reject such referrals for the most part, whereas hearing parents of deaf children may request referral.

It is helpful to be familiar with the literature that deals with both the grieving process and counseling families. The reader is referred to the writings of Kubler-Ross (1969, 1974), who has clearly identified and described the stages of grief. This information may help the audiologist recognize where parents may be in the process. Moses (1985) has addressed grief and counseling for parents of hearing-impaired infants. Luterman (1984, 1987) has addressed counseling and the effect of hearing impairment on the family of the impaired individual (also see chapter 13).

Parents' Groups

An effective means of both educating parents and helping them adjust to their child's hearing loss is a parents' group, conducted by parents and not professionals. The most common threads in such groups are their children's hearing losses and the decisions that need to be made about education and habilitation programs.

The parents of our hearing-impaired patients have formed such a group and have invited participation of parents from many different clinics and programs. It has proven to be an excellent resource for the parents, who determine when and how often they will meet and what their programs will consist of. Annually they include a panel of hearing-impaired children who discuss their feelings, opinions, and needs. Our professional staff does not participate except by invitation of the parents or as a learning experience for themselves. Included in the parents' group programs are periodic meetings described as "For Parents Only," which serve as "gripe sessions." Gripes may be directed toward school programs, physicians, audiologists, or any other issue felt to be important to members of the group.

By airing concerns and complaints, parents help each other resolve many conflicts. In addition, the group empowers individual members, enabling them to advocate for their child.

Early Intervention

Parents frequently relate feelings of helplessness in dealing with their hearing-impaired children. Their active involvement in the youngster's habilitation program is indispensable, for it helps them develop a communication system and feel that they are constructively engaged in helping their children. Intense parental participation is probably the most effective means of ensuring that amplification will yield positive reinforcement for the child—and for the parent as well.

The audiologist must be responsible for directing the early attempts at habilitation both by providing activities that can be joined in by all at home and by making referrals for other support services. Besides the necessary educational referrals, it is important—as part of a total program—that the child receive some type of hearing therapy, whether it is provided by a speech-language pathologist or an audiologist.

As part of management of the child, parents should observe the training sessions and be encouraged to reinforce the training at home. Positive reinforcement from the specialist treating the child provides support for the parents and serves as the stimulus to keep them working. Within our clinical settings, we advise all parents of infants and preschool children to contact the John Tracy Clinic to obtain the free-to-parents material that agency provides. Involvement in this type of program also serves to help parents feel useful. Parents are also provided with the names and addresses of other agencies and organizations whose primary function is service to the hearing impaired.

An excellent source of material for intervention—for audiologists, speech-language pathologists, and parents—is *Parent-Infant Communication: A Pro-*

gram of Clinical and Home Training for Parents and Hearing-Impaired Infants (Schuyler et al. 1985). It is a well-organized and thorough training program that is fairly easy to initiate and conducive to home training by parents. Audiologists working with hearing-impaired children should be familiar with this publication.

Educational Options

Choosing an educational program for a hearing-impaired child is often a difficult decision for parents. However, it must be the child's parents who make the choice and not the professionals who are or will be involved in the habilitation or education process. Input from the audiologist may be solicited, but information should always be provided as objectively as possible. It is the audiologist's responsibility to ensure that parents are aware of the choices available to them both within their local school districts and by state and federal mandate. Schwartz (1987) provides an excellent presentation for parents on educational options for hearing-impaired children.

Another excellent source of information for parents is *Beginnings for Parents of Hearing-Impaired Children* (Greene 1990). The Beginnings Program was instituted by and developed through the extensive effort of Art Mines, who was, for a time, its executive director, and through the input of many parents and professionals. Greene's publication is a resource that evolved from those efforts. It contains an excellent, objective presentation of educational choices. We recommend that parents have access to the material. The audiologist's professional responsibility includes ensuring that the parents are fully informed.

REFERENCES

Bentler, R. A. 1993. Amplification for the hearing impaired child. In *Rehabilitative audiology: Children and adults*, 2d ed., ed. J.G. Alpiner and P.A. McCarthy. Baltimore: Williams and Wilkins.

Bess, F.H., and A.M. Tharpe. (1984). Unilateral hearing impairment in children. *Pediatrics* 74:206–216.

Greene, J.C. 1990. *Beginnings for parents of hearing impaired children: A parent manual.* Durham, NC: The Beginnings for Parents of Hearing Impaired Children, Inc.

Harford, E.R., and J. Barry. 1965. A rehabilitative approach to the problems of unilateral hearing impairment: The contralateral routing of signals CROS. *Journal of Speech and Hearing Disorders* 30:121–128.

Hawkins, D.R. 1982. Overamplification: A well documented case report. *Journal of Speech and Hearing Disorders* 47:382–384.

Heffernan, H.P., and M.R. Simons. 1979. Temporary increase in sensorineural hearing loss with hearing aid use. *Annals of Otology, Rhinology and Laryngology* 88:86–91.

Hodgson, W.R., ed. 1986. *Hearing aid assessment and use in audiologic habilitation.* 3d ed. Baltimore: Williams and Wilkins.

Kubler-Ross, E. 1969. *On death and dying.* New York: Macmillan.

————. 1974. *Questions and answers on death and dying*. New York: Collier Books.

Langford, S.E., and W.L. Faires. 1973. Objective evaluation of monaural vs. binaural amplification for congenitally hard-of-hearing children. *Journal of Auditory Research* 13:263–267.

Lidén, G., and E.R. Harford. 1985. The pediatric audiologist: From magician to clinician. *Ear and Hearing* 6:6–9.

Luterman, D. 1984. *Counseling the communicatively disordered and their families*. Boston: Little, Brown and Co.

————. 1987. *Deafness in the family*. Boston: Little, Brown and Co.

Madell, J.R. 1992. FM systems for children birth to age five. In *FM auditory training systems: Characteristics, selections, and use*, ed. M.A.Ross. Timonium, MD: York Press.

Matkin, N.D., and J. Thomas. 1972. The utilization of CROS hearing aids in children. *Maico Audiological Library Series* 10:8.

Maxon, A.B. 1981. Binaural amplification of young children: A clinical application of Ross's theory. *Ear and Hearing* 2:215–219.

Moses, K.L. 1985. Infant deafness and parental grief: Psychosocial early intervention. In *Education of the hearing-impaired child*, ed. F. Powell, T. Fenitzo-Hieber, S.F. Friel-Patti, and D. Henderson. San Diego: College-Hill Press.

Mueller, H.G. 1986. Binaural amplification: Attitudinal factors. *The Hearing Journal* 39: 7–10.

Mueller, H.G., and D.B. Hawkins. 1990. Three important considerations in hearing aid selection. In *Handbook of hearing aid amplification*, ed. R. Sandlin. Boston: College-Hill Press.

Mueller, H.G., D. Hawkins, and J. Northern. 1992. *Probe microphone measurements: Hearing aid selection and assessment*. San Diego: Singular Publishing Group.

Musket, C.H. 1988. Maintenance of personal hearing aids. In *Auditory disorders in school children*, 2d ed., ed. R. Roeser and M. Downs. New York: Thieme Medical Publishers.

Northern, J.L., and M.P. Downs. 1991. *Hearing in children*. 4th ed. Baltimore: Williams and Wilkins.

Northern, J.L., S.A. Gabbard, and D.L. Kinder. 1990. Pediatric consideration in selecting and fitting hearing aids. In *Handbook of hearing aid amplification*, Vol. II, ed. R.E. Sandlin. Boston: College-Hill Press.

Pollack, M.C., ed. 1988. *Amplification for the hearing-impaired*. 3d ed. New York: Grune and Stratton.

Rintelmann, W.F., and F.H. Bess. 1988. High-level amplification and potential hearing loss in children. In *Hearing impairment in children*, ed. F.H. Bess. Parkton, MD: York Press.

Ross, M.A., ed. 1992. *FM auditory training systems: Characteristics, selections, and use*. Timonium, MD: York Press.

Schneider, P.K., J.A. Rich, and C. Bazell. 1989. The effect of SSPL setting on gain measurement in the soundfield in children: A pilot study. Poster session presented at MSHA Annual Conference, March.

Schuyler, V., N. Rushmer, R. Arpan, A. Melum, J. Sowers, and N. Kennedy. 1985. *Parent-infant communication: A program of clinical and home training for parents and hearing-impaired infants*. Portland, OR: Infant Hearing Resource Publications.

Schwartz, S., ed. 1987. *Choices in deafness: A parent's guide*. Kensington, MD: Woodbine House.

Skinner, M.W. 1988. *Hearing aid evaluation*. Englewood Cliffs, NJ: Prentice Hall.

For Parents of Hearing-Impaired Children
Prepared by the Staff
of the Marie Carls Communication Disorders Centers,
Children's Hospital of Michigan

LEARNING to listen—or auditory training—is one of your child's most important goals. You need to make sure that the child's hearing aid is always working well and that you do a lot of talking to the child. The responsible adult must be "in charge" of the hearing aids. This means that you will determine when they are put on and when they are removed from the ears. If your child pulls the hearing aids off, it is critical that you replace them immediately. If you think that your child has worn the instruments long enough for that period of the day, then remove the hearing aids yourself. Remember, you are in control.

In the Beginning

1. Practice putting the hearing aid on and adjusting its controls. Encourage the child—if old enough—to take care of the aid unassisted.
2. To put the earmold into the ear, place the canal part down into the ear canal. Gently push and rotate the earmold back and forth until it sits firmly in the ear.
3. Turn up the volume to the recommended setting. If you hear "whistling" (feedback), the earmold is probably not in correctly.
4. Always remember to turn the aid off before removing it to prevent feedback.
5. Children get used to their new hearing aids and earmold at different rates. In general, your child should begin wearing the aids for short periods of time and then gradually increase the length of these periods. Since the child has been living in a quiet world up until now, loud sounds and noise may bother the child. Start with quiet listening environments and work toward more difficult or noisy situations. Point out some of the familiar sounds in your house, such as the telephone, washing machine, and so on.

What to Do Every Day

Always listen to your child's hearing aid through your hearing aid stethoscope before the aids are worn. This procedure should be followed each day and any time your child does not seem to be hearing as well as usual.

1. Always use a battery at full strength. It is best to check the battery at night with a battery tester.
2. Put the battery into the battery compartment so the positive (+) side of the battery matches the positive (+) mark on the compartment.
3. With the hearing aid stethoscope attached to the earmold, turn the hearing aid on. If possible, listen to the aid at the recommended volume setting. As you turn the volume control, the hearing aid should gradually increase in loudness. Say the following five sounds into the microphone of the hearing aid: oo as in moon, ah as in father, ee as in key, sh as in shoe, s as in say.

These five sounds cover the frequency range for speech and will indicate whether speech sounds are being adequately picked up by the hearing aid. The vowel sounds should be clear. No hissing or other distortion should be present when saying "sh" or "s."

4. If you notice a problem, consult the "possible problems and their causes" sheet.

5. Turn the hearing aid on: If the child is too young or is unable to handle the aid alone, put it on for the child.

6. If old enough, the child should now put the aid in and turn it on. Note the volume setting. Did the child set it at the recommended setting? If not or if the child turns the volume all the way down during the day, call us, and we will check to see if all the internal settings are appropriate.

7. Do the five-sound test with your child facing you. Have your child indicate that the sounds are heard by clapping, pointing to the ear, or repeating the sound.

8. Ask your child to turn around and do the five-sound test again.

What to Do at Night

1. Always turn the aid off before taking it out of the ear.

2. Open the battery compartment and take the battery out. Check it on the battery tester. It is best to test the battery after it has been used all day. Discard any bad batteries.

3. Check the earmold for wax. Pick the wax out of the little hole that lets the sound into the ear. Pipe cleaners work very well for this. Wipe the outside with a damp cloth. Do not use alcohol because that will dry out the earmold material.

4. Put the hearing aid in a safe place away from extreme heat or cold, water, pets, and so on. It is wise to put the aids in an air-tight container along with a package of silica gel.

What to Do Yearly

Have the audiologist recheck your child's hearing.

What Never to Do

Never put the hearing aid back on your child after it has been repaired without first having the audiologist reset the internal settings.

Questions Asked Most Often

1. How can I get my child to wear the aid(s)?

Your child's self-concept and willingness to wear the hearing aid have a lot to do with parent attitude. Your acceptance and firm and consistent reinforcement will encourage the child to wear the aids just as shoes, socks, and glasses are worn.

2. Do hearing aids make my child hear normally?

No. A hearing aid does not work the same way for hearing as glasses do for seeing. It makes the speech sound that your child hears louder and tunes your child into environmental sounds that may not be heard without the aid. It does not make speech clearer, though. Consistent auditory training needs to be done to increase the child's ability to understand the sounds the child is hearing. The more you work with your child, the better off he/she will be.

3. When should my child wear the aid(s)?

The child needs to wear them all the time while awake, except when bathing, swimming, or playing in the sandbox. For parents of napping children: Some parents turn their child's aid off but leave them in during naptime, whereas others take the aids out. Always remember to put the hearing aids back in and turn them on.

4. How long does a battery last?

This depends on:

(a) the type of battery;
(b) how powerful the hearing aid is;
(c) how many hours the aid is worn during the day; and
(d) whether the aid is in good working order.

That is why it is so important to check the battery on the battery tester. A battery can build up power overnight and seem ok in the morning, so get into the habit of checking the battery when your child gets home from school or at night before bed. Battery testers can be purchased from a hearing aid dealer or from:

Hal-Hen Company
36–14 Eleven Street
Long Island City, NY 11106

5. How long will a hearing aid last?

Depending upon the daily care it is given, between two and four years, and sometimes longer.

6. What if the earmold seems to be bothering my child's ear?

Sometimes the ear can get irritated or sore from the earmold. If this happens, have your audiologist or the hearing aid dealer check how well the earmold fits. There are nonallergenic materials available if they have not been tried already. If the problem persists, take your child to an ear doctor (otolaryngologist or otologist) for evaluation and treatment. The child may have a skin disorder in the ear canal or other problems that need medical attention. Sometimes the problem does not have a medical cause nor is it the earmold. Your child may be sensitive to loud sounds. Call your audiologist in order to make sure the power controls are set appropriately.

7. Will my child learn to talk?

Children learn and progress at their own rate. (How far your child will go toward that goal depends on many factors, however.) Ask your audiologist to discuss this with you. One of the most important influences is *you*, the parent. Your son or daughter needs to develop listening skills as soon as possible. You need to encourage dependence on sound and do a lot of talking about the things that matter to the child. Daily activities such as dressing, bathing, eating, and playing are perfect opportunities. Ask your audiologist or your child's teacher for suggestions.

8. What if my child accidentally swallows a battery?

This could be dangerous. Call the National Button-Battery Ingestion Hotline, 1-202-625-3333, or your local poison control hotline.

9. In addition to my daily test check, how often should I have my child's hearing aids checked?

Two or three times each year (or more if a problem comes up). To help your child improve listening skills, here are some things to remember:

(a) Shouting distorts your voice and leads to frustration and irritability. Stay close to your child and talk in a normal voice.

(b) Do not touch the child to get his/her attention. If you speak first, your child will get used to listening and paying attention to your voice. If you act as though you don't expect to be heard, your child will become conditioned to not listening.

(c) Try sitting side-by-side or have the child on your lap when you talk about pictures in books or play games. This encourages more use of hearing.

(d) If you have not already contacted the John Tracy Clinic, we strongly recommend it. They will send good activities, free of charge, to help you work with your child. The address and form are in the back of this pamphlet.

DAILY CHECK LIST

1. Did you check the battery?
2. Did you check the earmold?
3. Did you listen to the hearing aid and check the volume control?
4. Did you do the five-sound test?

11

Cochlear Implants

Judith A. Brimacombe and Anne L. Beiter

COCHLEAR implants are state-of-the-art microelectronic devices designed to restore a level of auditory function to profoundly deafened individuals who do not benefit from conventional amplification. These biomedical mechanisms convert sound into electrical current and bypass the damaged receptive sensory end-organ to stimulate directly the remaining auditory nerve fibers. The resulting neural activity propagates along the auditory pathways to the cortex. In individuals who have had prior auditory experience, and thus have some auditory memory, the sensations are reported as hearing immediately. It is difficult to know how these sensations are interpreted initially by congenitally deaf children who have had no exposure to acoustic stimuli. However, with experience, these children also respond to auditory input and display the ability to use the information provided by the cochlear implant in a meaningful way. This chapter discusses the management of profoundly deaf children at different chronological ages and stages of auditory development who may be candidates for, or utilize, this technology.

Research on direct electrical stimulation of the auditory system has a long history. The first reported application of direct stimulation of the auditory system occurred in 1957 when two French physicians, Djourno and Eyries, placed an electrode on a segment of the auditory nerve during facial nerve reconstructive surgery. The patient reported hearing background sounds and found the device helpful with lipreading (Luxford and Brackmann 1985). Shortly after that, several investigators in the United States (e.g., House, Michelson, Simmons, and Eddington) began their investigations into the feasibility of direct electrical stimulation of the auditory system. Soon researchers in Australia (Clark) and Europe (Chouard, Douek, Fisch, Hochmair, and Hochmair-Desoyer) began their research studies. Other investigators followed in the 1980s. More detailed information on the historical development of cochlear prostheses can be found in House and Berliner (1991), Luxford and Brackmann (1985), Mecklenburg and Lehnhardt (1991), Mecklenburg and Shallop (1988), Shallop and Mecklenburg (1987), Simmons (1966), Staller (1985), and Tyler and Tye-Murray (1991).

Today, cochlear implants are considered a safe and effective medical treatment for profound, bilateral sensorineural hearing loss in appropriately selected adults and children. In November 1984, the United States Food and Drug Administration (FDA) approved the first cochlear implant for commercial use in adults. It was a single-channel device developed by House and his colleagues and manufactured by 3M Corporation, St. Paul, Minnesota. Soon after that, in October 1985, the FDA approved commercial distribution of the Nucleus 22-channel cochlear implant developed by Clark and his colleagues at the University of Melbourne and manufactured by Cochlear Pty. Ltd., Sydney, Australia. The FDA's approval of this multichannel device was restricted to adults. In 1980, the first child was implanted with the 3M/House single-channel cochlear implant (Eisenberg and House 1982). Multisite clinical trials with this device began in 1983 and 1984 (Berliner and Eisenberg 1985).

The first pediatric implantation of the Nucleus multichannel device took place in Melbourne, Australia, in 1985. A multisite clinical trial began in the United States in 1986 (Mecklenburg, Demorest, and Staller 1991). Before FDA approval of the single-channel cochlear implant in children, 3M Corporation ceased manufacture of the single-channel device. Final FDA approval was never achieved. In 1990, the FDA approved commercial distribution of the Nucleus multichannel cochlear implant in children, ages two to seventeen years.

These FDA approvals are the only ones granted for cochlear implants in the United States. Several cochlear prostheses are considered investigational in the United States. These include the Ineraid device, manufactured by Smith and Nephew Richards, Memphis, Tennessee (Dorman et al. 1989), and the Clarion device, manufactured by Advanced Bionics Corporation (formerly MiniMed Technologies, Ltd.), Sylmar, California (Schindler and Kessler, 1993). There are a number of other single-channel and multichannel devices that have been implanted in adults and children in Europe, where there are fewer regulatory constraints. Mecklenburg and Lehnhardt (1991) provide a thorough review of these devices, most of which are not available in the United States. The focus of this chapter is on the only commercially approved cochlear implant for children, the Nucleus 22-channel cochlear implant system.

DEVICE DESCRIPTION

THE Nucleus device consists of three basic components: the cochlear implant, the speech processor, and headset. The system is illustrated in Figure 11.1. The cochlear implant is composed of a receiver-stimulator and an electrode array. The receiver-stimulator contains a custom-designed integrated circuit and other passive components. The circuitry is sealed hermetically within a titanium capsule. Connected to the hermetic package is a platinum receiving coil with a samarium cobalt magnet seated in the middle of the coil. These components are coated with a biocompatible, medical grade, silicone rubber. A smoothly

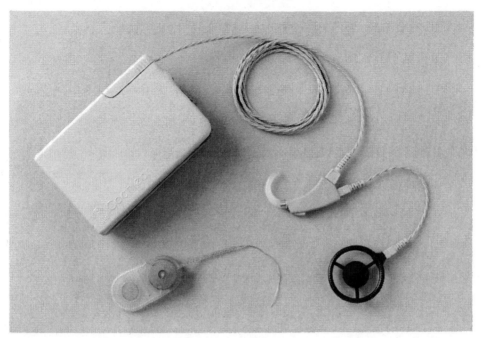

Figure 11.1. The Nucleus 22-channel cochlear implant system consists of the receiver-stimulator and electrode array, a miniaturized speech processor, an ear-level directional microphone, and transmitting coil.

tapered and flexible electrode array is connected to the receiver-stimulator via ceramic feedthroughs. It consists of thirty-two evenly spaced platinum bands supported on a silicone rubber carrier. The distal twenty-two bands are active and are used for electrical stimulation, whereas the proximal ten bands serve only as mechanical support rings, aiding in electrode array insertion into the scala tympani of the cochlea. The thirty-two bands vary in a smooth taper from 0.6 millimeter (mm) at the proximal end (closest to the receiver-stimulator) to 0.4 mm at the distal end. The bands are spaced equally at 0.75 mm intervals. For the active twenty-two electrodes, a separate, insulated platinum-iridium wire is connected to each electrode; these wires course through the silicone rubber carrier, connecting each electrode individually to the receiver-stimulator (Beiter and Brimacombe 1993; Brimacombe and Beiter 1994; Clark et al. 1987a; Patrick and Clark 1991).

The cochlear implant procedure is performed under general anesthesia. The receiver-stimulator is placed under the skin in a surgically created depression in the mastoid bone. The electrode array is placed up to 25 mm into the scala tympani, either through the round window or, more commonly, through a cochleostomy near the round window. More information about the surgical procedure can be found in Clark et al. (1987b); Clark, Franz et al. (1991); Clark, Cohen, and Shepherd (1991); Webb et al. (1990).

The speech processor and headset (microphone, transmitting coil, and cables) comprise the externally worn portion of the system. Sound from the environment is picked up by an ear-level, directional, electret microphone and is transmitted via cabling to the speech processor. The processor is a minature personal computer that uses a dedicated, custom-designed digital signal processor (DSP) for preemphasis, analog-to-digital conversion, and analysis of the incoming signal. The speech processor contains a random-access memory (RAM) that stores an individualized program. This program contains measurements of the amount of electrical current required to elicit a threshold and maximum acceptable listening level for each electrode pair to be used in the patient's program. These measurements vary across the electrode array and from individual to individual. Also stored is information that relates the frequency of spectral peaks in the acoustic signal to electrode position within the cochlea. Frequency information between 250 Hz and 6000 Hz is divided into the number of channels available for electrical stimulation (most commonly 20 to 22). Stimuli with a low-frequency component activate more apical electrode pairs, and those with a high-frequency component activate more basal electrode pairs. In this way, the cochlea is stimulated following the general tonotopic order of neural distribution.

Once the patient-specific program has been configured, it is accessed by the speech processor's encoder chip to generate a series of digital pulses that power and control the implanted receiver-stimulator. These pulses provide information regarding the stimulating and indifferent electrodes and the amount of current to be delivered. This digital code is sent by radio frequency (2.5 MHz) across the skin via the transmitting coil that is worn over the implant site. The transmitting coil is held in place with a rare-earth magnet identical to the one inside the cochlear implant. To start up the receiver-stimulator, power from the AA battery in the speech processor is also transmitted across the skin on the same link.

The speech processor is programmed using an IBM-compatible computer, two multibit interface cards, a specialized interface unit to hold the speech processor, and custom-designed software. The specialized interface unit allows the computer to control the electrical stimulation delivered by the speech processor. Electrical threshold and maximum acceptable listening level measurements are obtained for each electrode pair. Next, the electrode pairs are balanced for equal loudness (unless the patient is too young to understand this task), and the electrodes are stimulated in rapid sequence to assess place pitch perception. Then the patient-specific program is configured, tested using live-voice stimuli, and automatically placed on the speech processor's RAM.

Coding Strategies

In the Nucleus cochlear implant system, the primary function of the speech processor is to analyze and encode the incoming acoustic information and send it to the implanted receiver-stimulator. The processor has been designed to extract specific parameters of speech that are critical for speech recognition. This method of signal processing is called *speech feature extraction* and contrasts with a vocoder or filter bank approach, which divides the incoming signal into a series of bandwidths that are then assigned to specific electrode pairs.

The first speech processor encoded three parameters: the amplitude of the ongoing acoustic signal, the fundamental frequency (F0), and the second-formant frequency (F2) in the range of 800 to 4000 Hz (Tong et al. 1979, 1980, 1982). Later, the estimate of the first-formant frequency in the range of 280 to 1000 Hz was added to the encoding scheme (Blamey, Dowell, Brown et al. 1987; Blamey, Dowell, Clark et al. 1987; Blamey and Clark 1990; Dowell et al. 1987). In these strategies, amplitude information is encoded as the amount of electrical current delivered to an electrode pair. The amount of current delivered falls between the measured threshold and maximum acceptable listening level for each electrode pair and directly translates into perceived loudness. The place of stimulation within the cochlea varies and is dependent upon the estimates of the spectral peaks that are measured in the F1 and F2 range. Approximately the most apical one-third of the electrodes in the cochlea are assigned to track F1 information. Each of these electrodes is assigned a frequency bandwidth within the range of 280 to 1000 Hz. Thus, if the estimate of F1 is 300 Hz, the most apical F1 electrode would be stimulated. Conversely, if the F1 estimate is close to 1000 Hz, a more basal electrode in the apical one-third of the array would be stimulated.

The remaining two-thirds of the electrodes track frequency information in the F2 range. For inputs with a relatively high F2, one of the basally placed electrodes is stimulated. If the estimate of F2 is lower in frequency, then a more apically placed electrode in the F2 range would be stimulated. This strategy takes advantage of the tonotopic organization of the cochlea, with the result that different input frequencies generate different pitch perceptions for the listener.

The stimulus delivered to the selected F1 and F2 electrode pairs is pulsatile and rapidly sequential, with the F2 electrode pair stimulated first, followed by the F1 pair. Estimates of F1 and F2 are made in real time. The rate of pulsatile stimulation to the selected electrode pairs represents the fundamental frequency or voice pitch.

More recently, in an attempt to provide supplementary cues for consonant recognition, the extraction of further high-frequency information has been added to the parameters discussed above. This latest speech feature coding strategy is called Multipeak (MPEAK). This scheme extracts, encodes, and delivers the F1 and F2 estimates and the amplitudes in three high-frequency bands: 2000 to 2800 Hz (Band 3), 2800 to 4000 Hz (Band 4), and 4000 Hz and above (Band 5). A simplified block diagram of the speech processor is presented in Figure 11.2. Three fixed basal electrodes (one for each band) are stimulated according to the amount of energy detected in each of the three bands. The speech processor digitizes the information and sends it to the receiver-stimulator, where it is decoded. The stimulator delivers charge-balanced biphasic current pulses to four

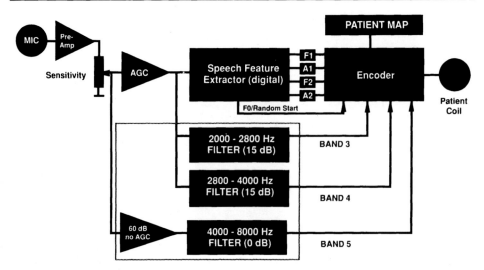

Figure 11.2. A simplified block diagram of the Mini Speech Processor with its custom-designed digital signal processor (DSP) and high-frequency filter chip.

specific pairs of electrodes along the implanted electrode array. These electrical current pulses directly stimulate remaining neural tissue (Dowell et al. 1990; Skinner et al. 1991; von Wallenberg and Battmer 1991).

A later development in speech coding research for the Nucleus device is based on studies conducted by McDermott, McKay, and their colleagues at the University of Melbourne using an experimental Spectral Maxima Sound Processor (SMSP) (McDermott, McKay, and Vandali 1992; McKay et al. 1991, 1992; McKay and McDermott 1993). These studies showed significantly improved speech recognition, especially in the presence of background noise, when the SMSP was compared to the commercially available MPEAK strategy.

Based on these findings, a new custom-designed CMOS integrated circuit (IC) was developed. This IC contains twenty digitally programmable bandpass filters that span the audio spectrum from 200 Hz to 10 kHz. A simplified block diagram of the new speech processor with its twenty programmable filters is presented in Figure 11.3. These twenty filters are assigned to twenty of the twenty-two electrodes on the Nucleus array in a tonotopic order. The programmable filters are repetitively scanned, and the largest outputs (or maxima) are selected and presented to their assigned electrodes. Typically four to ten maxima are selected for every scan cycle. Figure 11.4 illustrates the selection of six maxima from the twenty filter outputs.

The stimulation rate is adaptive in nature. When twenty stimulation sites are available, the pulse rate on each channel varies between approximately 180 and 300 Hz, depending upon the spectral composition, the intensity of the incoming acoustic signal, and the individual's speech processor program or MAP. For broad spectrum signals such as vowels, more maxima are present, and the stim-

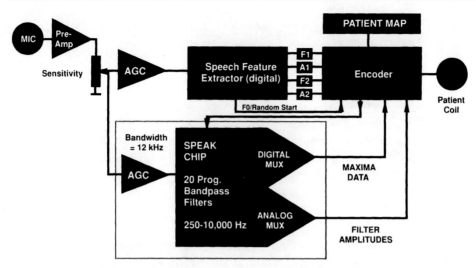

Figure 11.3. A simplified block diagram of the Spectra 22 processor with its custom-designed digital signal processor (DSP) and SPEAK chip.

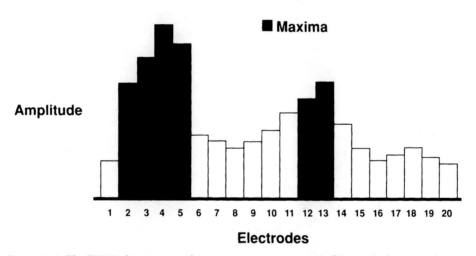

Figure 11.4. The SPEAK chip measures the energy in 20 programmable filters and selects a predetermined number of bands (typically six) with the greatest energy. The electrode pairs assigned to the filters with the largest maxima are then selected for stimulation.

ulation rate is reduced to allow a more detailed representation of the spectral content. For sounds with limited spectral content, such as high-frequency voiceless plosives or fricatives, fewer maxima are present, and the stimulation rate increases automatically to provide improved temporal resolution. This strategy is called Spectral Peak (SPEAK).

Application of Cochlear Implants to the Pediatric Population

Preoperative Evaluation

Cochlear implants are indicated for carefully selected, profoundly deaf children, ages two to seventeen years, who show little or no benefit from amplification. Table 11.1 provides the recommended selection criteria. The clinical evaluation of a pediatric candidate requires a team of professionals representing a variety of disciplines, including otolaryngology, audiology, speech-language pathology, psychology, and deaf education. In addition, the parents and family play an important role in the team process.

Medical-Surgical Evaluation

Preoperatively, the otolaryngologist conducts a detailed evaluation of the child's medical status. This consists of a comprehensive history, physical examination, and high-resolution CAT scans. The history should include information regarding the pregnancy, the child's developmental milestones, any postnatal complications, additional disabling conditions, and a family history related to hearing loss.

High-resolution CAT scans are used to estimate the degree of cochlear patency. In some instances, magnetic resonance imaging (MRI) has also been used (Yune, Miyamoto, and Yune 1991). Proper electrode placement may be impeded by fibrous or bony occlusions in the cochlea. Ossification of the cochlea is of greater concern in the pediatric population for several reasons. First, a large proportion (42 to 64%) of the children who have received cochlear implants have been deafened due to meningitis (Luxford and House 1985; Staller, Beiter, and Brimacombe 1991; Staller et al. 1991; Yune, Miyamoto, and Yune 1991). Secondly, studies have shown a higher incidence of ossification in individuals deafened by meningitis—and in meningitically deafened children in particular (Balkany, Gantz, and Nadol 1988; Eisenberg et al. 1984; Ketten 1994; Luxford and House 1985; Yune, Miyamoto, and Yune 1991).

Despite this concern, the average electrode insertion length of the Nucleus array was 17.32 mm for a group of 212 meningitically deafened children as

Table 11.1. Preoperative Selection Criteria

1. Profound sensorineural hearing loss, bilaterally.
2. At least two years of age.
3. Little or no benefit from hearing aids as defined by obtaining virtually zero on open-set measures or chance performance on closed-set segmental tasks.
4. No radiological contraindications.
5. No medical contraindications to undergoing the operation:
   a. No deafness due to lesions of the acoustic nerve or central auditory pathway;
   b. No active middle ear infection;
   c. No absence of cochlear development.
6. Appropriate trial period with hearing aids and a tactile device (when necessary).
7. Recommend enrollment in educational settings that emphasize oral-aural training.
8. Families and candidates (if possible) should be psychologically and motivationally suitable.

compared to 20.03 mm for a group of 294 nonmeningitically deafened children. Studies have shown that, when the new bone formation is limited to the inferior segment of the basal turn of the cochlea, a full insertion of all thirty-two bands (approximately 25 mm) can be achieved. When ossification extends throughout the cochlea, it is possible to drill a bony trough and insert the electrode array up to 9 mm (Balkany, Gantz, and Nadol 1988).

High-resolution CAT scans are also used to determine whether cochlear malformations are present. This type of malformation, often called Mondini dysplasia, may include a small cochlear bud, an incomplete cochlear partition, or a common cavity. For a complete classification of the different categories of Mondini dysplasia, see Jackler, Luxford, and House (1987). When these congenital malformations are identified, a partial insertion of the electrode may be anticipated due to the incomplete development of the sensory end-organ. In addition, electrode array insertion may be impeded by a perilymph gusher when the scala is opened (Clark, Cohen, and Shepherd 1991; Cohen and Hoffman 1993; Webb et al. 1990). Despite these concerns, 24 deaf children with congenital malformations had been implanted by 1994 with the Nucleus multichannel device. The average electrode insertion length was 17.88 mm for this group.

Cochlear agenesis and the absence of an eighth nerve are contraindications to cochlear implantation (Jackler, Luxford, and House 1987). These conditions are rare. When the Organ of Corti is severely damaged due to infectious, traumatic, metabolic, or genetic causes, some reduction in spiral ganglion cells may be expected. The extent of spiral ganglion cell degeneration may have an impact on the degree of benefit that can be derived from a multichannel cochlear implant (Hinojosa and Marion 1983; Otte, Schuknecht, and Kerr 1978).

The general status of the auditory nerve can be evaluated using preoperative electrical stimulation of the promontory or round window. For this procedure, a transtympanic needle electrode is placed on the promontory and a ground electrode on the cheek. Alternatively, a tympanomeatal flap can be raised and a ball electrode placed in the round window niche. In either case, small amounts of electrical current are delivered, and the patient is asked to indicate when sound is perceived. Although this technique has been used extensively with profoundly deafened adults, it is difficult to test young children using this behavioral method (Rickards et al. 1990).

Kileny (1991, 1994) has reported a modification of the procedure that involves sedation of young children and the recording of electrically elicited auditory brainstem and middle latency (where appropriate) responses while stimulating the promontory(Kileny and Kemink 1987). This procedure is not done on a routine clinical basis. One drawback is the difficulty in controlling the electrical stimulus artifact generated, which can easily contaminate the evoked responses (Gardi 1985; Kileny 1991; Shallop et al. 1990; Waring, Don, and Brimacombe 1985). Another concern is the sedation of young children. In addition, experience has shown that the incidence of nonstimulability in profoundly deafened children is very low. Of 126 children implanted with the 3M/House single-channel cochlear implant, only two did not obtain auditory sensations (Thiele-meir et al. 1985). For the Nucleus multichannel device, only 3 of 1905 children (0.15%) did not display behavioral responses to electrical stimulation. Interestingly, three meningitically deafened children who received the Nucleus device did not respond initially to electrical stimulation. Following five to twelve months of device use, reliable behavioral responses were noted (Geier et al. 1993).

The medical evaluation for candidacy should also include an assessment of middle ear pathology. Otitis media is as prevalent in profoundly deafened children as it is in the general pediatric population. If an active condition is found, surgery may need to be postponed until the sequelae of the otitis media have been resolved (Clark, Cohen, and Shepherd 1991). In the past, there was concern that the development of otitis media in children with cochlear implants might lead to potentially life-threatening complications such as labrynthitis and meningitis. Several studies have shown that the presence of a cochlear implant does not increase the incidence or severity of otitis media in children. In addition, no complications were reported when otitis media occurred in the implanted ear (Clark, Cohen, and Shepherd 1991; Cohen and Hoffman 1993; House, Luxford, and Courtney 1985).

In summary, cochlear implantation of young children is a safe procedure when performed by a well-trained otolaryngologist. The overall medical-surgical complication rate in children has been acceptably low and is less than that reported for adults.

Audiological Evaluation

The initial objective of the audiological evaluation is to determine the extent of the hearing loss and whether any middle ear pathology exists. Standard audiometric measures should be obtained; these include unaided pure-tone thresholds under headphones for frequencies ranging from 125 Hz to 8000 Hz, as well as bone conduction, immittance, and acoustic reflex testing. The immittance battery is administered to rule out significant middle ear pathology, and acoustic reflexes should be consistent with a profound bilateral sensorineural hearing loss. Electrophysiological tests may also be performed to confirm the behavioral findings.

Once a profound bilateral sensorineural hearing loss has been determined, the degree of benefit obtained from amplification should be assessed. First, sound field detection thresholds using warble tones or narrow bands of noise should be obtained with high-gain amplification. To ensure accuracy, measurements in decibels (dB) sound pressure level (SPL) are made using a microphone placed at ear level (close to the hearing aid microphone) and connected to a sound level meter. To verify the appropriateness of the hearing aid fitting, real ear measurements are recommended. For a thorough discussion of hearing aid selection and evaluation, see chapter 10 and Skinner (1988).

For children who have not worn appropriately fitted hearing aids, an extended trial with amplification should be undertaken. Generally, at least a six-month trial is recommended. During this time, the child should be enrolled in a (re)habilitation program that emphasizes the development of auditory skills for communication. The training should incorporate diagnostic therapy to assess the child's use of amplified sound. For very young children, the training should emphasize basic auditory concepts and the development of specific vocabulary that will later be used in the assessment of aided speech perception. The specific tests and methods for assessing speech perception abilities in children of different age groups are described in the sections that follow.

Speech-Language Evaluation

The primary benefits of cochlear implantation relate to the restoration of hearing sensation and the improvement in speech perception abilities. Important secondary benefits involve the development of improved speech production and oral language skills, provided adequate training is received. The speech-language pathologist on the team should evaluate the child's general communication, with special emphasis on speech production and receptive and expressive oral language abilities. Although speech and language skills typically do not determine a child's candidacy for implantation, the speech-language pathologist may recommend additional habilitation before surgery if a young child cannot communicate at a basic level using either oral or manual means.

The objective of the speech production assessment is to evaluate the fundamental skills that underlie expressive communication and to measure more complex processes such as overall speech intelligibility (Tobey and Hasenstab 1991). Speech production should be evaluated using standardized tests whenever possible. The child's ability to imitate nonsegmental contours and segmental speech patterns can be assessed using the Ling Phonetic Level Speech Evaluation (Ling 1976). The Ling evaluation also provides logical sequences for training speech production skills. The child's use of speech for communicative purposes can be assessed using the Phonologic Level Speech Evaluation (Ling 1976). An elicited or spontaneous language sample is gathered while the child is engaged in play, enabling the specialist to evaluate the child's speech skills, language abilities, and general intelligibility.

The choice of test measures for evaluating receptive and expressive language depends upon the child's chronologic age, mode of communication, general linguistic competence, and cognitive development. Standardized tests should be used whenever possible; instruments that have norms for hearing-impaired children are preferred. Two such tests are the Grammatical Analysis of Elicited Language (GAEL) (Moog and Geers 1979, 1980) and the Rhode Island Test of Language Structures (RITLS) (Engen and Engen 1983). Both tests provide normative data for children in total communication settings; the GAEL also has norms for children using oral communication. A commonly used test of receptive vocabulary is the Peabody Picture Vocabulary Test–Revised (Dunn 1981).

Educational Assessment

The cochlear implant team may include an educational consultant whose role is to interact with the child's teachers to determine the child's current academic, auditory, cognitive, linguistic, and social functioning in school (Nevins et al. 1991). Following implantation, the educational consultant may conduct periodic school visits to observe the child in the classroom and to give suggestions to the classroom teachers regarding techniques for maximizing auditory skill development. The child's teachers also should play an important role in advising the cochlear implant team on the educational suitability of a particular child for implantation. Postoperatively, the classroom teacher plays a significant role in documenting changes in the child's use of hearing as well as any changes in speech and language. It is vital that the teachers communicate this information, including any problems they observe, to the cochlear implant team.

Psychological Evaluation

The psychologist may provide meaningful information about cognitive, social, and emotional development. It is critical to rule out any significant organic abnormalities or personality disorders. Typically, the psychologist interviews the parents and, when appropriate, the older child to determine their motivation for considering implantation and whether their expectations regarding potential benefit are realistic. Tests of nonverbal intelligence may be administered, such as the Wechsler Preschool and Primary Scale of Intelligence (WPPSI), Wechsler Performance Scale for children (Wechsler 1967), the Wechsler Intelligence Scale for Children–Revised (WISC-R) (Wechsler 1974), and the Central Institute for the Deaf (CID) Preschool Performance Scale (Geers and Lane 1984).

Family

The family plays a vital role in the evaluation and habilitation process and is regarded as an integral part of the team. The parents provide information regarding the child's communication skills within the home and family environment. If a cochlear implant is considered, it is imperative that the family realizes the long-term commitment and support required for any child to achieve maximum potential.

CHILDREN UNDER THE AGE OF TWO YEARS

FDA indications for device use exclude children under the age of two years. This age constraint has been set for several reasons. Although the cochlea is adult size at birth, the mastoid bone of the skull is not sufficiently developed to accommodate the receiver-stimulator package. Significant skull growth takes place within the first two years of life (Mangham et al. 1986). The distance from the cochlear promontory to the mastoid cortex increases approximately 1.7 cm from birth to adulthood; half of this growth occurs during the first two years (O'Donoghue et al. 1986). In addition, when hearing loss has been diagnosed within the first two years of life, there must be sufficient time to confirm the degree of loss, the amount of aidable residual hearing, and the extent to which hearing aids will be beneficial before making a recommendation for cochlear implantation (Northern et al. 1986).

It is critical that young children with hearing loss be identified as early as possible and fitted with appropriate amplification (see chapter 10). Once this has been done, the child and parents should be enrolled in a parent-infant stimulation program. One aim of the program should be to facilitate the development of age-appropriate auditory skills, leading to the child's use of oral language. The parents have the greatest contact with the child and serve as the primary facilitators of auditory skill development. Typically, the parent-infant program offers the parents instruction and guidance in using daily activities to teach listening skills and early language development. Hasenstab and Horner (1982), Pollack (1985), and Schuyler and Rushmer (1987) provide comprehensive reviews of parent-infant habilitation.

Throughout the habilitation period, there should be an ongoing assessment of the child's utilization of amplified sound. For those children who, after an appropriate trial period, do not show responses to acoustic stimuli when using high-gain amplification, a tactile device should be used in conjunction with the hearing aids. The tactile device is added to facilitate stimulus-response conditioning. One device used is the Tactaid 7 (Audiological Engineering Corporation). This multichannel vibrotactile device extracts estimates of the first and second formants and delivers the output to seven vibratory stimulators worn on the back of the neck or on the sternum. More information on other single-channel and multichannel vibrotactile and electrotactile devices can be found in Weisenberger and Kozma-Spytek (1991).

PRESCHOOL CHILDREN (TWO TO FIVE YEARS OF AGE)

THE evaluation and selection of young, profoundly deafened children for cochlear implantation presents challenges concerning candidate selection, device fitting, (re)habilitation, and determination of postoperative outcome. These challenges are outweighed by the long-term potential benefit derived from early intervention with a multichannel cochlear implant.

If the child has been diagnosed recently with a profound sensorineural hearing loss, a minimum six-month trial period with high-gain amplification should be undertaken. During this period, the parent and child should be enrolled in a parent-infant program for developing auditory skills and conditioned responses. If the child was diagnosed earlier in life and is making minimal progress with traditional amplification, a determination must be made whether the child understands the concepts underlying stimulus-response testing. If the child is not yet showing conditioned responses to acoustic stimulation, a tactile aid should be used to teach or verify that the child understands the stimulus-response paradigm. Once this has been established, the tactile device should be removed for the purpose of assessment only. The child should be tested again in the unaided condition under earphones and in the aided condition (hearing aids only) in sound field to determine unaided (individual ear) and aided detection levels across the frequency range.

Figure 11.5 illustrates typical preoperative unaided and aided detection thresholds across the frequency range for pediatric cochlear implant recipients. Also shown are the aided detection thresholds postoperatively with the cochlear implant. For the unaided condition, mean thresholds are shown. For the aided conditions, both means and standard deviations are presented. Preoperatively, with high-gain amplification, these children had limited access to sound within the normal conversational speech spectrum, especially above 1000 Hz. Postoperatively, detection thresholds improved, falling well within the normal conversational speech range.

Following audiometric testing, a determination of aided speech perception abilities should be made. Establishing the degree of benefit a young child receives from hearing aids or a tactile device can be challenging because young

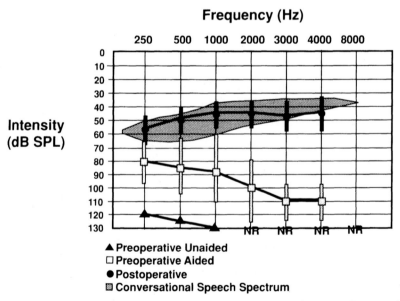

Figure 11.5. Mean preoperative unaided thresholds obtained under headphones as a function of frequency for 284 children. Also shown, are mean (± one standard deviation) aided thresholds measured in the sound field, preoperatively with hearing aids, and at the first annual postoperative evaluation with the cochlear implant. The conversational speech spectrum is illustrated by the shaded gray area.

deaf children have limited linguistic abilities. Therefore, most standard speech perception measures are inappropriate.

The Discrimination after Training (DAT) test was developed for use with very young, profoundly deaf children who were evaluated for the 3M/House single-channel cochlear implant (Thielemeir 1984). This test, which is administered using monitored live-voice, consists of twelve levels and progresses in a hierarchy of difficulty. It begins with the discrimination of a long versus short sound while lipreading to determine that the child understands the task (level 1). It proceeds to auditory-only detection of sound (level 2), auditory-only discrimination of nonlinguistic speech stimuli of various temporal patterns (levels 3 to 5), auditory-only discrimination of linguistic speech stimuli of various patterns (levels 6 to 8), and auditory-only discrimination of spondees in small sets (levels 9 to 12). Levels 9 through 12 require the perception of spectral cues at a segmental level.

Figure 11.6 presents longitudinal mean scores on the DAT, both preoperatively and at five annual postoperative test intervals. These data show clinically significant gains from preoperative to postoperative conditions. Preoperatively, only 5 of 86 children (6%) achieved level 9 or higher. Scores at this level would indicate some ability to process spectral cues. Postoperatively, at the twelve-month test interval, 43 of 77 children (56%) achieved level 9 or higher; 21 of these children (49%) reached level 12. At the 24-month test session, 43 of 59 children (73%) achieved level 9 or higher; 33 of these children (77%) reached level 12. Clearly, this test is too easy for many young children who use a multichannel cochlear implant.

Another test that was developed specifically for young, profoundly deaf children is the Central Institute for the Deaf (CID) Early Speech Perception (ESP)

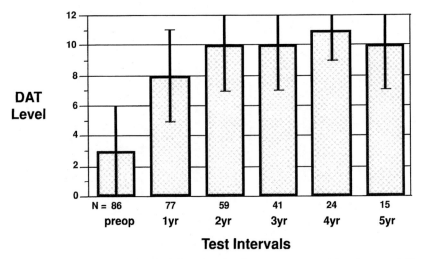

Figure 11.6. Mean scores (± one standard deviation) for the Discrimination After Training (DAT) test, preoperatively and at five annual postoperative intervals, for children ages two to five years.

Test–Standard Version (Geers and Moog 1992; Moog and Geers 1990). This test consists of three subtests administered in the auditory-only condition: pattern perception, spondee identification, and monosyllable identification. The twelve-item pattern perception subtest is the easiest and requires the child to identify words based on the number of syllables (one, two, or three) and the stress patterns (trochee versus spondee). The spondee and monosyllable subtests require the identification of a specific stimulus item out of a set of twelve alternatives. Each of the subtests requires a picture pointing response. In addition, there is a low-verbal version of the ESP designed for children ages two to three years who are unable to take the standard version of the test (Moog and Geers 1990). The low-verbal version incorporates the same three subtests as the standard version but uses objects instead of pictures. The child is required to select the stimulus item from a set of four alternatives.

Figures 11.7, 11.8, and 11.9 present pre- and postoperative mean scores on the pattern perception, spondee identification, and monosyllable identification subtests of the ESP battery. Scores obtained on the two versions of the test have been combined. Preoperatively, when the child is younger and vocabulary is more limited, the low-verbal version may be used. Postoperatively, as the child matures and vocabulary increases, the standard version is more likely to be administered. The number of children who were administered the spondee and monosyllable identification subtests preoperatively is rather small. This is most likely because the test is criterion based, and it is recommended that the more difficult subtests not be given if the child does not demonstrate pattern perception (8 out of 12 items correct on the low-verbal version or 17 out of 24 items correct on the standard version).

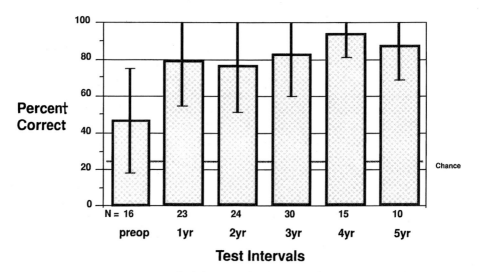

Figure 11.7. Mean scores (± one standard deviation) for the pattern perception subtest of the Early Speech Perception (ESP) test, preoperatively and at five annual postoperative intervals, for children ages two to five years.

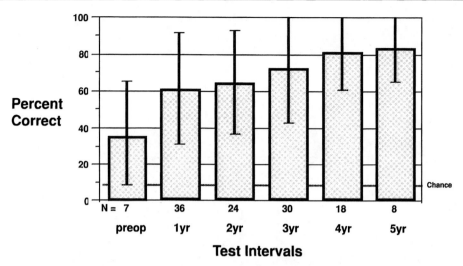

Figure 11.8. Mean scores (± one standard deviation) for the spondee subtest of the Early Speech Perception (ESP) test, preoperatively and at five annual postoperative intervals, for children ages two to five years.

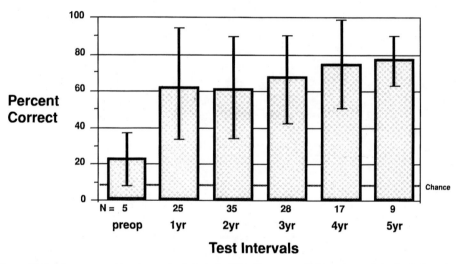

Figure 11.9. Mean scores (± one standard deviation) for the monosyllable subtest of the Early Speech Perception (ESP) test, preoperatively and at five annual postoperative intervals, for children ages two to five years.

Preoperatively, only three of 16 children (19%) showed pattern perception. After twelve months of device use, 17 of 23 children (74%) had this skill; 52% of the children scored 90% or higher on the pattern perception subtest. On the more difficult subtests, after one year of cochlear implant experience, 25% of the children scored 90% or higher on spondee identification, and 36% scored 90% or higher on monosyllable identification. Despite the small sample size preoperatively, there is a clear trend toward improvement on all three subtests after at least twelve months of cochlear implant use. There was also a trend toward improvement over time, postoperatively.

Another test developed for use with young hearing-impaired children is the Monosyllable, Trochee, Spondee (MTS) test (Erber and Alencewicz 1976). It predates the ESP test and uses twelve pictured stimuli consisting of four monosyllables, four trochees, and four spondees. It assesses pattern perception and word identification. This test is also administered in the auditory-only condition. The longitudinal mean data for pattern perception and word identification are presented in Figures 11.10 and 11.11, respectively. These data show improve-

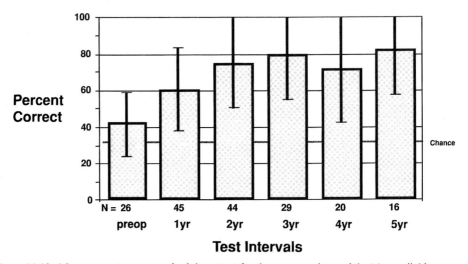

Figure 11.10. Mean scores (± one standard deviation) for the pattern subtest of the Monosyllable, Trochee, Spondee (MTS) test, preoperatively and at five annual postoperative intervals, for children ages two to five years.

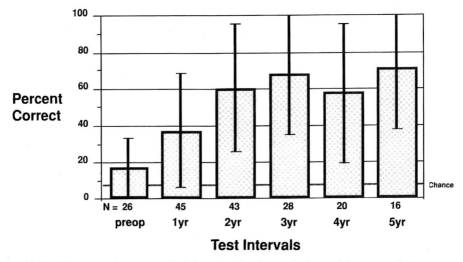

Figure 11.11. Mean scores (± one standard deviation) for the word subtest of the Monosyllable, Trochee, Spondee (MTS) test, preoperatively and at five annual postoperative intervals, for children ages two to five years.

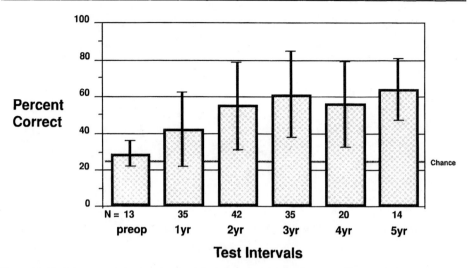

Figure 11.12. Mean scores (± one standard deviation) for the Northwestern University Children's Perception of Speech (NU-CHIPS) test, preoperatively and at five annual postoperative intervals, for children ages two to five years.

ments from the preoperative to the postoperative conditions. Repeated measures analyses of variance revealed statistically significant improvements in performance over time for twelve children who were tested preoperatively, and at the first three annual postoperative test intervals (F=12.97; P<.0001). The mean scores for this group were not different from the data for all children tested (see Figures 11.10 and 11.11).

Another pediatric test of speech perception is the Northwestern University Children's Perception of Speech (NU-CHIPS) test developed by Elliott and Katz (1980) (see chapter 5). It is a more difficult closed-set measure appropriate for children with more sophisticated vocabularies. The test consists of monosyllabic words in a four-alternative picture paradigm. There are fifty items, administered auditory-only. Figure 11.12 presents longitudinal mean data for the NU-CHIPS test. Preoperatively, on average, the children did not score significantly above chance. At the one year postoperative test interval, mean performance was significantly above chance. A significant improvement between the first and second annual postoperative test periods was also noted (t = 3.67; p <.002).

There are few tests of open-set word recognition that are appropriate for young deaf children. One closed-set test that has been adapted for administration in an open-set format is the Glendonald Auditory Screening Procedure (GASP) (Erber 1982; Thielemeir et al. 1985). This twelve-item test measures word recognition using simple vocabulary that varies in syllable length (e.g. fish, toothbrush, Santa Claus). Figure 11.13 presents longitudinal mean data on this measure, preoperatively and at five annual postoperative intervals. Few young children have been given this test preoperatively (N = 6 in our sample). The mean score for these six children was less than one word correct. A child who

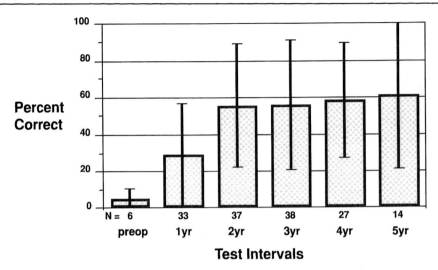

Figure 11.13. Mean scores (± one standard deviation) for the Glendonald Auditory Screening Procedure (GASP), preoperatively and at five annual postoperative intervals, for children ages two to five years.

recognizes more than one word on the GASP typically would not be considered for cochlear implantation.

Postoperatively, there was a clear trend toward improved performance between the first and second annual test sessions. For a group of thirteen children who were tested at both the one- and two-year test periods, mean scores were significantly better at the two-year interval (mean = 35%, S.D. = 32% at one year; mean = 60%, S.D. = 38% at two years; t = 4.12; p <0.001). These average scores at the one- and two-year intervals were very similar to the mean scores of all children tested. After one year of cochlear implant experience, 17 of 33 children (52%) showed no open-set word recognition; 16 of the children (48%) scored 25% or greater on this simple open-set test. In contrast, after two years of implant use, only five of 37 children (14%) had no open-set word recognition; 30 of these children (81%) scored 25% or higher.

Summary: Preschool Children

Regarding the audiological evaluation of the young child, the typical candidate presents with a profound sensorineural hearing loss and little residual hearing above 1000 Hz. These children do not detect conversational speech levels even with appropriately fit high-gain amplification. For those children who have detection thresholds within the average conversational speech spectrum, detection is most likely limited to the low-frequency region.

During the aided speech perception evaluation, these children may demonstrate above chance performance on the easiest subtest of the ESP (pattern) but may not score high enough to be considered pattern perceivers (17 out of 24 items correct). On the more difficult spondee subtest of the ESP, these children may score above chance, but average performance typically falls below the criterion level for demonstration of some word identification ability (8 out of 24 spondees). On the most difficult subtest of the ESP (monosyllables), these children may score at chance levels. If above chance scores are achieved, the typical cochlear implant recipient will score well below 54% (the criterion level for consistent word identification). If performance on the monosyllables subtest exceeds 50%, the child most likely is receiving too much benefit from hearing aids to be considered a cochlear implant candidate. It is unlikely that a young child who is being considered for cochlear implantation would score above chance preoperatively on the NU-CHIPS or MTS tests, in part due to the more difficult vocabulary. Similarly, scores on the open-set GASP test would most likely be below 10% (one out of 12 words correct).

School-Age Children (Six to Seventeen Years of Age)

WHEN determining candidacy for a cochlear implant, the young school-age child presents similar challenges to the preschool child. Most likely, the profound nature of these children's hearing loss has been confirmed already, and they have been wearing hearing aids. However, they may not have gained enough benefit from amplification to develop auditory skills beyond basic detection or simple discrimination. Oral language for communication purposes may be very limited.

For children in this age group, standard audiometric testing techniques should be used to confirm the amount of residual hearing, bilaterally. For children under the age of ten years, the tests of speech perception described in the section on Preschool Children will be administered to assess benefit from amplification. If the child's vocabulary is sufficiently developed and test scores on the ESP are high, the NU-CHIPS test or the Word Intelligibility by Picture Identification (WIPI) test (Ross and Lerman 1971) should be administered. The WIPI is a twenty-five-item monosyllabic word test, using a six-alternative picture-pointing paradigm. It can be administered in three conditions: auditory-only, speech-reading only, and the bimodal condition. Whenever possible, it is helpful to obtain a measure of speechreading ability with and without amplification to help in the determination of general hearing aid benefit.

Another test that can be used to measure speechreading abilities is the Craig Lipreading Inventory–Word Recognition (Cochlear Corporation 1990a; Craig 1964; Jeffers and Barley 1977). It is a thirty-three-item monosyllabic word test, using a four-alternative picture-pointing paradigm. The Craig Lipreading Inventory is administered in the speechreading-only and auditory-speechreading conditions.

To assess open-set word recognition abilities, the GASP (described in the section on Preschool Children) or the Kindergarten Phonetically Balanced Word List (PBK) (Haskins 1949) can be administered. The PBK is a very difficult test.

The stimulus items are monosyllabic, the vocabulary is more advanced, and there are more test items than the GASP (50 versus 12). If a child achieves a score of two or more words correct on the GASP or PBK tests, some benefit from amplification is evident, and the child would not be considered a cochlear implant candidate.

For older children, it is also beneficial to assess open-set sentence recognition. Few sentence tests have been developed for children. Consequently, measures typically administered to adults may be given if the child's vocabulary is fairly well developed. Examples of open-set sentence recognition measures include the CID Sentences of Everyday Speech test (Davis and Silverman 1978), the Bamford-Kowal-Bench (BKB) Sentences (Bench and Bamford 1979), and the Iowa Sentence Understanding With and Without Context, which is an adaptation of the BKB Sentences test (Tyler, Preece, and Lowder 1983). If the child is older and postlinguistically deafened, a battery of tests may be used that has been developed for the assessment of adults (Cochlear Corporation 1986). It includes three closed-set measures: the Four-Choice Spondee subtest of the Minimal Auditory Capabilities (MAC) Battery (Owens et al. 1985), and the Iowa Vowel and Medial Consonant tests (Tyler, Preece, and Lowder 1983). The Four-Choice Spondee test is the easiest in the battery. It consists of 20 spondaic word items in a 4-alternative format. The Iowa Vowel test assesses the identification of the nine pure vowels in American English within a /hVd/ context. It is a 45-item, 9-alternative task. The Iowa Medial Consonant test is the hardest closed-set measure in this battery. It consists of nonsense syllables in an /aCa/ context. It is a 70-item 14-alternative test.

Three open-set measures are included in this battery. The CID Sentences of Everyday Speech and the Iowa Sentence Understanding Without Context assess open-set sentence recognition. The CID Sentences test consists of twenty sentences. It is scored by the number of key words correctly identified out of one hundred. The Iowa Sentences test contains thirty sentences and eighty-eight key words. The Northwestern University No. 6 (NU #6) Monosyllabic Word test (Tillman and Carhart 1966) assesses open-set word recognition and is the most difficult test in the battery. It consists of fifty items and is scored for the number of words and phonemes correctly identified.

Several tests have been developed by Osberger and colleagues (Osberger et al., 1991). These include the Change/No Change, Minimal Pairs, Hoosier Auditory Visual Enhancement, and Common Phrases tests. These measures assess speech perception from simple discrimination (Change/No Change) through open-set word recognition (Common Phrases). They are used primarily with school-age children and are not commercially available.

The speech perception battery for assessing benefit from amplification will most likely begin with the administration of the ESP, unless the child is much older and postlinguistically deafened. Figures 11.14, 11.15, and 11.16 present mean scores obtained on the pattern, spondee, and monosyllable subtests of the

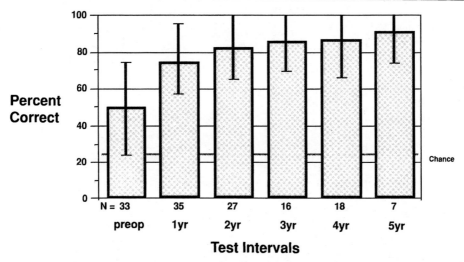

Figure 11.14. Mean scores (± one standard deviation) for the pattern subtest of the Early Speech Perception (ESP) test, preoperatively and at the five annual postoperative intervals, for children ages six to seventeen years.

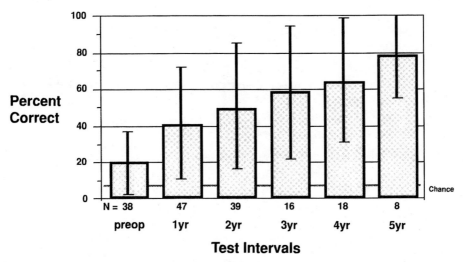

Figure 11.15. Mean scores (± one standard deviation) for the spondee subtest of the Early Speech Perception (ESP) test, preoperatively and at the five annual postoperative intervals, for children ages six to seventeen years.

ESP, preoperatively and at five annual postoperative evaluations. The data are strikingly similar to the data on the two- to five-year-old children.

Other tests of closed-set pattern and word identification include the MTS and NU-CHIPs tests. Figures 11.17 and 11.18 provide mean scores for these two measures, preoperatively and at five annual postoperative test intervals. Again, the data are very similar to the average performance achieved by the preschool children. For the school-age children, a statistically significant improvement on all closed-set measures was observed between the preoperative

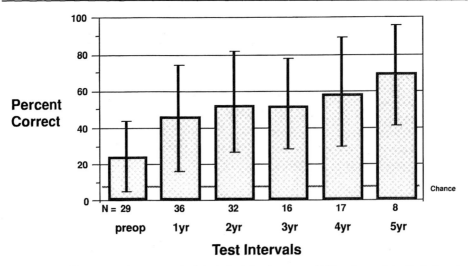

Figure 11.16. Mean scores (± one standard deviation) for the monosyllable subtest of the Early Speech Perception (ESP) test, preoperatively and at the five annual postoperative intervals, for children ages six to seventeen years.

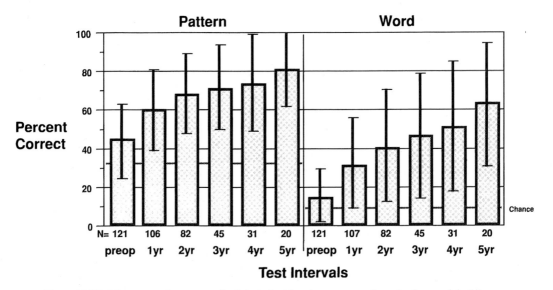

Figure 11.17. Mean scores (± one standard deviation) for the pattern and word subtests of the Monosyllable, Trochee, Spondee (MTS) test, preoperatively and at the five annual postoperative intervals, for children ages six to seventeen years.

and the first annual postoperative test session. In addition, repeated measures analyses of variance revealed a statistically significant main effect of length of cochlear implant use for several test measures (MTS pattern, ESP pattern, NU-CHIPS). For the NU-CHIPS test, mean scores were found to be significantly improved over the first four postoperative intervals for a group of nineteen children (F = 12.33, p <.0001). For these nineteen children, mean scores were 36% at

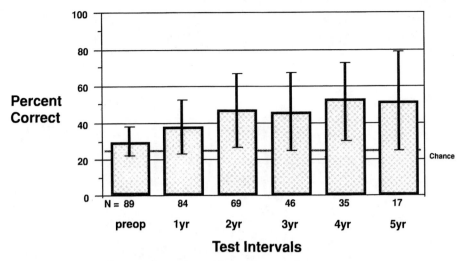

Figure 11.18. Mean scores (± one standard deviation) for the Northwestern University Children's Perception of Speech (NU-CHIPS) test, preoperatively and at the five annual postoperative intervals, for children ages six to seventeen years.

one year, 42% at two years, 48% at three years, and 54% at four years, postimplantation. These mean scores are all significantly above chance levels.

Several measures of open-set word and sentence recognition have been administered to school-age children, including the GASP, PBK monosyllables, and CID Sentences of Everyday Speech tests. Mean scores on each of these measures can be found in Figures 11.19, 11.20, and 11.21, respectively. For the GASP test, the mean scores for the school-age children were very similar to those obtained for the preschool children at the preoperative test interval, but were poorer at each of the annual evaluations, postoperatively. At the preoperative test interval, 41 of 45 (91%) of the children tested scored zero or one word correct. At the one-year postoperative evaluation, 45 of 81 children tested (56%) scored zero or one word correct, whereas 26 of 81 children tested (32%) scored 25% or higher. At the second year evaluation, 38 of 80 children tested (48%) scored zero or one word correct, whereas 34 of 80 children tested (43%) scored 25% or higher.

Mean scores for the GASP, PBK monosyllables, and CID Sentences tests were near zero preoperatively, and paired t-tests revealed a statistically significant improvement in performance from the preoperative to the first postoperative evaluations for all three measures (GASP: $n=26$, $t=3.71$, $P<.001$; PBK: $n=19$, $t=2.32$, $p<.03$; CID Sentences $n=27$, $t=2.95$, $p<.007$). In addition, repeated measures analyses of variance revealed a main effect of length of cochlear implant use for the CID Sentences test ($F=9.87$, $p<.001$), but not the PBK monosyllables. For 11 children who had been evaluated on the CID Sentences test at each of the first three postoperative evaluations, mean scores improved from 17% at one year, to 29% at two years, and 34% after three years of implant use.

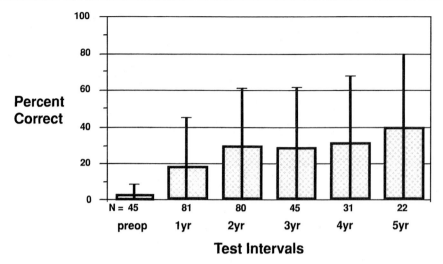

Figure 11.19. Mean scores (± one standard deviation) for the Glendonald Auditory Screening Procedure (GASP), preoperatively and at the five annual postoperative intervals, for children ages six to seventeen years.

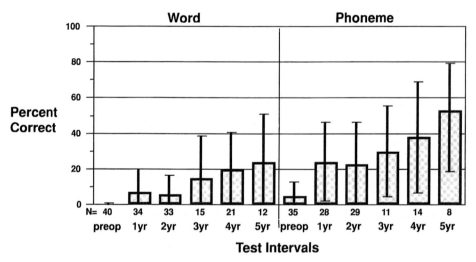

Figure 11.20. Mean word and phoneme scores (± one standard deviation) for the Phonetically Balanced Kindergarten Word List (PBK), preoperatively and at the five annual postoperative intervals, for children ages six to seventeen years.

Summary: School-Age Children

The school-age child has a preoperative audiologic profile that is very similar to that of the preschool child. One advantage in the assessment of the school-age child is the wider range of tests available. For example, speechreading measures may have been given to the older school-age child, unlike the preschool child, who rarely has the visual attention necessary to take such a test. If a speechreading measure has been given, scores for the bimodal condition are often very simi-

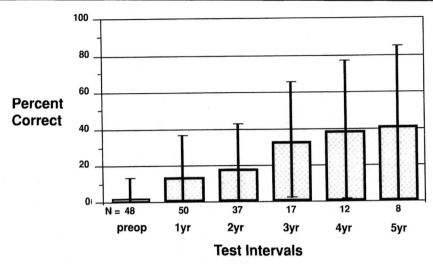

Figure 11.21. Mean scores (± one standard deviation) for the Central Institute for the Deaf (CID) Sentences of Everyday Speech test, preoperatively and at the five annual postoperative intervals, for children ages six to seventeen years.

lar to the speechreading-only condition. If the child's vocabulary is more advanced and an open-set word or sentence recognition test has been administered, the typical cochlear implant candidate will score near zero on these measures preoperatively.

DEVICE FITTING

WHEN the pediatric clinical trial began with the Nucleus multichannel device, concern was raised over the feasibility of measuring electrical thresholds and maximum acceptable listening levels for very young children whose exposure to auditory information had been limited. Clinical experience has proven that with adequate stimulus-response training preoperatively, even two-year-old children can be successfully fit with the device.

A typical programming session for a young child involves the use of play audiometry techniques to determine the electrical threshold levels for each electrode pair, using an ascending stimulus presentation technique. For assessment of maximum acceptable listening levels, it is important to increase slowly the amount of electrical stimulation to avoid an aversion response from the child. When working with younger children who are developing the concepts of loudness scaling, clinicians may use behavioral observation to establish thresholds for hearing and to ensure that the device is set at comfortable levels. These behavioral changes might include quieting or subtle changes in facial expression (see chapter 4). Cochlear Corporation (1990b) has developed programming cards for older children that allow them to associate a soft or loud, but comfortable, sound with a particular picture; other cards have also been developed to teach the concept of high and low pitch.

For the very young child, the clinician may obtain measurements on only a few electrode pairs during the initial programming session. These measurements are configured into a program for the child to wear home. Additional measurements will be made, and electrode pairs added to the child's program at subsequent sessions. Typically, the measurements for all electrode pairs can be made during the first two or three programming sessions, even for very young children. As the child gains experience listening through the cochlear implant, these measurements are refined.

Educational Setting

For years, there has been ongoing debate concerning the most appropriate method of educating deaf children. Several methods have been advocated: total communication, auditory-oral, and manual (see chapter 12). All auditory-oral programs emphasize the importance of developing audition; they vary in the amount of speechreading support utilized. Total communication (TC) aims to combine the use of auditory-oral and signed communication. In reality, many TC programs do not emphasize the auditory-oral component and are primarily manual in nature. Strictly manual programs use American Sign Language (ASL) rather than signed English systems.

Educators have speculated that children with cochlear implants might derive more benefit from them when they are placed in programs that emphasize the use of audition and spoken language for communication (Boothroyd, Geers, and Moog 1991). Over a period of years, implanted children have been placed in both TC and auditory-oral environments. Postoperative GASP data were reviewed to determine whether differences existed between the open-set word recognition abilities of congenitally deafened children in oral and TC programs. Data from the most recent postoperative evaluation period (most often the second or third annual interval) were analyzed for seventy children. Twenty-six children were educated in oral settings. For this group, 77% had open-set word recognition (two or more words correct); 42% scored 50% or greater. The remaining forty-four children were in TC programs. For these children, 34% showed open-set word recognition; 18% scored 50% or higher.

Figures 11.22 and 11.23 present individual data on the GASP for congenitally deaf children as a function of age at implant and educational setting. In general, children implanted before the age of seven years displayed better speech recognition abilities, despite educational setting. Of the 26 children in oral programs, 13 were implanted before the age of seven years, and 12 of these children scored greater than 30% on the GASP. Of the 13 children implanted after the age of seven, eight developed some open-set word recognition abilities. Of the 44 children educated in TC programs, 17 were implanted before the age of seven years, and 9 of them achieved open-set scores of 25% or greater. Of the 27 children implanted after the age of seven, only 5 children demonstrated any open-

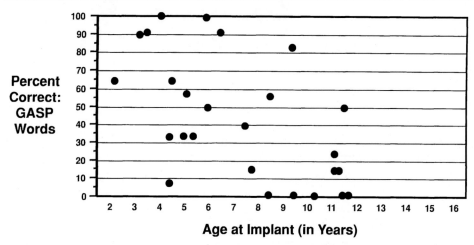

Figure 11.22. Individual postoperative scores on the Glendonald Auditory Screening Procedure (GASP) for congenitally deafened children, educated in auditory-oral settings, as a function of the age at implantation.

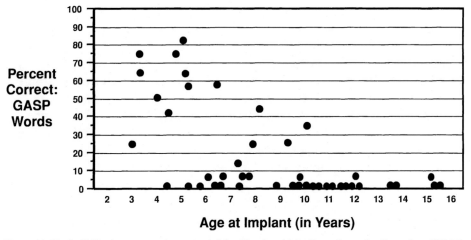

Figure 11.23. Individual postoperative scores of the Glendonald Auditory Screening Procedure (GASP) for congenitally deafened children, educated in total communication settings, as a function of the age at implantation.

set word recognition. It appears that children implanted at an early age are more likely to achieve open-set word recognition. In addition, children in oral environments may reach higher levels of performance with the cochlear implant than children in total communication programs.

CONTROVERSIES

ETHICAL issues have been raised by the Deaf community regarding the use of cochlear implants in children (see chapter 13). Specifically, the National Association for the Deaf (NAD) takes exception to the decision of the FDA regarding its approval of the Nucleus multichannel device for children. The NAD position paper, prepared by the Task Force on Cochlear Implants in Children (Lane et al. 1991), raises several issues concerning the scientific merit, clinical protocol and procedures, and the social implications of cochlear implantation. The NAD position paper makes general statements about the lack of scientific evidence of benefit from the device, without citing any data to support their position. The position paper criticizes the fact that no one from the Deaf community was a member of the FDA's Ear, Nose, and Throat Advisory Panel, which voted unanimously to approve the device.

One of the group's main concerns is that parents who are making the decision to proceed with a cochlear implant for their child may be poorly informed about the Deaf Culture. Lane (1992) believes that the child's inability to give informed consent for cochlear implantation is a serious ethical issue. He implies that parents should not be allowed to assume this responsibility. He further states that even if cochlear implants provided essentially normal hearing, young deaf children should not be implanted. What seems to be at the heart of the controversy is the perception that the Deaf Culture will be eliminated by the advent of widespread cochlear implantation in children.

The NAD has taken an extreme position on the issue of pediatric cochlear implantation. Cohen (1994) argues strongly that there is a substantial body of scientific evidence regarding the merits of cochlear implantation, especially with early intervention. In addition, he believes that it is the parents' responsibility to choose any medical treatment that they believe is in the best interests of their child. According to Cohen, deaf children of hearing parents are not members of the Deaf community until they willingly choose to become members or until their parents make that decision for them before the age of consent. There is a growing body of data supporting Cohen's assertion that there is a window of opportunity within which early intervention will allow young deaf children to achieve optimal benefit from cochlear implantation. To defer implantation until the child can make the decision for himself decreases the likelihood of a successful outcome.

FUTURE DIRECTIONS

MANY improvements in cochlear implant design have been studied, and some have been introduced. As more complex speech encoding strategies have been developed, providing greater redundancy in the electrical signal delivered, open-set speech recognition has improved (Dowell et al. 1987, 1990; McDermott, McKay, and Vandali 1992; McKay et al. 1991, 1992; McKay and McDermott 1993; Skinner et al. 1991, 1994; Tye-Murray, Lowder, and Tyler 1990; von Wallenberg and Battmer 1991; Wilson et al. 1991).

The growing body of evidence suggests that performance can be enhanced further by additional developments in signal processing technology. The use of a greater number of channels of electrical stimulation to provide more spectral information shows promise. For example, the new SPEAK strategy described earlier uses six to eight channels within one scan cycle to convey additional information about the highest amplitude spectral energy. A study of sixty-five postlinguistically deafened adults comparing speech perception with the SPEAK and current MPEAK coding strategies has shown improved performance for test measures in quiet and especially in noise (Skinner et al. 1994).

Ongoing research also suggests that the delivery of higher stimulation rates, which may better represent the temporal fine structure of speech, has the potential to enhance speech understanding. Wilson and his colleagues (1991) have shown improved open-set speech recognition when using a six-channel continuous interleaved sampling (CIS) strategy. A key feature of this strategy is its high rate of stimulation on each channel, usually above 800 Hz.

Improvements in digital signal processing may enable greater preservation of important amplitude and spectral cues in speech and environmental sounds such as music. Improved noise reduction techniques may allow even better speech comprehension in the presence of background noise. As microelectronic technology develops, devices will become smaller.

In the future, the selection criteria for cochlear implantation may be broadened slightly. Miyamoto et al. (1993) and Osberger (1994) have studied profoundly deaf children who obtained limited benefit of various degrees from their hearing aids and compared their performance to that of children with the Nucleus device. These data suggest that children with cochlear implants often perform as well as, or better than, the children who used hearing aids. The Nucleus device has been studied in postlinguistically deafened adults who have small amounts of residual hearing and derive some benefit from hearing aids. Results of this multisite clinical trial have shown that speech perception abilities are significantly improved with the use of the multichannel device (Brimacombe et al. 1993). As cochlear implant technology improves and provides ever greater levels of speech recognition, more children with severe-to-profound hearing losses and marginal benefit from amplification may be considered for cochlear implantation.

References

Audiological Engineering Corporation, 35 Medford Street, Somerville, MA.

Balkany, T., B.J. Gantz, and J.B. Nadol. 1988. Multichannel cochlear implants in partially ossified cochleas. *Annals of Otology, Rhinology, and Laryngology* (Suppl. 135) 97:3–7.

Beiter, A.L., and J.A. Brimacombe. 1993. Cochlear implants. In *Rehabilitative audiology: Children and adults*, ed. J.G. Alpiner and P.A. McCarthy, 417–440. Baltimore, MD: Williams and Wilkins.

Bench, J., and J. Bamford, eds. 1979. *Speech-hearing tests and the spoken language of hearing-impaired children*. London: Academic Press.

Berliner, K.I., and L.S. Eisenberg. 1985. Methods and issues in the cochlear implantation of children: An overview. The cochlear implant: An auditory prosthesis for the profoundly deaf child. *Ear and Hearing* (Suppl. 6) 3:6S–13S.

Blamey, P.J., and G.M. Clark. 1990. Place coding of vowel formants for cochlear implant patients. *Journal of the Acoustical Society of America* 88:667–673.

Blamey, P.J., R.C. Dowell, A.M. Brown, G.M. Clark, and P.M. Seligman. 1987. Vowel and consonant recognition of cochlear implant patients using formant-estimating speech processors. *Journal of the Acoustical Society of America* 82:48–57.

Blamey, P.J., R.C. Dowell, G.M. Clark, and P.M. Seligman. 1987. Acoustic parameters measured by a formant-estimating speech processor for a multiple-channel cochlear implant. *Journal of the Acoustical Society of America* 82:38–47.

Boothroyd, A., A.E. Geers, and J.S. Moog. 1991. Practical implications of cochlear implants in children. In *Multichannel cochlear implants in children*, ed. S.J. Staller. *Ear and Hearing* (Suppl. 12) 4:81S–89S.

Brimacombe, J.A., P.L. Arndt, S.J. Staller, and A.L. Beiter. 1993. Multichannel cochlear implantation in adults with severe-to-profound sensorineural hearing loss. Paper presented at the Third International Cochlear Implant Conference, April 4–7. Innsbruck, Austria.

Brimacombe, J.A., and A.L. Beiter. 1994. The application of digital technology to cochlear implants. In *Understanding digitally programmable hearing aids*, ed. R.E. Sandlin. Boston: Allyn and Bacon.

Clark, G.M., P.J. Blamey, A.M. Brown, et al. 1987a. The engineering of the receiver/stimulator and speech processor. In *The University of Melbourne-Nucleus multielectrode cochlear implant*, ed. C.R. Pfaltz. *Advances in Otorhinolaryngology* 38:63–84. Basel: Karger.

———. The surgery. 1987b. In The University of Melbourne-Nucleus multielectrode cochlear implant, ed. C.R. Pfaltz. *Advances in Otorhinolaryngology* 38:93–112.

Clark, G.M., N.L. Cohen, and R.K. Shepherd. 1991. Surgical safety considerations of multichannel cochlear implants in children. In *Multichannel cochlear implants in children*, ed. S.J. Staller. *Ear and Hearing* (Suppl. 12) 4:15S–24S.

Clark, G.M., B.K.-H. Franz, B.C. Pyman, and R.L. Webb. 1991. Surgery for multichannel cochlear implantation. In *Cochlear implants: A practical guide*, ed. H. Cooper. London: Whurr Publishers Ltd.

Cochlear Corporation. 1986. *Cochlear Corporation/University of Iowa cochlear implant test battery*. Englewood, CO: Resource Point.

———. 1990a. *Craig lipreading inventory-word recognition*. Englewood, CO: Resource Point.

———. 1990b. *Pediatric test materials and programming kit*. Englewood, CO: Resource Point.

Cohen, N.L. 1994. The ethics of cochlear implants in young children. *American Journal of Otology* 15:1–2.

Cohen, N.L., and R.A. Hoffman. 1993. Complications of cochlear implant surgery. In *Complications in head and neck surgery*, ed. D.W. Eisele. St Louis: Mosby.

Craig, W.N. 1964. Effects of preschool training on the development of reading and lipreading skills of deaf children. *American Annals of the Deaf* 109:280–296.

Davis, H., and S.R. Silverman. 1978. *Hearing and deafness*. 3rd ed. New York: Holt, Rinehart, and Winston.

Dorman, M.F., M.T. Hannley, K. Dankowski, L. Smith, and G. McCandless. 1989. Word recognition by 50 patients fitted with the Symbion multichannel cochlear implant. *Ear and Hearing* 10:44–49.

Dowell, R.C., P.M. Seligman, P.J. Blamey, and G.M. Clark. 1987. Speech perception using a two-formant 22-electrode cochlear prosthesis in quiet and in noise. *Acta Oto-Laryngologica* 104:439–446.

Dowell, R.C., L.A. Whitford, P.M. Seligman, B.K.-H. Franz, and G.M. Clark. 1990. Preliminary results with a miniature speech processor for the 22-electrode Melbourne cochlear hearing prosthesis. *Otolaryngology—Head and Neck Surgery* 98:1167–1173.

Dunn, L. 1981. *Peabody picture vocabulary test* (Revised). Circle Pines, MN: American Guidance Services.

Eisenberg, L.S., and W.F. House. 1982. Initial experience with the cochlear implant in children. In *Cochlear implants: Progress and perspectives*, ed. W.F. House and K.I. Berliner. *Annals of Otology, Rhinology, and Laryngology* (Suppl.) 91:67–73.

Eisenberg, L.S., W.M. Luxford, T.S. Becker, and W.F. House. 1984. Electrical stimulation of the auditory system in children deafened by meningitis. *Otolaryngology—Head and Neck Surgery* 92:700–705.

Elliott, L., and D. Katz. 1980. Northwestern University children's perception of speech (NU-CHIPS). St. Louis: Auditec.

Engen, E., and T. Engen. 1983. *Rhode Island test of language structure*. Baltimore: University Park Press.

Erber, N.P. 1982. *Auditory training*. Washington, D.C.: Alexander Graham Bell Association for the Deaf.

Erber, N.P., and C.M. Alencewicz. 1976. Audiologic evaluation of deaf children. *Journal of Speech and Hearing Disorders* 41:256–267.

Gardi, J.N. 1985. Human brain stem and middle latency responses to electrical stimulation: Preliminary observations. In *Cochlear implants*, ed. R.A. Schindler and M.M. Merzenich. New York: Raven Press.

Geers, A.E., and H.S. Lane. 1984. *The CID preschool performance scale*. Chicago: Stoelting.

Geers, A.E., and J.S. Moog. 1992. The Central Institute for the Deaf cochlear implant study: A progress report. *Journal of Speech-Language Pathology and Audiology* 16:129–140.

Geier, L., J. Gilden, C. Luetje, and H. Maddox. 1993. Delayed perception of cochlear implant stimulation in children with postmeningitic ossified cochleae. *American Journal of Otolaryngology* 14:556–561.

Hasenstab, M.S., and J.S. Horner. 1982. *Comprehensive intervention with hearing-impaired infants and preschool children*. Rockville: Aspen Systems.

Haskins, J. 1949. Kindergarten phonetically balanced word lists (PBK). St Louis: Auditec.

Hinojosa, R., and M. Marion. 1983. Histopathology of profound sensorineural deafness. In *Cochlear prostheses: An international symposium*, ed. C.W. Parkins and S.W. Anderson. New York: New York Academy of Sciences.

House, W.F., and K.I. Berliner. 1991. Cochlear implants: From idea to clinical practice. In *Cochlear implants: A practical guide*, ed. H. Cooper. London: Whurr Publishers Ltd.

House, W.F., W.M. Luxford, and B. Courtney. 1985. Otitis media in children following the cochlear implant. *Ear and Hearing* (Suppl.) 6:24S–26S.

Jackler, R.K., W.M. Luxford, and W.F. House. 1987. Congenital malformations of the inner ear: A classification based on embryogenesis. *Laryngoscope* (Suppl. 40) 90:2–14.

Jeffers, J., and M. Barley. 1977. *Speech reading: "Lipreading."* Springfield, IL: Charles C. Thomas.

Ketten, D.R. 1994. Differences in postmeningitic inner ear occlusions in children vs. adults. Paper presented at the Fifth Symposium on Cochlear Implants in Children, February 4–5. New York.

Kileny, P. 1991. Use of electrophysiologic measures in the management of children with cochlear implants: Brainstem, middle latency, and cognitive (P300) responses. In *Cochlear implants in children,* ed. R.T. Miyamoto and M.J. Osberger. *American Journal of Otolaryngology* (Suppl.) 12:37–42.

———. 1994. Objective measures: Evoked potentials as indicators of auditory electrical excitability. Paper presented at the Fifth Symposium on Cochlear Implants in Children, February 4–5. New York.

Kileny, P., and J.L. Kemink. 1987. Electrically evoked middle-latency auditory potentials in cochlear implant candidates. *Archives of Otolaryngology—Head and Neck Surgery* 113:1072–1077.

Lane, H. 1992. *The mask of benevolence.* New York: Alfred A. Knopf.

Lane, H., B. Brauer, L. Fleischer, J. Groode, N. Marbury, and M. Schwartz. 1991. Cochlear implants in children: A position paper of the National Association of the Deaf. *NAD Broadcaster* (March).

Ling, D. 1976. *Speech and the hearing impaired child: Theory and practice.* Washington, D.C.: Alexander Graham Bell Association.

Luxford, W.M., and D.E. Brackmann. 1985. The history of cochlear implants. In *Cochlear implants,* ed. R.F. Gray. San Diego: College-Hill Press.

Luxford, W.M., and W.F. House. 1985. Cochlear implants in children: Medical and surgical considerations. *Ear and Hearing* (Suppl) 6:20S–23S.

Mangham, C.A., W.M. Luxford, T.J. Balkany, F.O. Black, N.L. Cohen, B.J. Gantz, M.S. Hirshorn, J.L. House, S.A. Martinez, R.E. Mischke, R.T. Miyamoto, M. Novak, and J.J. Shea. 1986. Cochlear prosthesis surgery in children. In *Cochlear implants in children,* ed. D.J. Mecklenburg. *Seminars in Hearing* 7:361–369.

McDermott, H.J., C.M. McKay, and A.E. Vandali. 1992. A new portable sound processor for the University of Melbourne-Nucleus limited multielectrode cochlear implant. *Journal of the Acoustical Society of America* 91:3367–3371.

McKay, C.M., and H.J. McDermott. 1993. Perceptual performance of subjects with cochlear implants using the spectral maxima sound processor (SMSP) and the mini speech processor (MSP). *Ear and Hearing* 14:350–367.

McKay, C.M., H.J. McDermott, A.E. Vandali, and G.M. Clark. 1991. Preliminary results with a six spectral maxima sound processor for the University of Melbourne-Nucleus multiple-electrode cochlear implant. *Journal of the Otolaryngological Society of Australia* 6:354–359.

———. 1992. A comparison of speech perception of cochlear implantees using the spectral maxima sound processor (SMSP) and the MSP (multipeak) processor. *Acta Oto-Laryngologica* 112:752–761.

Mecklenburg, D.J., M.E. Demorest, and S.J. Staller. 1991. Scope and design of the clinical trial of the Nucleus multichannel cochlear implant in children. In *Multichannel cochlear implants in children,* ed. S.J. Staller. *Ear and Hearing* (Suppl.) 12(4):10S–14S.

Mecklenburg, D.J., and E. Lehnhardt. 1991. The development of cochlear implants in Europe, Asia, and Australia. In *Cochlear implants: A practical guide,* ed. H. Cooper. London: Whurr Publishers Ltd.

Mecklenburg, D.J., and J.K. Shallop. 1988. Cochlear implants. In *Handbook of speech-language pathology and audiology,* ed. N.J. Lass, L.V. McReynolds, J.L. Northern, and D.E. Yoder. Toronto: B.C. Decker.

Miyamoto, R.T., M.J. Osberger, S.L. Todd, and A.M. Robbins. 1993. Speech perception skills of children with multichannel cochlear implants. Paper presented at the Third International Cochlear Implant Conference, April 4–7. Innsbruck, Austria.

Moog, J., and A. Geers. 1979. *Grammatical analysis of elicited language: Simple sentence level.* St. Louis: Central Institute for the Deaf.

————. 1980. *Grammatical analysis of elicited language: Complex sentence level.* St. Louis: Central Institute for the Deaf.

————. 1990. *Early speech perception test for profoundly hearing-impaired children.* St. Louis: Central Institute for the Deaf.

Nevins, M.E., R.E. Kretschmer, P.M. Chute, S.A. Hellman, and S.C. Parisier. 1991. The role of an educational consultant in a pediatric cochlear implant program. *Volta Review* 93: 197–204.

Northern J.L., F.O. Black, J.A. Brimacombe, N.L. Cohen, L.S. Eisenberg, S.V. Kuprenas, S.A. Martinez, and R.E. Mischke. 1986. Selection of children for cochlear implantation. In *Cochlear implants in children,* ed. D.J. Mecklenburg. *Seminars in Hearing* 7:341–347.

O'Donoghue, G.M., R.K. Jackler, W.M. Jenkins, and R.A. Schindler. 1986. Cochlear implantation in children: The problem of head growth. *Otolaryngology—Head and Neck Surgery* 94:78–81.

Osberger, M.J. 1994. Auditory perception and speech production results. Paper presented at the Fifth Symposium on Cochlear Implants in Children, April 4–5, New York.

Osberger, M.J., A.M. Robbins, R.T. Miyamoto, S.W. Berry, W.A. Myres, K.S. Kessler, and M.L. Pope. 1991. Speech perception abilities of children with cochlear implants, tactile aids, or hearing aids. In *Cochlear implants in children,* ed. R.T. Miyamoto and M.J. Osberger. *American Journal of Otology* (Suppl.) 12:105–115.

Otte, J., H.F. Schuknecht, and A.G. Kerr. 1978. Ganglion cell populations in normal and pathological human cochlea: Implications for cochlear implantation. *Laryngoscope* 88: 1231–1246.

Owens, E., D. Kessler, C. Telleen, M. Raggio, and E. Schubert. 1985. *The minimal auditory capabilities battery.* St. Louis: Auditec.

Patrick, J.F., and G.M. Clark. 1991. The Nucleus 22-channel cochlear implant system. In *Multichannel cochlear implants in children,* ed. S.J. Staller. *Ear and Hearing* (Suppl.) 12(4):3S–9S.

Pollack, D. 1985. *Educational audiology for the limited-hearing infant and preschooler.* 2d ed. Springfield: Charles C. Thomas.

Rickards, F.W., S.J. Dettman, P.A. Busby, R.L. Webb, R.C. Dowell, S.E. Dennehy, and T.G. Nienhuys. 1990. Preoperative evaluation and selection of children and teenagers. In *Cochlear prostheses,* ed. G.M. Clark, Y.C. Tong, and J.F. Patrick. Edinburgh: Churchill Livingstone.

Ross, M., and J. Lerman. 1971. *Word intelligibility by picture identification.* Pittsburgh: Stanwix House.

Schindler, R.A., and D.K. Kessler. 1993. Clarion cochlear implant: Phase I investigational results. *American Journal of Otology* 14:263–272.

Schuyler, V., and N. Rushmer. 1987. *Parent-infant habilitation.* Portland: IHR Publications.

Shallop, J.K., A.L. Beiter, D.W. Goin, and R.E. Mischke. 1990. Electrically evoked auditory brain stem responses (EABR) and middle latency responses (EMLR) obtained from patients with the Nucleus multichannel cochlear implant. *Ear and Hearing* 11: 5–15.

Shallop, J.K., and D. J. Mecklenburg. 1987. Technical aspects of cochlear implants. In *Handbook of hearing aid amplification*, ed. R.E. Sandlin. San Diego: College-Hill Press.

Simmons, F.B. 1966. Electrical stimulation of the auditory nerve in man. *Archives of Otolaryngology* 84:2–54.

Skinner, M.W. 1988. *Hearing aid evaluation*. Englewood Cliffs, NJ: Prentice-Hall.

Skinner, M.W., G.M. Clark, L.A. Whitford, P.M. Seligman, S.J. Staller, D.B. Shipp, J.K. Shallop, C. Everingham, C.M. Menapace, P.L. Arndt, T. Antogenelli, J.A. Brimacombe, S. Pijl, P. Daniels, C.R. George, H.J. McDermott, and A.L. Beiter. 1994. Evaluation of a new spectral peak coding strategy for the Nucleus 22 channel cochlear implant system. *American Journal of Otolaryngology* 15 (Suppl. 2): 15–27.

Skinner, M.W., L.K. Holden, T.A. Holden, R.C. Dowell, P.M. Seligman, J.A. Brimacombe, and A.L. Beiter. 1991. Performance of postlinguistically deaf adults with the wearable speech processor (WSPIII) and mini speech processor (MSP) of the Nucleus multielectrode cochlear implant. *Ear and Hearing* 12:3–22.

Staller, S.J. 1985. Cochlear implant characteristics: A review of current technology. In *Cochlear implants*, ed. G.A. McCandless. *Seminars in Hearing* 23–32.

Staller, S.J., A.L. Beiter, and J.A. Brimacombe. 1991. Children and multichannel cochlear implants. In *Cochlear implants: A practical guide*, ed. H. Cooper, 283–3221. London: Whurr Publishers Ltd.

Staller, S.J., R.C. Dowell, A.L. Beiter, and J.A. Brimacombe. 1991. Perceptual abilities of children with the Nucleus 22-channel cochlear implant. In *Multichannel cochlear implants in children*, ed. S.J. Staller. *Seminars in Hearing* (Suppl.) 12(4):34S–47S.

Thielemeir, M.A. 1984. *The discrimination after training test*. Los Angeles: House Ear Institute.

Thielemeir, M.A., L.L. Tonokawa, B. Petersen, and L.S. Eisenberg. 1985. Audiological results in children with a cochlear implant. *Ear and Hearing* (Suppl.) 6:27S–35S.

Tillman, T.W., and R. Carhart. 1966. An expanded test for speech discrimination utilizing CNC monosyllabic words (Northwestern University auditory test no. 6). Technical report, SAM-TR-66–55, USAF School of Aerospace Medicine. Aerospace Medical Division (AFSC), Brooks Air Force Base, Texas.

Tobey, E.A., and M.S. Hasenstab. 1991. Effects of a Nucleus multichannel cochlear implant upon speech production in children. In *Multichannel cochlear implants in children*, ed. S.J. Staller. *Ear and Hearing* (Suppl.) 12(4):48S–54S.

Tong, Y.C., R.C. Black, G.M. Clark, I.C. Forster, J.B. Millar, B.J. O'Loughlin, and J.F. Patrick. 1979. A preliminary report on a multiple-channel cochlear implant operation. *Journal of Laryngology and Otology* 93:7:679–695.

Tong, Y.C., G.M. Clark, P.J. Blamey, P.A. Busby, and R.C. Dowell. 1982. Psychophysical studies for two multiple-channel cochlear implant patients. *Journal of the Acoustical Society of America* 71:153–160.

Tong, Y.C., G.M. Clark, P.M. Seligman, and J.F. Patrick. 1980. Speech processing for a multiple-electrode cochlear implant prosthesis. *Journal of the Acoustical Society of America* 68:1897–1899.

Tye-Murray, N., M. Lowder, and R.S. Tyler. 1990. Comparison of the FOF2 and FOF1F2 processing strategies for the Cochlear Corporation cochlear implant. *Ear and Hearing* 11:195–200.

Tyler, R.S., J. Preece, and M. Lowder. 1983. *The Iowa cochlear implant tests*. Iowa City: University of Iowa, Department of Otolaryngology, Head and Neck Surgery.

Tyler, R.S., and N. Tye-Murray. 1991. Cochlear implant signal-processing strategies and patient perception of speech and environmental sounds. In *Cochlear implants: A practical guide*, ed. H. Cooper. London: Whurr Publishers Ltd.

von Wallenberg, E.L., and R.D. Battmer. 1991. Comparative speech recognition results in eight subjects using two different coding strategies with the Nucleus 22-channel cochlear implant. *British Journal of Audiology* 25:371–380.

Waring, M.D., M. Don, and J.A. Brimacombe. 1985. ABR assessment of stimulation in induction coil implant patients. In *Cochlear implants*, ed. R.A. Schindler and M.M. Merzenich. New York: Raven Press.

Webb, R.L., B.C. Pyman, B.K.-H. Franz, and G.M. Clark. 1990. The surgery of cochlear implantation. In *Cochlear prostheses*, ed. G.M. Clark, Y.C. Tong, and J.F. Patrick. Edinburgh: Churchill Livingstone.

Wechsler, D. 1967. *Wechsler primary and preschool intelligence scale*. New York: Psychological Corp.

———. 1974. *Wechsler intelligence scale for children* (Revised). New York: Psychological Corp.

Weisenberger, J.M., and L. Kozma-Spytek. 1991. Evaluating tactile aids for speech perception and production by hearing-impaired adults and children. In *Cochlear implants in children*, ed. R.T. Miyamoto and M.J. Osberger. *American Journal of Otolaryngology* (Suppl.) 12:188–200.

Wilson, B.S., C.C. Finley, D.T. Lawson, R.D. Wolford, D.K. Eddington, and W.M. Rabinowitz. 1991. Better speech recognition with cochlear implants. *Nature* 352:236–238.

Yune, H.Y., R.T. Miyamoto, and M.E. Yune. 1991. Medical imaging in cochlear implant candidates. In *Cochlear implants in children*, ed. R.T. Miyamoto and M.J. Osberger. *American Journal of Otolaryngology* (Suppl.) 12:11–17.

12

Audiology and Education

E. Harris Nober

DEFINITIONS OF HEARING IMPAIRMENT

THE generic term "hearing-impaired" denotes an auditory pure tone average (PTA) threshold that exceeds the designated 26-decibel average over the speech frequencies 500, 1000, and 2000 Hz (AAO-ACO 1979). For young children, it is more appropriate to assume that a PTA threshold of 15 decibels can interfere with the normal development of auditory communication and the skills needed for the educational process. About 8 to 10% of the U.S. population has some level of auditory impairment that may interfere with communication. If the hearing impairment is severe (70–90 dB) or profound (91 dB or more), the individual is often considered deaf, particularly if the individual is a child. The 91-dB PTA is considered the upper limit for the auditory system to serve a child effectively in educational and social settings even with amplification (Paul and Quigley 1990).

Definitions of human function and performance are always complex and relate to an array of intrinsic and extrinsic factors. When the auditory processing mechanism is defective, several parameters are pertinent to educational management: (1) age of onset, identification, and intervention; (2) degree, type, and locus of the hearing impairment; (3) etiology; (4) intellectual and linguistic abilities; (5) family and caregivers' communication mode and emotional support; (6) socioeconomic status; (7) cultural diversity; (8) psychological profile; (9) prevention activities; (10) general integrity of the auditory and related mechanisms; and (11) other physical aberrations.

There are additional factors, to be sure, but the issue of prelingual (two years or younger) and postlingual onset (two years or older) will have an impact on the educational plans for management and transition into the workplace despite delineations for terms such as hard-of-hearing and deaf. Over 90% of children attending special schools for the hearing-impaired have a prelingual onset (Allen and Osborn 1984; Paul and Quigley 1990). Many children with multiple disabilities at special schools for the deaf show hearing thresholds that are below a 70-dB PTA threshold level at speech frequencies 500, 1000, and 2000 Hz.

Advocates of deaf culture (e.g., Lane 1988) contend that hearing threshold levels connote a clinical or pathological perspective that dwells falaciously on auditory deprivation and a set of behavioral performance consequences relating to a hearing norm. Whereas proponents of the clinical view cite research that presents speech, language, academic, cultural, and social deficits, Lane contended that the methods of these studies were flawed because the standards and norms were set by normal-hearing control groups. Furthermore, he asserted that the research should be conducted by trained deaf researchers. Proponents of the clinical view (e.g., Myklebust 1964) have proposed that the lack of bona fide language development precluded normal learning mainly because of the inability to use abstract thought effectively.

EARLY INTERVENTION

WHEN deafness is first confirmed in an infant, considerations about the form of communication become a preoccupation for the family as communication is a formidable bonding process with the family and environment.

Family acceptance of the deafness, in itself, is a traumatic and consuming event for parents and siblings who have normal hearing and few or no experiences with congenital hearing loss. These parents, who represent 90% of the parent population of deaf children, go through a grieving process involving shock, denial, guilt, depression, anger, anxiety, and (we hope) full acceptance and confidence in various degrees (see chapter 13). Frequently, these stages overlap and linger for extended periods. Hearing-impaired infants in this family constellation are usually delayed in language and social development as emotional issues are resolved and future educational decisions are formulated (Meadow-Orlans 1990). This is a major adjustment period for the family and other caregivers.

When a deaf infant is born into a hearing family, it is most often the audiologist who confirms the deafness and notifies the parents. Accordingly, the audiologist monitors early intervention strategies and may play an integral role in the individual family service plan (IFSP) now required by law. This role is crucial as the audiologist is often the person to discuss the benefits of oral language vs. manual language. During this initial crisis period, the audiologist works with a team of professionals to counsel the family.

For the 10% of deaf infants born to deaf parents, the lack of hearing may be welcome and a relief. In these families, the communication process is predetermined and enables the infant to become an integral part of the family from the outset. For these all-deaf families, American Sign Language (ASL) is the prevailing operational language; the result is an immediate and strong family and cultural identity and cohesiveness. These deaf infants acquire language by signing in a developmental pattern similar to that of a normal-hearing infant using the auditory processing mechanism (Meadow-Orlans 1990).

Prevention

Prevention of secondary communication impairment is a formidable goal of early intervention. From the outset, a normal-hearing infant learns that crying brings the parent or caregiver, and an initial bond of trust and love quickly forms between the two. This author believes that most mothers start the bonding-love process while the baby is in utero, followed by instant adoration when the baby is first brought to them and the other family members. The bonding process with the deaf baby involves a considerable amount of vision constrained to the immediate field. Loss of auditory input impedes the protective benefits ascribed to the normal hearing mechanism. With early intervention, maximum use of the critical years for language development is accomplished, thus diminishing social isolation despite the mode of communication. Deaf children learn sign language at an accelerated rate during the formative language years. Often, early identification of a hearing loss abates negative attitudes and perceptions in school and among family members. Secondary prevention also has a significant impact on long-range total educational costs (Bricker 1986).

The birth-to-two-years early management program is necessarily shared with the parent or caregiver. Sometimes clinic visits are scheduled after working hours to accommodate single-parent working families. Group counseling and technical training intervention sessions foster team consistency. Many larger clinic settings have mini-apartment facilities to demonstrate kitchen, bathroom, bedroom, and play techniques. Because of the rapid changes in multicultural dynamics, some centers include cultural issues in the training agenda.

FEDERAL LAWS FOR THE DISABLED AND EDUCATIONAL MANAGEMENT

NATIONAL legislation for the education of hearing-impaired individuals in the United States dates to 1827 when Public Law 19-8 approved the purchase of land in Florida and Kentucky to establish "Asylums for the Deaf and Dumb." However, this law was not funded until 1847 as PL 29-1; other states quickly followed suit. Thirty years later, in 1857, Congress passed Public Law 34-36, establishing the Columbia Institution for the Deaf and Dumb. The school was renamed Gallaudet College in 1954 (PL 83-420) and 32 years later, Gallaudet University, as part of the 1986 Education of the Deaf Act. The National Technical Institute for the Deaf was also established in this act. The 1986 Education of the Deaf Act was reauthorized as Public Law 102-421 in October of 1992. The reauthorization included funds for Gallaudet University and the National Technical Institute for the Deaf, interpreters for schools, research, and scholarships for deaf-minority students majoring in special education.

Within twenty to thirty years after the establishment of the Columbia Institution, schools for the deaf, blind, mentally retarded, and other disabled persons
were established in New York, Boston, Philadelphia, Providence, and Hartford.
By the end of the 1800s, there were about fourteen federal laws with improved
or expanded entitlements to aid the disabled. Federal priorities for disabled children exceeded those for disabled adults. In 1965, Public Law 89-10, the Elementary and Secondary Education Act (ESEA), was enacted. A local education
agency (LEA) is a school district (e.g., the Boston Public Schools). A state education agency (SEA) denotes an agency such as the Massachusetts Board of Education. Under PL-89-10, LEAs and SEAs are to provide special education for
low-income, educationally-deprived children, many with hearing impairments.

In 1960, the Captioned Film for the Deaf Act (PL 89-258) was passed. In the
sixties, the Title I program (PL 89-313) was established with a plethora of other
federal legislative acts including:

1. creation of the National Technical Institute for the Deaf;
2. mental retardation and mental health and community health center construction;
3. extended federal assistance for state-operated and state-supported
schools for the disabled;
4. the Vocational Rehabilitation Act (PL 89-333) and its amendments;
5. the Model Secondary School for the Deaf Act (PL 89-694), with amendments to the Elementary and Secondary Education Act;
6. the National Eye Institute;
7. the Disabled Children Early Education Assistance Act (PL 90-538); and
8. the National Center in Educational Media for the Disabled (PL 91-61).

The first major law to affect directly the educational management of disabled children was Public Law 94-142, the Education for All Handicapped Children's Act, passed in 1975. This act entitled all school-aged children to an appropriate and free education; it also established due process state requirements
and nondiscriminatory testing. Public Law 94-142 did not emerge from a vac-
uum; indeed, it was nearly the two hundredth federal law for disabled persons
or social entitlements.

Over a decade later, in 1986, PL 94-142 was amended by PL 99-457, the
Education of the Handicapped Act Amendments, which changed the management and education of disabled infants, toddlers, preschool children, and their
families. It added two significant segments: a program for handicapped infants
and toddlers and preschool grant program. Shortly afterward, in 1991, PL 101-
476, the Individuals with Disabilities Education Act (IDEA), reauthorized PL
99-457. It adopted the term "disabled" instead of "handicapped," changed the
term "children" to "individuals," added autism and traumatic brain injury, and
installed a transition requirement to assist adolescents. Also in 1991, PL 102-
119, the Early Childhood Amendments Act, was passed to provide full rights to

infants, toddlers, children three to five, and any other children determined to be at risk. One milestone, the Elementary and Secondary Education Act (ESEA) in 1965 (PL 89-10), supplemented costs for LEA programs designed for educationally-deprived children. During a ten-year period, fifty-four laws relating to the disabled were enacted—an impressive fact compared to the fifty-one acts between 1920 and 1959, a period of nearly forty years.

The Education for All Handicapped Children Act (PL 94-142) of 1975 is often called the Educational Bill of Rights for Handicapped Children or the Quiet Revolution. This law included a revision of Part B of a prior Education of the Handicapped Act (PL 91-230) that had a significant impact on all phases of educational management of disabled children. To comply, a massive cooperative effort evolved among agencies throughout the country. Compliance included accountability and direct family involvement for all disabled children aged three to twenty-one years. Public Law 94-142 ensures:

1. a constitutional right to a free (no cost to parents) and appropriate education;
2. a redistribution of resources and revenue sharing;
3. due process;
4. nondiscriminatory testing and evaluation;
5. an individualized education program (IEP) to provide a unique special education;
6. a least-restrictive-environment (LRE) educational placement;
7. teams that include parents or advocate substitutes;
8. funding schedules including a schedule of SEA's and LEA's responsibilities;
9. well-trained and competent vendors;
10. self-contained and required in-service programs;
11. classrooms, physical education, home instruction, hospitals, and institutions.

When PL 94-142 was first implemented, in 1977, 800,000 children were identified as hearing impaired, and the prevalence growth was 2 to 3% a year. It is noteworthy that, between 1976–1977, mental retardation prevalence decreased by 38% because of reclassification to "learning disability." In 1992, the U.S. Department of Education Fourteenth Annual Report to Congress on the Implementation of the Individuals with Disabilities Education Act recounted that, of the 12% of school-aged children who were disabled, four of the ten disability types accounted for 96% of the total group:

1. learning disabled: 49.1% of the total, involved 2,144,377 children in the U.S.;
2. speech impaired: 22.7% of the total, involved 990,185 children in the U.S.;
3. mentally retarded: 12.7% of the total, involved 552,658 children in the U.S.;

4. seriously emotionally disturbed: 9.0% of the total, involved 393,300 children in the U.S.

The remaining 6.5%—the low incidence six categories (multiply handicapped, orthopedically impaired, hard of hearing, visually impaired, deaf-blind, and other health problems)—composed this group. The 1992 report revealed that 6.7% of the general population between three and twenty-one years of age received special education and related services in a regular class, resource room, separate class, residential facility, or a homebound or hospital environment. Serving these four million children were 300,000 full-time special teachers and paraprofessional nonteachers; the latter group is 53.4% of the total. Learning disability teachers are 32.1% of the workforce; speech and hearing clinicians, 13.7%; teachers of the mentally retarded, 17.7%; and teachers of children with severe emotional disturbance, 10% of the workforce.

The Education of the Handicapped Act Amendments (PL 99-457) passed in 1986. It required significant changes in the management and education of disabled infants, toddlers, preschool children, and their families. Many of these provisions were comprehensive and required significant preparation and effort by educational agencies. One new segment, the "Handicapped Infants and Toddlers Program," focused on the birth through two years age group, while another new feature, the "Preschool Grant Program," targeted the three- to five-year-old age group. As both age groups required different services, creative changes within educational and healthcare institutions were required. States were required to implement PL 99-457 by September 1, 1991. By that date, each state governor had appointed an "Interagency Coordinating Council" and identified the "Lead Agency" in that state to guarantee the following:

1. a definition of developmentally delayed;
2. establishment of a service timetable;
3. provision for multidisciplinary assessment of child and family needs;
4. preparation of an Individual Family Service Plan (IFSP) with a case manager;
5. development of "Child Find" and other operational referral systems;
6. promulgation of a public awareness program;
7. development of a Central Directory of resources, services, experts, and programs;
8. development of a "Comprehensive Service Personnel Development" (CSPD) plan;
9. activation of a "Lead Agency" to oversee the activities;
10. development of procedures for contracting with local providers;
11. establishment of a fiscal payment timetable;
12. provision of "Due Process" protection;
13. establishment of personnel standards and requirements for service providers;
14. maintenance of a data bank of early intervention programs;

15. creation of a Disabled Infants and Toddlers Program for children from birth through two years; and

16. creation of a Preschool Grant Program for children from three through five years of age.

The Handicapped Infants and Toddlers Program (birth through two years) advanced the need for an early intervention Case Manager for closer and more efficient family and professional interdisciplinary coordination. Early intervention, a planned element, required a detailed and comprehensive multidisciplinary Individual Family Service Plan (IFSP) for any infant suspect of or identified as at risk from the case history, developmental delays in physical and mental maturity, cognition, or speech and language communication.

The Preschool Grant Program for children of ages three to five years did not require the usual categorical labels for treatment eligibility to facilitate ongoing diagnostic exploration. Funds for innovative family training programs were made available along with funds to access health care and other social services for disabled children and their families. This provision included environmentally abused and deprived children and their families.

PL 99-457 provided financial support for early identification using at-risk registers and other systems. Ideally, hearing-impaired infants would be identified during the first few months rather than at 2 to 2½ years, the national average for identifying hearing impairment (Stein, Clark, and Kraus 1983). Early identification ensures an early IFSP with extended family-focused training and interagency collaboration. The early childhood literature abounds with evidence that early intervention has significant long-standing beneficial effects on maturation and development. Despite these innovations, there was considerable unrest about the specific accountability of deaf education, so a special Commission on Education of the Deaf was appointed. As expected, the commission determined that deaf education was poor, and serious changes were critical.

In 1991, the Individuals with Disabilities Education Act (PL 101-476) was passed. Fundamentally, it reauthorized PL 99-457 and changed the word "children" to "individuals" and the word "handicapped" to "disabled," thus earning its acronym, IDEA. The act added autism and traumatic brain injury (TBI) and required transition for adolescents into the workplace. The law also stipulated that an attention deficit disorder (ADD) was not a separate category of disability but a symptom of a learning disability or a TBI, enabling these children to receive aid. The act defined a TBI as: "an acquired injury to the brain caused by an external physical force, resulting in total or partial functional disability or psychosocial impairment, or both, that adversely affects educational performance . . . resulting in impairment in one or more areas such as cognition; language; memory; attention; reasoning; abstract thinking; judgment; problem solving; sensory, perceptual, and motor abilities; psychosocial behavior; physical functions; information processing; and speech." The term excludes congenital and birth trauma defects.

The Americans with Disabilities Act 1990 (PL 101-366) was enacted and became effective in July of 1992. It is a sweeping bill that protects forty million Americans with regard to employment, public service, transportation, public accommodations, and telecommunications, with an emphasis on "assistive technology" and "reasonable accommodation." Even the term *disability* was redefined into three components (*Americans with Disabilities Act*, Section 3, Summary of Existing Legislation Affecting People with Disabilities, U.S. Department of Education, Office of Special Education and Rehabilitation Services, Washington, D.C., June 1992):

(a) a physical or mental impairment that substantially limits one or more of the major life activities of such individual;

(b) a record of such an impairment; or

(c) being regarded as having such an impairment.

Two other noteworthy terms were defined: a "reasonable accommodation" and "undue hardship." The former includes modifying existing facilities, policies, examinations, work schedules, assignment to vacant positions, new technology, and use of qualified readers and interpreters. Undue hardship denotes a significant expense on the total cost to an employer, the type of operation, and the number affected.

The ADA evolved from decades of legislative bills enacted to protect the disabled, based on the Fourteenth Amendment to the U.S. Constitution. The collective benefits from preceding bills offered disabled children and adults medical treatment, protection from abuse, accessibility to public and private facilities, and protection against employment discrimination. The ADA contains five titles:

Title I prohibits employment discrimination via employment tests, hiring practices, advancement, discharge, compensation, job training, and other conditions by denying reasonable accommodations to the limitations of the disability.

Title II prohibits discrimination in public services, transportation vehicles, and buildings (including new construction) by making all state and local activities subject to the ADA. This sweeping protection was not afforded by the earlier Section 504 of the Rehabilitation Act.

Title III prohibits discrimination of private services open to the public or with public accommodations. The latter includes food, clothing and other stores, hotels, restaurants, bars, movies, theaters, concert halls, stadiums, auditoriums, shopping centers, gas stations, health facilities, museums, libraries, parks, schools, nurseries, day care centers, and exercise and recreation centers.

Title IV mandates that telephone companies install telecommunication equipment for the disabled with speech and hearing disorders.

Title V specifies that no other laws, particularly state or local laws, can be construed to invalidate, negate, or reduce the scope of this act. The federal government has a central role to enforce these titles using congressional authority based on the Fourteenth Amendment to the U.S. Constitution. This act waives immunity under the Eleventh Amendment to the U.S. Constitution, prohibiting retaliation. It also authorizes the Architectural and Transportation Barriers Compliance Board to issue minimum accessibility guidelines and authorizes the Attorney General and the National Council on Disability to spell out and enforce their procedures.

Educational Models and Settings for Severely Hearing-Impaired Children

THERE are several educational setting prototypes for children with a hearing disability. Very young children can be treated in a clinical or home-based setting, a preschool setting, special programs in agencies, day or residential schools for the deaf, special resource settings for children in inclusion programs, public schools with a variety of options that cascade the child toward the least restrictive environment, and so on. These programs can be located in private clinics, universities, public or private schools, community and governmental agencies, and professional agency clinics. Age is one parameter for eligibility, but other parameters are considered for the programs below.

Preschool

Children with hearing disability, ages three to five years, are entitled to a preschool education. Children can be placed in these classes with normal-hearing children to avail themselves of a wholesome interactive mix of speech and language. Frequently, the parent or caregiver participates in the structured activities. These classes are part of the ongoing evaluation and assessment continuum and involve numerous trial and error tasks during a crucial developmental stage. A variety of support services can be made available to the child and the parent to facilitate the communication process. During this period of development, various options such as amplification, auditory training, and combined technologies are tried in an effort to produce oral speech. Caregivers are also trained during this period.

Mainstreaming

This term receives surprisingly broad attention in the literature despite a paucity of definitions for it. It is probable that *mainstreaming* was widely popularized for academic placement of disabled children when PL 94-142 was enacted, but the term was never actually used in the act. The phrase found in PL 94-142 was "least restrictive environment," which conceptualized the idea of assimilating a disabled child into the regular or normal classroom setting. Thus, mainstream connotes a regular, normal, or standard school setting. It also connotes a movement toward the norm- and criterion-referenced standards, with placement in a regular classroom as the ultimate goal.

This paradigm precludes manual communication. Ross, Brackett, and Maxon (1982, 1991) reported an increase in the oral mode of communication because of the mainstreamed school setting. Some school programs attempted to use total communication as the intermediary model in the school setting (Moores, Cerney, and Garcia 1990; Reagan 1990). An even greater restriction on the communication model of choice is imposed by the "inclusion" paradigm that swept the United States (Heward and Orlansky 1992).

A goal of PL 94-142 was to enable disabled children to share experiences with nondisabled peers to maximize experiences. It enables the family to remain intact and the children to attend the same school as their siblings. These experiences need to be socially and psychologically sound within the educational and academic framework of the normal school environment. Indeed, the very title of PL 94-142 includes the phrase "appropriate education." One mainstreaming goal is to provide the most appropriate integrated education for the disabled child using support services.

"Appropriate" relates to the performance ability of the child and determines how restrictive the placement needs to be at a particular time and development level. It applies to preschool as well as school-aged children. Because learning is a dynamic process, what is appropriate will vary over time; hence, a hard-of-hearing child who shows language benefits with amplification may require only minimal support services.

Depending on the student's ability, mainstream can range from full classroom inclusion to placement into a special class located in a regular school setting. Optimal benefits are expected if the mainstreamed child was chronologically within two years of the classmates or one year in language, reading, and writing skills at time of placement. These benefits are also expected if the child had good auditory skills, was able to follow the regular curriculum, was socially mature, and had a strong self-image.

The range of services reflects the scope of the restriction. Ross, Brackett, and Maxon (1991) referred to full- and partial-mainstreaming. In a full-mainstreamed program, the regular classroom teacher assumes full responsibility for the academic and social activities with special services providing help to the child in special-needs areas such as language, speech, reading, and so on. They described partial-mainstreaming as the resource room instruction that follows the classroom curriculum in academic areas with which the child is having difficulty. Finally, these authors referred to social-mainstreaming as the placement of a child in a regular school setting but separation for special academic instruction. The special academic setting may be a class within the same building or class instruction contracted at a school for the deaf for part of the day, if the child is hearing-impaired.

Inclusion

Inclusion is one component of the educational school reform movement. The term refers to placement of the disabled child in the regular class with the regular classroom teacher as the instructor. Full inclusion means that there is no tracking or placement of students into sections based on test scores or performance. The classroom teacher alone is responsible for the disabled student along with all the other children in the class.

This issue has political implications. The National Joint Committee on Learning Disabilities (ASHA 1993) questioned whether all students with learning disabilities should be served solely in the regular education classroom. Many leaders in the special education, speech-language pathology, and deaf communities oppose full inclusion. The NJCLD asserted that the unique needs of the LD child require an individualized program to achieve maximum performance. The responsibility for developing the IEP rests with the combined efforts of regular and special educators, parents, and student consumers of the services (American Speech-Language-Hearing Association 1993; Council for Exceptional Children 1993; Heward and Orlansky 1992).

A draft statement from the Council for Exceptional Children (1993) supported a "rich variety of educational and vocational program options and experiences, available in community based, nonschool environments, special schools, and options for individual or small group instruction in 'regular' or 'home' schools." The CEC stressed the importance of placement in mainstream classes for part of the day. It views inclusive schools as the "first and foremost call for a change in attitudes and values. . . a new ethos that celebrates diversity; promotes accountability, culturalism, and professional collaboration; values the strengthening of social relationships among children; and explores strategies for pursuing excellence without sacrificing equity."

Classroom Acoustics, Noise, and Speech Perception

The physical characteristics of the classroom environment (room size, reverberation, absorption, reflection) modify the sound energy and subsequently affect perception of the speech signal for hearing-impaired students. Whereas the adverse acoustic effects may be minimal for the normal-hearing student with full language development, the hearing-impaired student with diminished speech perception and language development will have difficulty in a poor acoustic environment. The audiologist is expected to analyze the acoustic situation and make suggestions to minimize adverse acoustic conditions and thus enhance speech perception in the classroom (Madell 1992).

Transmitted sound will (1) penetrate an object, (2) reverberate or reflect off the object, and (3) circumscribe the object. Usually, all three occur to various degrees, depending on a room's structural characteristics and its contents. Soft items absorb sound better than hard items because they have a higher absorption coefficient. An empty or perfectly rectangular or square room will reflect and produce more standing wave patterns than rooms with multidimensional walls. Pictures on walls and other decorative objects in the room will disrupt standing wave patterns. High frequency sounds with short wavelengths are more direct than low frequency sounds with longer wavelengths that can circumscribe an object. Sound intensity diminishes with distance and as it penetrates an object; the intensity reduction is called transmission loss.

Thus, reverberation or sound reflection depends on the interaction between the acoustic composition of the room and the sound signals. It is measured as reverberation time (RT), the fraction of a second it takes for a sound stimulus to diminish 60 decibels after the sound has stopped. The greater the RT, the more the initial sound lingers and interferes with successive sounds. Reverberation can cause the energy of an early sound to augment a later sound and increase the combined sound intensity. If the two sounds are out of phase, reverberation can diminish intensity or even cancel the energy if the two conflicting sounds are precisely in opposite phase direction and of equal magnitude. Acoustic changes ("smearing of the time domain") from reverberation essentially alter the characteristics of combined sounds, reducing signal fidelity. Thus, increased reverberation time increases signal distortion. The perception of consonants is more susceptible to auditory error than the perception of vowels because consonants are of shorter duration and have less intensity than vowels. Earlier vowel signals mask later or successive consonants during continuous speech output (Berg 1986). As a longer RT increases speech signal distortion, there is a notable speech perception reduction in the auditory discrimination of the hearing impaired.

Speech signal reverberation of 0.02 to 0.03 second can induce "coloration," which enhances timbre or quality and sometimes perception (Lochner and Burger 1961; Nabalek and Robinette 1978). Reflected sound greater than the incident sound by .03 second will diminish speech perception for any listener and with significantly greater disruption to the hearing impaired. The critical RT for the hearing impaired appears to be near 1.2 seconds where word recognition performance can diminish to less than half (Finitzo-Hieber 1981; Olsen 1981). In general, audiologists (Bess and McConnell 1981; Crandell and Bess 1986, 1987; Olsen 1981) recommend that the ideal classroom RT should not exceed 0.4 second, a criterion that is met in only 22% of classrooms.

Clearly, extraneous noise will reduce speech perception further in a reverberant room that exceeds 0.3 second RT. When the teacher's (or student's) speech is the acoustic signal, all other sound is designated as noise, and the relative levels of the two sound sources are the signal-to-noise (S/N) ratio for that classroom. There is no absolute classroom S/N ratio setting. Rather there is a dynamic interactive continuum of sound changes. Therefore, only best estimates can be determined from sampling ongoing conditions (e.g., student presence and movement, period of the day, subject matter, age and class levels, classroom location, internal and external noise such as ventilation, mechanical and traffic noise, and so on) (Finitzo-Hieber 1981; Nober and Nober 1977). As unwanted sound, noise masks the signal when its intensity approaches or supersedes the signal intensity; furthermore, the frequency spectrum of the signal and noise affects the auditory perceptual masking impact on both normal and hearing-impaired listeners. A reduced S/N ratio has a greater negative impact with increased RT for hearing and hearing-impaired listeners, but the impact is greater on the hearing impaired; this deficit in auditory discrimination increases as the hearing loss increases.

On average, the traditional classroom noise level with twenty-five students and a teacher ranges from 56 dBA to 63 dBA with the mean around 60 dBA (Finitzo-Hieber 1981; Nober and Nober 1962, 1977; Ross and Giolas 1971; Sanders 1965). The traditional classroom, with the teacher three feet from the students, has a speech signal intensity of 60 to 65 dBA (Madell 1992); in addition, the teacher's speech level is about 60 dBA. Thus, with ambient classroom noise at 60 dBA, the S/N is 0 dB. Their intensity levels are similar, but frequency composition differs. In this typical classroom listening condition, normal hearing students perceive well. Crandell (1993) showed sentence recognition scores of 93.2% for students with normal hearing, whereas students with a mild hearing loss scored 25% lower. These score differences increase precipitously as the S/N diminishes and hearing loss increases. As noise is disproportionally more detrimental to speech perception of the hearing impaired, a S/N of +20 dB is often recommended for these students in the mainstreamed classroom (Finitzo-Hieber and Tillman 1978; Tillman, Carhart, and Olsen 1970). To ensure favorable listening conditions for the hearing-impaired student in the classroom during the day as signal and noise conditions change, Bess and McConnell (1981) recommended an empty-classroom ambient noise maximum of 35 dBA.

The S/N ratio is influenced directly by the acoustic distance between the speaker and the listener (in this instance, the teacher and the student). On average, the teacher's speech level is about 66 dB at three feet from the student (Ross, Brackett, and Maxon 1982), and the typical classroom ambient noise level can be estimated at 60 dBA, as indicated earlier. With these values, Ross et al. determined the S/N was +6 dB; at twelve feet the speech level was 54 decibels, so the S/N was -6 dB with corresponding S/N decreases as teacher-student distance and noise levels increased. Speech perception performance is improved by increasing the S/N ratio (i.e., by reducing the teacher-student distance).

Maintaining a favorable S/N can be difficult, particularly in preschool and earlier grades. Amplification using an FM device or a regular hearing aid will not alter the detrimental effects of reverberation but will improve the S/N ratio to counterbalance reverberation (see chapter 10). With the teacher wearing a microphone and the student wearing a receiver, the teacher-student distance is reduced to a three- to four-inch span between the teacher's (or student's) microphone and the mouth. With this amplification setup, background noise and reverberation have less of a deleterious impact on the speech perception of the hearing-impaired child. With a microphone-to-mouth distance of about

4.5 inches, speech can reach 84 dB, or a favorable S/N ratio of +24 dB if the background classroom noise is estimated at 60 dBA.

The interaction of distance and reverberation can yield a critical distance situation for the hearing impaired because the two are inversely related (i.e., as RT increases, critical distance decreases). Critical distance occurs when the amounts of incident and reflected sound reaching the ear are equal. A listener receives more direct sound within this critical distance and more reflected sound when beyond it (Niemoeller 1981). The hearing-impaired child should be seated closer to the teacher to facilitate direct reception of speech.

COMMUNICATION ALTERNATIVES

Oral Communication

ORAL communication dates from the seventeenth and eighteenth centuries and is based on the premise that the natural auditory route is preferred despite severe damage to the auditory system. Oral communication uses vision to read the oral movements of the speaker. The combination of speechreading and audition is preferred by devoted oralists for multisensory stimulation that discourages manual input during communication. The rationale is to avoid isolation of the hearing-impaired from the hearing community.

In the 1960s, the efficacy of oralism was challenged because of low academic performance by deaf students in the United States—30% were unable to pass literacy tests and 60% scored at the fifth grade reading level (Evans 1982)—resulting in a corresponding drift back to manualism. The preferred choice was American Sign Language (ASL). By 1994, the oral approach was the sole communication system in only a few schools in the United States, whereas two decades earlier, only a few facilities had used a manual system as the exclusive mode of communication and teaching.

Manual Sign Systems

Manual (or nonverbal) systems also were developed during the seventeenth and eighteenth centuries. There are several of these hand-gesture systems, some used as auxiliaries to other approaches. Deaf children naturally gesture to each other to communicate (Charrow 1975); indeed, a manual system is so natural to the prelingual deaf child with deaf parents that these children even dream in sign language. In some normal-hearing cultures, manual movements provide a secondary source of information. A manual sign system is considered different from a manual sign language. The former creates an equivalent to oral language (fingerspelling), whereas the latter (ASL) is a distinctively different language with its own vocabulary, syntax, and lexical components (Wilcox 1988, 1990).

There are many similarities between manual and oral language. Both are a form of communication and can serve as a primary language. Both have structured information codes such as phonetic (or cheremic) elements, syntactic, and lexical (or semantic) elements. Both have group similarities and differences that reflect cultural and social patterns. Vocabulary, however, is quite different. In ASL, there are about 6000 signs vs. 600,000 dictionary words, although only about 3000 words are used orally in conversation with hearing people. There are other differences as well: Because the hands and body are much larger than the tongue and oral cavity, signs take twice as long to produce as speech; however, the expression of ideas is transmitted at the same speed. Signed language is sometimes influenced by oral language, but the reverse does not occur.

Fingerspelling (Rochester Method)

Fingerspelling is a supplemental manual system. The Rochester method, a modification of a single-handed letter-spelling approach, was developed at the Rochester (NY) School for the Deaf. It is based on a letter alphabet of finger signs (twenty-six positions in English) used with speechreading to aid students in elementary school. When it became apparent that preschool-age children using oralism could also benefit from fingerspelling, the Rochester method was adopted to facilitate the total communication approach (Evans 1982).

Words are spelled out on the fingers, often with ASL (which has borrowed signs from fingerspelling), and is used to convey technical information, new terms, and proper nouns. This manual system became an integral peg in the development of the Total Communication (TC) model. Although fingerspelling is about three times slower than other signed communication, it is precise and has minimal ambiguity. Fingerspelling has been found to improve the reading and writing skills of elementary and secondary deaf students (Quigley 1969) as well as their Stanford Achievement Test scores (Braverman-Callahan and Radzirwicz 1989). Most people who use ASL will occasionally supplement information using fingerspelling (Moores 1987, 1991).

Cued Speech

Because it was slow, the Rochester method was largely replaced by cued speech (Cornett 1967), a set of manual signs used to indicate speech movements. Furthermore, it is easier for hearing parents to learn because it is dependent on lip movements and follows the syllable flow. The hands are used to supplement lip movements that are not visible; cued speech is not carried out in isolation (Bench 1992). It has been found effective for teaching speech to deaf children (Quenin and Blood 1989).

American Sign Language (ASL)

American Sign Language is the language system most used by the deaf community in the United States. It is a system of gestures with its own unique vocabulary, grammar, and prosodic features. Variations of movements convey the equivalence of intensity, frequency, continuation, movement, and so on (King and Quigley 1985). Toddlers learn the hand, facial, and body gestures during their formative years with the same facility their hearing counterparts learn language using the auditory route (Stokoe 1960). Not until the 1970s did educators and psycholinguists take serious note of Stokoe's research (1960, 1975) that established ASL as a formidable and distinct language with the equivalence of the phonology, syntax, and semantic components that constitute standard English.

The impact of ASL manifested itself in two major ways: English was regarded as a second language for the deaf, and a representative deaf culture began to emerge. These ideas spread throughout the world where deaf signed language was the first language and the national language of the normal-hearing was the second language (Gerber and Prutting 1981; Kyle and Woll 1985). Part of the reemergent success of ASL as the preeminent communication mode is that it "depathologizes" deafness and is itself treated as a bona fide first language (Paul and Jackson 1993). The signed systems of various nations differ so significantly that a deaf person in England using the British Sign Language (BSL) does not communicate well with an American using ASL, despite the equivalence of the two spoken languages. Because ASL lacks a written form, written information is borrowed from English. Many deaf individuals are from multi-cultural-multilinguistic groups (e.g., ASL and English).

American Sign Language has ties to French Sign Language but not to British Sign Language. A sign is the equivalent of the spoken word in most sign systems. In ASL, one dominant hand is manipulated in space from the top of the head to the bottom of the hands. There are three components of ASL, called cheremes, that are roughly equivalent to syllables: (1) place on the body where the sign is made (tab); (2) shape of the hand making the sign (dez); and (3) the movement of the hands (sig). Altogether, there are 55 cheremes: 12 tab, 19 dez, and 24 sig; a change in any of these elements alters the meaning. Cheremes provide the distinctive features of ASL and foster a dynamic interplay with social and political forces, just as oral language responds to societal forces. In ASL, prosodic or suprasegmental characteristics are conveyed by breadth of movement to connote intensity; intonation is conveyed by hand movement sharpness, facial expressions, and general body language. Dialectal cheremes occur culturally (Stokoe 1975).

A conference on ASL at Gallaudet University (October 28–30, 1992) concluded that, for the deaf:

1. ASL should be the primary language, and English, the secondary;

2. ASL should be used for communication and instruction because it is easier to learn than oral English; it facilitates language acquisition, whereas English inhibits communication;

3. When oral and TC methods fail, ASL is the preferred alternative;

4. Deaf children with hearing parents have difficulty with ASL and may not want to learn English;

5. Speech-language pathologists and audiologists have to reconsider (a) use of amplification for children who use ASL and (b) whether speech is advised.

While the Gallaudet meeting was taking place, a policy statement was issued by the U.S. Department of Education (October 30, 1992) about deaf education with reference to section 504 of the Rehabilitation Act and IDEA. The statement said that schools must consider these issues:

1. Communication needs of the child and family and their preferred communication mode;

2. Linguistic needs and academic level of performance;

3. Social, emotional, and cultural needs and peer interactions;

4. Curriculum, content, and method of teaching;

5. Least restrictive environment plus supplemental aids must meet student needs; otherwise, it is not a least restrictive environment;

6. Some deaf children can be placed in regular classes with supplements to provide the least restrictive environment;

7. SEA and LEA must fully inform parents of rights, alternatives, procedures, and the school's obligations.

Signed English; Manual English (ME)

Many educators prefer to use these supplemental systems early because they are based on regular English grammar and enable the child to read and write with greater ease and clarity. In both systems, signs and fingerspelling are combined with ASL as an aid to language reception. Using different formats, these systems offer a variety of ways to assist communication by positioning the hand near the lips to sign words, vowels, consonants, intensity, and so on. There is little or no effect on spoken language.

Seeing Essential English 1 (SEE 1)

This manual language system uses formal rules to alter ASL so that it is more like English. There is a different sign for English words with the same English spelling but different meaning. The semantic boundaries of the signs are adjusted to meet English. At the syntactic level, SEE 1 has pronouns that follow English word order. This system is easier for hearing parents to learn because it follows the structure of oral English (Anthony 1971).

Signing Exact English 2 (SEE 2)

Developed by Gustason (1983), this system superseded SEE 1. The rules in this manual language system are very similar to SEE 1 but are simpler and less rigorous. Because it is closer to ASL than to English and uses signs to represent the whole word (not just a component), it is more easily used by younger deaf children and their parents (Bench 1992).

Total Communication (TC)

Developed by a graduate of Gallaudet University in the mid-seventies, TC adapts signed systems (usually not ASL) to employ the vocabulary and syntax of written standard English and concurrently use and watch spoken English. Controversy has raged over whether a combined (oral-manual) or "simultaneous" approach is more effective than a straight manual approach (Ling 1984; Schlesinger 1972). Total Communication was tried for several years but never achieved its goal of improving English language competence because it is difficult to use the spoken language route and the visual ASL route simultaneously (Moores 1987).

The two different language strategies (reading the hand and lip movements concurrently) were better suited for younger deaf children, who naturally default to the signed system, which is easier and learned faster. TC did not produce the academic benefits, improved self-concept, and improved speech projected in the original rationale for the combined system. Some claimed it diminished speech production (Nix 1983). Another problem with TC is the difficulty of identifying what TC really means. A specific definition of TC is construed differently by oralists and manualists. The differences have to do with the stress given the different approaches in the communication interplay (Eagney 1987).

LANGUAGE DEVELOPMENT AND HEARING IMPAIRMENT

LANGUAGE is a form of communication and, as speech, is a coded set of verbal symbols, manual gestures, facial expressions, body language, and other prosodic features. Communication is interpersonal where thoughts, ideas, meaning, and social intercourse are shared among people (Bench 1992). Normally, human communication consists of several forms, starting with the birth cry, progressing shortly afterward to infant coos, smiles, and reflexive and purposeful vocalizations. Within a short period, vocabulary zooms to hundreds, then thousands, of words and, by young adulthood, can reach 50,000 words.

An integral part of language development is found in the context of social interaction. This setting intertwines syntax and semantics in a relationship known as *pragmatics*. Pragmatics in deafness is not the same as for normal-hearing children. This skill base of perceptual and cognitive language enables the hearing child to learn to read and write and is a major educational and social deterrent for the deaf child who did not develop oral language.

SPEECH DEVELOPMENT AND PRODUCTION

SPEECH is the product of several integrated physiologic processes: articulation (the molding of sounds into phonetic units); phonation (the vocal tones); respiration (the basic air stream); and resonance (the modification of the acoustic parameters). Speech is cognitive verbal language, an intellectual event. In speech development, the normal-hearing infant associates the sounds of speech with surrounding activities, particularly the facial movements of the caregiver and the infant's own articulatory sounds. A child unable to hear the speech of the caregiver does not automatically associate facial movements with speech. As normal speech production is acquired by a normal-hearing toddler, the pattern is stabilized via the auditory feedback (or servo feedback mechanism). But clear and articulate speech is always dependent on auditory feedback monitoring; therefore, a loss of hearing is rapidly reflected in speech output even if the speech was once fully developed.

Speech deterioration occurs quickly (Waldstein 1990). In general, the speech production errors that characterize hard-of-hearing vs. deaf speakers are quantitative rather than qualitative: The errors may be similar, but deaf people have more of them. Furthermore, the greater the hearing loss, the greater the number of speech errors because motor speech production is inextricably related to sensory perception of the speech signal.

An improvement in speech audibility quickly results in improved speech (Levitt 1989). Hence, an individual with a conductive loss shows changes in speech output intensity by diminishing the vocal intensity output. On the other hand, persons with a sensorineural loss of hearing may speak with greater intensity to compensate for the auditory feedback reduction and an intrinsic need to balance the input feedback homeostasis level with the speech output level. The relationship between auditory threshold level and speech output level is frequency-dependent as well. Hearing loss in the high frequencies is quickly translated into deterioration of high frequency consonant production in adults with normal speech.

Age of onset of the hearing impairment is crucial: The dichotomy is prelingual vs. postlingual onset. The earlier a prelingual onset and the later a postlingual onset, the greater are the differences in speech and language development. During the first four years, speech is easily and rapidly acquired by normal or near-normal-hearing infants and toddlers who attend to the comprehension of speech, not the acoustic event (Ross, Brackett, and Maxon 1991). With mild hearing loss (down to fifteen decibel thresholds), speech may be delayed or slightly defective, but it is absent in a deaf child. As hearing diminishes, the defective speech elements increase until total deafness and complete lack of speech development are reached. Total or near total lack of speech development is characteristic of prelingual onset and a better ear threshold of eighty decibels or more.

Deaf speech is often unintelligible to the average listener. During infant development, reflexive babbling occurs, possibly from tactile exteroception and kinesthetic proprioception, but this jabbering disappears. Deaf speech is distinctive: It has flawed articulation, breathing, phonation, rhythm, intonation, and phrasing due to a lack of segmental perception. The difference in speech errors between a hard-of-hearing and a deaf child is more quantitative than qualitative.

Listener perception and speaker intelligibility are aided by the intrinsic redundancy in language. Deaf speech does not encode the complex array of neuromotor synergy that reflects normal emotion and is consequently less intelligible. Children with severe hearing loss have defective spoken language as well as defective speech output and therefore generate a speech product with fewer of the redundant features that are inherent in the basic structure and delivery of language. The loss of redundancy is evidenced in reduced language comprehension, speech recognition, and speech perception in the prelingually deaf child. Oralists attempt to minimize poor speech production in deaf children by using residual hearing and reinforcement from tactile, visual, and kinesthetic modalities; early intervention auditory training programs are initiated to enhance speech intelligibility.

Deaf children lack the full range of phonologic, phonemic, and suprasegmental distinctive elements (Boothroyd 1984; Geers and Moog 1987; Kretschmer and Kretschmer 1978; Nober 1967; Oller, Jensen, and Lafayette 1978). As a result, individual sounds and syllables are omitted and distorted; sound order is incorrect; intonation, stress, rate, and temporal patterns are faulty. Breathing incoordination is apparent as intensity distortion. Vowel and consonant phonemes may be neutralized where one sound replaces several other sounds. Even articulatory coordination and suprasegmental features of deaf children differ (Robb and Saxman 1985; Tye-Murray 1987). More than half a century ago, Hudgins and Numbers (1942) depicted "deaf speech" with five type-of-vowel errors and seven type-of-consonant errors. Among other problems, they were the first to note excessive breath; slow, labored, and arhythmical speech; a voice quality that is colorless, monotonous, and lacks sufficient volume; inappropriate manipulation of the articulators; defective resonance and nasality. Deaf individuals use more vowels than consonants in a ratio of 2:1; such instances involve substitutions, omissions, distortions, improper relative durations among phonemes, and confusion of voiced and voiceless cognates (Nober 1967).

Nober (1967) studied the articulation of deaf children. He ranked the errors following a developmental pattern in which the easiest to produce, most visible, and most intense sounds (learned first by normal-hearing infants) were the most intelligible and least distorted by deaf children. A review relative to placement, manner of articulation, and voicing exhibited that the more visible, more intense, and easiest consonants to produce were the least defective and most intelligible.

Nober also reviewed literature relating to the rank order of phonetic development and intelligibility for children with other congenital disabilities such as mental retardation (developmental disabilities), cerebral palsy, and cleft palate. Collectively, these children represent disabilities that encompass sensory, motor, cognitive, and structural areas, but the developmental profile of each followed the normal maturational sequence of normal sound development. Usually the first sounds developed are more visible and easier to produce accurately.

ACADEMIC PROFILE OF THE HEARING-IMPAIRED CHILD

LANGUAGE skills are preparatory to the education of the young child. All other things equal, the magnitude of the hearing impairment will have a significant impact on the development of language skills and, subsequently, educational achievement in reading, writing, mathematics, social areas, and general academic skills (Paul and Jackson 1993). Variations always occur, but, in the continuum of development, hearing loss is detrimental to academic achievement in a young child. Clearly, one functional and major difference between the deaf and the hard-of-hearing child, regardless of hearing thresholds, is the language learned by the hard-of-hearing child by the auditory route, perhaps with amplification and some visual assistance. The deaf child uses a different language base (i.e., ASL) that is not replicated in written form.

Reading

Literacy in hearing students is said to be a translation of oral language from a repository of information, often called inner language or inner speech. Research shows that, when children and adults read, there is concomitant subvocal muscular activity (as during speech) as the written information is decoded. This covert and silent phonological coding (Rayner and Pollatsek 1989) is extended into adulthood (Conrad 1979; Hanson, Goodell, and Perfetti 1991). Deaf children use a visual-imagery code rather than a phonological code (Hirsh-Pasek and Treiman 1982; Locke 1978). Reading is ordinarily the major vehicle for educating children and extending their knowledge of world of events. When the deaf child is taught to read in the second language, there are often problems with multiple meaning, idioms, metaphors, and syntax because the words have a different syntactic and semantic system (Webster and Ellwood 1985).

Research has not demonstrated a clear benefit of any one mode of communication used by severely deaf students learning to read, but reading proficiency is related to the nature of the texts. There is evidence that most good deaf readers use primarily a speech-based code rather than a visual-based code to mediate print (Cohen, Fishgrund, and Redding 1990). Despite the reading mechanism, most deaf students who complete high school attain the reading level of a nine- to eleven-year-old normal-hearing student (Furth 1966; Quigley and Kretchmer 1982), and this gap increases with age and experience.

It is noteworthy that prelingually deaf students with deaf parents who signed achieved better reading scores than deaf children with hearing parents (Kampfe and Turecheck 1987). We assume that this is due to earlier acquisition of language. Another factor that contributes to the poor reading levels of deaf children is their qualitatively poorer skills involving short- and long-term memory. Both are essential components for reading, and short-term memory needs to be recoded into long-term memory (Hanson 1990; Paul and Jackson 1993). Additional issues include the cerebral dominance of the deaf child and its relationship to language development, reading, and writing.

Writing

Writing is the graphic expression of verbal discourse and reading material; hence, it is derived from the same verbal syntax and semantic context. Because there is a strong correlation to reading comprehension ability, hearing-impaired students manifest significant writing problems. The difficulty is related to the degree of hearing impairment among other factors. Because of the wide range of intervening variables, Quigley and Paul (1984) contended that sentences must be taught at a "broader pragmatic context" level dealing with the structure of the text. Many reasons have been ascribed as causative to the writing limitations of hearing-impaired students. There is controversy about structural aberrations and whether the writing is at an arrested level of writing development (Bench 1992; Gormley and Sarachan-Deily 1987; McAfee, Kelly, and Samar 1990).

PSYCHOSOCIAL ATTRIBUTES OF HEARING IMPAIRMENT

THERE is one school of thought that claims severe hearing impairment does not qualitatively alter the cognitive processes of the severely hearing-impaired child (Furth 1966). Other researchers, however, believe that severe hearing impairment causes language imbalance and precludes normal cognitive development (Myklebust 1964), such as an inner language that a normal-hearing child develops to engage in abstract thought. The latter group contends that the use of alternative sensory input establishes a qualitatively different type of short- and long-term memory ability. Hence, severely hearing-impaired children cannot be educated in a fashion described as normal.

Substantively, the question is one of language delay or language difference. Studies indicate that memory skills based on auditory codes will be troublesome to deaf students who use visual input. Nevertheless, deaf students will perform as well as normal-hearing children when the memory items are based on visual coding (Paul and Jackson 1993). Information processing speed is also a factor for children with a severe hearing disability who use alternative forms of communication.

Researchers often refer to the "deaf personality" (Lane 1988; Levine 1960, 1981). Some depict social immaturity, dependence, low self-image, low self-esteem, aggression, paranoia, and reduced intelligence. Research using variables such as degree of hearing loss, age of onset, parent attitudes, language mode, educational setting, and so on demonstrate conflicting results. Research in this area began over three-quarters of a century ago with the pioneering work of Pintner and Patterson (1916), whose findings are still used as a viable reference. Myklebust (1964) confirmed some of the earlier findings of Pintner and Patterson and added that he found more psychopathology in deaf adults than in hearing adults. An updated, detailed theoretical and pragmatic review on the psychology of deaf individuals can be found in Paul and Jackson (1993).

Deaf Culture

HELEN Keller said "blindness cuts people off from things, deafness cuts people off from people." More recently, the deaf culture movement has become a powerful influence in connecting deaf people socially and in shaping educational reform. Deaf power advocates describe the Deaf as an ethnic group biologically equipped to do everything but hear. These proponents contend that deaf culture is a shared affirmation, not a denial of their condition. In the September 1993 issue of the *Atlantic Monthly*, Edward Dolnick writes that the "new" deaf culture claims to be distinctive, rewarding, and worth preserving. Deaf power activists insist that deafness is not deprivation; consequently, they do not perceive deafness as a disability such as blindness.

Deaf culture thrives on the pride of deaf people, and some deaf power advocates claim to prefer a deaf baby over a hearing baby for maintaining family identity and harmony. Some even claim "ownership" of a deaf child born to hearing parents for educational management because the deafness will make the deaf child a linguistic minority in the hearing family. Over 90% of children born deaf will have hearing parents and siblings. Dolnick further states that deaf power activists vehemently reject alteration by assistive devices such as hearing aids or—worse still—cochlear implants wired into the inner ear, indeed, "a retrofit to nature's choice . . . the ultimate invasion of the ear."

Furthermore, deaf power advocates contend that the mainstream movement isolates deaf children in the classroom because of their low incidence and because the deaf student may be alone or older than other students in the class. However, mainstreaming is recommended by this author for the hard-of-hearing or deaf child who is postlingually deaf (after three years of age) and who has developed spoken language proficiency before the loss of hearing.

Multicultural Issues and Deafness

BY the year 2000, about half of the population of inner cities (and about one third of the nation) will be multicultural (Christensen and Delgado 1993). There has been a serious educational and psycholinguistic movement for educational reform for students who require bilingual education. For these culturally diverse students, English represents their second language. From this linguistic perspective, minority and multicultural students who are severely hearing-impaired would be trilingual. They are indeed linguistically different from the mainstream. The issues involving their communication barriers are reflected in standardized test scores, below grade-level academic performance, and arrested reading and writing proficiency.

The drive to reduce the inequities prompted sensitivity to multicultural education concerns. Part of the movement toward equity was the development of child-centered, individualized curricula and programs to improve the self-esteem and social profiles of minority groups. Federal reform laws have facilitated enlightened multicultural and multiethnic teaching programs. Diversity plans fostered the growth of students' natural strengths and the acquisition of new education and social skills.

The deaf population is historically a "minority" group, although the federal term has been "low incidence." Low incidence serves to temper the perceived responsibility of society although deaf culture advocates historically have professed a more functional and utilitarian perspective. To deaf culturalists, deaf communication needs require two languages: the ASL manual language based on visual-spatial perception and the auditory-oral written language of English (Christensen and Delgado 1993). Some believe strongly that ASL is the native or natural visual-feedback language system of the deaf (Paul and Jackson 1993; Stokoe 1975).

Significantly depressed achievement of deaf children from ethnic, linguistic, and racial minority backgrounds relative to Anglo deaf peers was reported by Cohen, Fishgrund, and Redding (1990). They reported that deaf students from African-American and Hispanic groups were less likely to be placed in mainstreamed settings with their Anglo counterparts, were exposed to less curriculum content, and were more likely to be placed in lower grade levels (Holt and Allen 1989). This imposes serious implications for "educational assessment, placement, student expectations, curriculum development, staffing, and policy making." This critical situation gave rise to the first national conference on the needs of African-American and Hispanic children, sponsored by the Committee on Ethnic and Multicultural Concerns of the Conference of Educational Administrators Serving the Deaf (CEASD) at Gallaudet University in March of 1989. To improve the education of minority deaf children, the conference focused on four areas: (1) home-school relations; (2) staff development; (3) curriculum and instruction; (4) assessment and placement. Although minority children with normal hearing generally have more educational problems than their white peers for a variety of reasons, African-American and Hispanic children have had more severe problems.

In a study of 3,866 students in twenty-three schools and programs for severe-to-profound hearing-impaired students, Nober (1993) reported that only 3% of the teachers were themselves deaf. Cohen, Fishgrund, and Redding (1990) reported that 6.8% of the minority teachers treated 35.6% of the minority deaf students in the deaf school population. The situation is unlikely to improve in the future. Only 8.7% of the undergraduate students and 7.8% of the Master's level students who are in training programs in the field of speech-language-hearing disorders are minority, culturally diverse, or disabled themselves. In the larger inner-city areas, 70 to 90% of the children in the special needs programs represent racial, linguistic, and ethnic minority backgrounds. In schools for the deaf, minority and other multicultural students constitute 36% of the student population. Reform will require a national effort that includes the audiologist in a major role.

REFERENCES

Allen, T., and T. Osborn. 1984. Academic integration of hearing-impaired students: Demographic, handicapping, and achievement factors. *American Annals of the Deaf* 129: 100–113.

American Academy of Otolaryngology and American Council of Otolaryngology. 1979. *Guide to evaluation of hearing handicap.* 241:2055–2059.

American Speech-Language-Hearing Association and National Joint Committee on Learning Disabilities. 1993. *Reaction to "full inclusion": A reaffirmation of the rights of students with learning disabilities to a continuum of services* (November):63.

Anthony, D.A. 1971. *Seeing essential English.* Anaheim: Anaheim Union High School District.

Bench, J. 1992. *Communication skills in hearing-impaired children.* San Diego: Singular Publishing Group, Inc.

Berg, F. 1986. Classroom acoustics and signal transmission. In *Educational audiology for the hard of hearing child*, ed. F. Berg, J. Blair, S. Viehweg, and A. Wilson-Vlotman. Orlando: Grune and Stratton.

Bess, F., and F. McConnell. 1981. *Audiology, education, and the hearing impaired child.* St. Louis: C.V. Mosby.

Boothroyd, A. 1984. Auditory perception of speech contrasts by subjects with sensorineural hearing loss. *Journal of Speech and Hearing Research* 27:134–144.

Braverman-Callahan, J., and C.K. Radzirwicz. 1989. Hearing impaired children: Language acquisition and remediation. In *Language and communication disorders in children*, ed. D.K. Bernstein and E. Tiegerman. Columbus: Merrill Publishing Co.

Bricker, D. 1986. *Early education of at-risk and handicapped infants, toddlers, and preschool children.* Glenville, IL: Scott, Foresman.

Charrow, V.R. 1975. A psycholinguistic analysis of "deaf" English. *Sign Language Studies* 7:139–150.

Christensen, K., and G. Delgado. 1993. *Multicultural issues in deafness.* New York: Longman.

Cohen, O.P., J.E. Fishgrund, and R. Redding. 1990. Deaf children from ethnic, linguistic, and racial minorities backgrounds: An overview. *American Annals of the Deaf* 135: 67–73.

Conrad, R. 1979. *The deaf school child.* London: Harper and Row.

Cornett, O. 1967. Cued speech. *American Annals of the Deaf* 112:3–13.

Council for Exceptional Children. 1993. *The council for exceptional children's draft statement on inclusive schools.* Reprinted in *Masstream* (Spring).

Crandell, C. 1993. Speech recognition in noise by children with minimal degrees of sensori-neural hearing loss. *Ear and Hearing* 14:210–216.

Crandell, C., and F. Bess. 1986. Speech recognition of children in a "typical" classroom setting. *Asha* 28:82.

———. 1987. Sound field amplification in the classroom setting. *Asha* 29:87.

Dolnick, E. 1993. Deafness and culture. *Atlantic Monthly* September, 37–53.

Eagney, P. 1987. ASL? English? Which? Comparing comprehension. *American Annals of the Deaf* 132:272–275.

Evans, L. 1982. *Total communication*. Washington, D.C.: Gallaudet University Press.

Finitzo-Hieber, T. 1981. Classroom acoustics. In *Auditory disorders in school children*, ed. R.J. Roeser and M.P. Downs. New York: Thieme-Stratton.

Finitzo-Hieber, T., and T. Tillman. 1978. Room acoustics effects on monosyllabic word discrimination ability for normal and children with hearing impairments. *Journal of Speech and Hearing Research* 21:440–458.

Furth, H.G. 1966. A comparison of reading test norms of deaf and hearing children. *American Annals of the Deaf* 111:461–462.

Geers, A., and J. Moog. 1987. Predicting spoken language acquisition of profoundly hearing impaired children. *Journal of Speech and Hearing Disorders* 52:84–94.

Gerber, S.E., and C.A. Prutting. 1981. Bilingualism: An environment for the deaf infant. In *Early management of hearing loss*, ed. G.T. Mencher and S.E. Gerber. New York: Grune and Stratton.

Gormley, K., and A.B. Sarachan-Deily. 1987. Evaluating hearing-impaired students: A practical approach. *Volta Review* 89:157–169.

Gustason, G. 1983. *Teaching and learning signing exact English*. Los Alamitos, CA: Modern Signs Press.

Hanson, V.L. 1990. Recall of order information of deaf signers: Phonetic coding in temporal order recall. *Memory and Cognition* 18:604–610.

Hanson,V.L., E.W. Goodell, and C.A. Perfetti. 1991. Tongue-twister effects in the silent reading of hearing and deaf college students. *Journal of Memory and Language* 30:319–330.

Heward, W., and M. Orlansky. 1992. *Exceptional children: An introductory survey to special education*. 4th ed. Columbus: Merrill Publishing Co.

Hirsh-Pasek, K., and R. Treiman. 1982. Recoding in silent reading: Can the deaf child translate print into a more manageable form? *Volta Review* 84:71–82.

Holt, J.A., and T. Allen. 1989. The effects of schools and their curricula on the reading and mathematics achievement of hearing impaired students. *International Journal of Educational Research*. 13:547–562.

Hudgins, R., and F. Numbers. 1942. An investigation of intelligibility of speech of the deaf. *Genetic Psychology Monographs* 25:289–392.

Kampfe, C.M., and A.G. Turecheck. 1987. Reading achievement of prelingually deaf students and its relationship to parental method of communication: A review of the literature. *American Annals of the Deaf* 132:11–15.

King, C., and S. Quigley. 1985. *Reading and deafness*. San Diego: College-Hill Press.

Kretschmer, R., and L. Kretschmer. 1978. *Language development and intervention with the hearing impaired*. Baltimore: University Park Press.

Kyle, J., and B. Woll. 1985. *Sign language: The study of deaf people and their language*. Cambridge: Cambridge University Press.

Lane, H. 1988. Is there a "psychology of the deaf"? *Exceptional Children* 55:7–19.

Levine, E. 1960. *The psychology of deafness: Techniques of appraisal for rehabilitation*. New York: Columbia University Press.

———. 1981. *The ecology of early deafness: Guides to fashioning environments and psychological assessment*. New York: Columbia University Press.

Levitt, H. 1989. Speech and hearing in communication. In *The handbook of special education: Research and practice*. Vol. 3, ed. M. Wang, M. Reynolds, and H. Waldberg. Oxford: Pergamon Press.

Ling, D., ed. 1984. *Early intervention of hearing impaired children: Total communication options*. San Diego: College-Hill Press.

Lochner, J., and J. Burger. 1961. The intelligibility of speech under reverberant conditions. *Acustica* 11:195–200.

Locke, J.L. 1978. Phonemic effects in the silent reading of hearing and deaf students. *Cognition* 6:185–187.

Madell, J.R. 1992. FM systems for children birth to age five. In *FM auditory training systems: Characteristics, selections, and use*, ed. M.A. Ross. Timonium, MD: York Press.

McAfee, M.C., J.F. Kelly, and V.J. Samar. 1990. Spoken and written English errors of postsecondary students with severe hearing impairment. *Journal of Speech and Hearing Disorders* 55:528–634.

Meadow-Orlans, K. 1990. Research in developmental aspects of deafness. In *Educational and developmental aspects of deafness*, ed. D. Moores and K. Meadow-Orlans. Washington, D.C.: Gallaudet University Press.

Moores, D.F. 1987. *Educating the deaf: Psychology, principles, and practices*. 3d ed. Boston: Houghton Mifflin.

———. 1991. The great debate: Where, how and what to teach deaf children. *American Annals of the Deaf* 135:35–37.

Moores, D.F., B. Cerney, and M. Garcia. 1990. School placement and least restrictive environment. In *Educational and developmental aspects of deafness*, ed. D.F. Moores and K. Meadow-Orlans. Washington, D.C.: Gallaudet University Press.

Myklebust, H. 1964. *The psychology of deafness: Sensory deprivation, learning, and adjustment*. 2d ed. New York: Grune and Stratton.

Nabalek, A., and L. Robinette. 1978. Influences of the precedence effect on word identification by normally hearing and hearing impaired subjects. *Journal of the Acoustical Society of America* 63:187–194.

Niemoeller, A. 1981. Physical concepts of speech communication in classrooms for the deaf. In *Amplification in education*, ed. F. Bess, B. Freeman, and J. Sinclair. Washington, D.C.: A.G. Bell Association for the Deaf.

Nix, G.W. 1983. How total is total communication? *Journal of the British Association of Teachers of the Deaf* 7:177–181.

Nober, E.H. 1967. Articulation of the deaf. *Exceptional Children* 33:611–621.

———. 1993. *Section IV. P.L. 99-457 and its effects on educational management of hearing impaired children*. Presented to in-service, training, research, and assistive warning device programs for the hearing impaired in Australia and New Zealand. Durham, NH: University of New Hampshire, International Exchange of Experts and Information in Rehabilitation.

Nober, E.H., and L.W. Nober. 1962. Speech reception thresholds and discrimination scores as a function of method of presentation and frequency response. *Journal of Auditory Research* 2:1–4.

———. 1977. Effects of hearing loss on speech and language in the post-babbling stage. In *Hearing loss in children*, ed. B. Jaffe. Baltimore: University Park Press.

Oller, D.K., H. Jensen, and R. Lafayette. 1978. The relatedness of phonological processes of a hearing-impaired child. *Journal of Communication Disorders* 11:97–105.

Olsen, W. 1981. The effects of noise and reverberation on speech intelligibility. In *Amplification in education*, ed. F. Bess, B. Freeman, and J. Sinclair. Washington, D.C.: A.G. Bell Association for the Deaf.

Paul, P., and D. Jackson. 1993. *Toward a psychology of deafness*. Boston: Allyn and Bacon.

Paul, P., and S. Quigley. 1990. *Education and deafness*. New York: Longman.

Peterson, N. 1987. *Early intervention for handicapped and at-risk children*. Denver: Love Publishing.

Pintner, R., and D. Patterson. 1916. A measurement of the language ability of deaf children. *Psychological Review* 23:413–436.

Quenin, C.S., and I. Blood. 1989. A national survey of cued speech programs. *Volta Review* 91:283–289.

Quigley, S. 1969. *The influence of fingerspelling on the development of language, communication and educational achievement in deaf children*. Urbana: University of Illinois, Institute for Research on Exceptional Children.

Quigley S., and R. Kretschmer. 1982. *The education of deaf children: Issues, theory and practice*. Austin: Pro-Ed.

Quigley, S., and P. Paul. 1984. *Language and deafness*. San Diego: College-Hill Press.

Rayner, K., and A. Pollatsek. 1989. *The psychology of reading*. Englewood Cliffs, NJ: Prentice-Hall.

Reagan, T. 1990. Cultural considerations in the education of deaf children. In *Educational and developmental aspects of deafness*, ed. D. Moores and K. Meadow-Orlans. Washington, D.C.: Gallaudet University Press.

Robb, M., and J. Saxman. 1985. Developmental trends in vocal fundamental frequency of young children. *Journal of Speech and Hearing Research* 28:421–427.

Ross, M., D. Brackett, and A. Maxon. 1982. *Hard of hearing children in the regular schools*. Englewood Cliffs, NJ: Prentice-Hall.

———. 1991. *Assessment and management of mainstreamed hearing impaired children*. Austin: Pro-Ed.

Ross, M., and T. Giolas. 1971. Effects of three classroom listening conditions on speech intelligibility. *American Annals of the Deaf* 116:580–584.

———. 1978. *Auditory management of hearing-impaired children: Principles and prerequisites for intervention*. Baltimore: University Park Press.

Sanders, D. 1965. Noise conditions in normal school classrooms. *Exceptional Children* 31:344–353.

Schlesinger, H. 1972. A developmental model applied to problems of deafness. In *Sound and sign: Childhood deafness and mental health*, ed. H. Schlesinger and K. Meadow. Berkeley: University of California Press.

Stein, L., S. Clark, and N. Kraus. 1983. The hearing-impaired infant: Patterns of identification and habilitation. *Ear and Hearing* 4:232–236.

Stokoe, W. 1960. Sign language structure: An outline of the visual communication systems of the American deaf. *Studies in Linguistics*. Occasional Papers no. 8. Buffalo: University of Buffalo Department of Anthropology and Linguistics.

———. 1975. The use of sign language in teaching English. *American Annals of the Deaf* 120:417–421.

Tillman, T., R. Carhart, and W. Olsen. 1970. Hearing aid efficiency in a competing speech situation. *Journal of Speech and Hearing Research* 13:789–811.

Tye-Murray, N. 1987. Effects of vowel context on the articulatory closure postures of deaf speakers. *Journal of Speech and Hearing Research* 30:99–104.

U.S. Department of Education. 1992. *To assure the free appropriate education of all handicapped children.* Fourteenth annual report to Congress on the implementation of P.L. 94–142: The education for all handicapped children act. Washington, D.C.: U.S. Government Printing Office.

Waldstein, R. 1990. Effects of postlingual deafness on speech production: Implications for the role of auditory feedback. *Journal of the Acoustical Society of America* 88:2099–2114.

Webster, A., and J. Elwood. 1985. *The hearing impaired child in the ordinary school.* London: Croom Helm.

Wilcox, S. 1988. Introduction: Academic acceptance of American Sign Language. *Sign Language Studies* 59:101–108.

———. 1990. The structure of signed and spoken languages. *Sign Language Studies* 67:141–151.

13

Counseling Families of Hearing-Impaired Children: Suggestions for the Audiologist

George T. Mencher

INTRODUCTION

IF we could remain healthy, wealthy, and wise, many of us would like to live forever. Well, we can't. So the next best thing is to live as long as we can and, when our time has come, let our children keep us alive through their memories and their contributions. To many of us, our children are our immortality. We want them to do more than we did, have more than we had, and achieve more than we achieved. Our children are extensions of us; they truly give us a chance to continue and to relive our lives. Given that relationship, it is easy to see why parents have dreams and sometimes even fantasies about their children's achievements.

The birth of a disabled child usually shatters those dreams. It denies parents the opportunity to extend and relive their lives through their children. This is a serious blow to the ego and usually triggers a grieving process. Grieving is not abnormal, nor is it pathological. It is a normal process through which an individual may recognize a situation, seek support from others, cope with the difficulty, adjust to change, and then move on to other things. One of the most important roles the audiologist plays is in explaining the diagnosis of hearing impairment to parents and then supporting them as they adjust to the impact of that diagnosis through grieving.

Three critical elements should be kept in mind as parents begin to recognize that their concerns about their child are realized. First, some parents begin to see a hearing loss or handicap foremost, and then a child. Second, many are confronted with a sense of overwhelming self-doubt and fear about their ability to care for a disabled child. Finally, the bonding necessary for personal and

343

psychological growth may be interrupted. Bonding requires interaction between parent and child. The parents' reaction to the child and the child's inability to react to the parents because of its impairment may lead to serious difficulties and delays in language, cognition, and emotional development.

The diagnosis itself is rarely a single-step procedure. Most children undergo several appointments with a variety of practitioners before a loss is confirmed. Because most parents have a sense of the hearing deficit long before the final word is given, the grieving process usually begins before that fateful day. Consequently, at the time of final confirmation of a loss, clinicians may be the recipients of a flood of anguish or hostility that has been building and waiting for an opportunity for expression. The response parents receive to that outpouring will often determine the patient-clinician relationship in the future and may strongly influence the parents' response to their child. A responsive, empathetic, and knowledgeable clinician can establish a level of trust with the family that can serve the child for a lifetime. A key element in the clinician's response is a full understanding of the nature of the grieving process.

BREAKING THE NEWS

ONE of the most uncomfortable situations for any human being is to tell another bad news. It is reasonable, therefore, that clinicians may have difficulty informing parents that their child is hearing impaired. Tales are often repeated about the physician who bluntly notifies someone they will die and then moves hurriedly on to the next patient. This hit-and-run approach allows the clinician to report the diagnosis quickly and then escape before the patient has a chance to react. That way, the clinician does not have to deal with the patient's pain or anger. Of course, the patient is left confused, wondering what happened and what to do next.

Sometimes, to soften the blow, a caring clinician may exaggerate the potentially positive outcome of the situation. Statements such as "With the use of hearing aids, special schooling, and a little hard work, your child will grow up to be normal" can result in a parent having false expectations or unreasonable goals for the child.

Other clinicians may take a different tack. In an effort to be thorough and professional, the clinician explains every nuance of the audiogram and indeed of human hearing. The benefits of hearing aids are outlined, and the options available for educational programming are detailed to the Nth degree. In these situations, the parent rarely says anything, hears little, and understands even less, and the clinician manages to avoid listening to the parent by monopolizing the session.

To ensure that parents get off on a good footing, some clinicians present a set of organized tasks for them to pursue. Even before the diagnosis has been completed, the parent is given a list of instructions to follow and places to visit or call. Although, on the surface, this approach may appear to be helpful by providing specific assignments and a focus for a parent's activity, it does not provide an opportunity to express feelings or to focus thoughts and emotions. Often more important to the parent-child relationship and the child's well-being are these latter activities, for they are an essential part of grieving and the healing process.

An appropriate counseling session includes a complete explanation of what the audiogram means and, more importantly, what the child hears and does not hear. It is sometimes helpful to present a tone at the parent's hearing threshold level as a baseline and then the lowest intensity tone the child hears in contrast. Parents are often astounded at the difference, and it really brings home the extent of the pure tone loss to them.

The most frequent questions often focus on medical treatments available to cure the problem. A clear picture of medical options, if any, is vital. Information concerning psychological support groups for parents in the area is very important. If the parent asks for and is ready to receive additional information, an explanation of educational programs (auditory, oral, and so on) in the community is quite worthwhile. It helps to establish in the parent's mind that there is a variety of resources they can turn to for help.

Before the initial session ends, both the parents and the clinician should restate any agreements reached. Finally, phone numbers to call in case of emergency are exchanged, and the clinician offers reassurance about future meetings and ongoing support. Note that a hearing aid fitting has not even been mentioned. It takes an unusual parent to accept that step so early in the process, and the clinician should wish to avoid focusing the grieving process on the amplification device.

THE GRIEVING PROCESS

KUBLER-ROSS (1969) described grieving in her book, *On Death and Dying*. Moses and Van Hecke-Wulatin (1981) adapted her work and applied it to understanding the actions and reactions of families of disabled children. They suggested that grieving consists of a series of affective states, each of which is independent, but all of which can be felt at the same time. These states allow individuals to grow, to reconstruct their internal affective world, and to adjust to the new reality. The reactions are healthy and spontaneous and should not be judged or "treated." Briefly, the states are denial, guilt, depression, anger, and anxiety. This chapter examines each of these attitudes and then discusses how to cope with and move beyond them.

Denial

There are two reasons to deny something. First, because you believe it is not true; and second, because you may recognize intellectually that something is true but are simply not ready to accept it. Through denial, parents can hope against hope that things will change, while simultaneously providing themselves with the time and opportunity to build the inner strength necessary to accept reality. Parents do this by searching for and finding people and ideas that reinforce and strengthen belief in one's own abilities. Parents need time to search out these community resources. The audiologist is a major source of support and information but is also the entry to additional resources. Empathy, trust, and appropriate information in proper doses and according to parental need will go a long way toward helping a family move from denial to acceptance of their child and the hearing impairment.

There are several classic manifestations of denial. "Shopping for a new diagnosis" is a frequent one. This often occurs when parents refuse to accept the accuracy of the results at one institution and travel to another for a second opinion. This is not to suggest that seeking a second opinion is wrong or inappropriate. Many clinics recommend that families do so. However, shoppers sometimes seek a second, third, and even a fourth evaluation to confirm results. They find fault with equipment, competence, clinical manner, and so on if they do not like what they are told. But those are the extremes. For most families, a second opinion is sufficient. By that time, they have begun to accept the hearing loss and have read enough and met enough people with relevant information to begin to develop a sense of understanding.

A second frequently seen denial mechanism is inactivity or inconsistent activity. Parents may bring a child to appointments and agree to many things; however, they seem never to accomplish them. The child never seems to be wearing a hearing aid, or the batteries are always dead. Speech or sign lessons are missed or incomplete. Excuses are plentiful, but effort is sparse. The behavior is, in reality, a passive resistance. It is easy for the clinician to engage in a tug of war with the parents over this lack of activity. However, doing so misses the essence of the problem. There is no room for criticism in this situation. The good clinician recognizes the behavior for what it is—denial—and helps the parents by moving them toward acceptance through education, counseling, and modeling.

Guilt

It is frustrating and annoying for human beings to have a mystery and no solution. The lack of closure leaves one feeling incomplete. Thus it is to be expected that, when a child is diagnosed with a disorder, the parents want to know "Why?" Because it is normal for parents to feel protective of their child, it is reasonable for them to wonder if they are responsible for the child's predicament. If the parents have even the slightest doubt about their situation relating to the child, this may be expressed as guilt. Parents in this situation have been heard to say things such as "If I hadn't gone here" or "done that," "I could have avoided this." Carried to the extreme, parents have even reported, "This is my cross to bear for. . . ."

Sometimes parents channel their feelings of guilt into constructive efforts. For example, they may become active in church. However, religious activity based solely on the notion of penitence or receiving forgiveness for causing a child's disability is clearly an expression of grief and guilt that requires special care. Occasionally, effort is channeled into other constructive avenues such as parents' groups or school activities. However, sometimes the parents' participation is so dominant it interferes with the effectiveness of the group. These are parents who must be present to guide their child in every activity and who are so overprotective that the child lacks a life of his/her own. These are parents who take guilt to heart and seem to give up their lives to atone for it. Often these are angry, militant people.

Again, it is important to stress that these are not abnormal or pathological responses that require treatment. They are normal feelings triggered by the parents' need to know the etiology of the hearing loss and by their need for reassurance that they have not harmed their child. The clinician's role is to help define the etiology whenever possible by utilizing the available resources. Opinions are no substitute for facts. The clinician should seek help from the experts, including all the many appointments and investigations that may entail. For some parents, the act of arriving at a conclusion themselves, after exhausting all avenues of inquiry, serves as a major step in the healing process.

Sometimes a parent could have prevented a hearing loss. Typically, this involves failure to immunize or exposure to drugs, diseases, or disorders known to cause hearing loss. The clinician must be sensitive to the parents' remarks and attitudes and react accordingly. The wise clinician knows when to let the grieving process continue as a normal part of healing and when the client needs outside help. Referral for appropriate professionals for counseling is always a good idea.

Depression

For most people, depression is a disconcerting phenomenon to observe. We sense the futility and frustration, and we often regard the inactivity as pitiful. What we need to do, however, is look beyond the external signs and explore the roots of those symptoms. People who are depressed feel powerless to control their lives or the events around them. The parents of a disabled child are no different. They have prepared themselves to be the protectors of their newborn; they want to defend that child from evil. Suddenly, they discover they have failed. The child is not perfect; it is flawed. They—the guardians—did not prevent a problem nor can they cure it. Their internal definitions of their own potency and competence have been destroyed and must now be altered, unfortunately, in a negative direction. For some people, this is devastating.

A classic sign of depression is inactivity based on a sense of futility and powerlessness. Overtly, the behavior is similar to that seen in denial. After all, if one can deny something has occurred, one does not have to take action to fix it.

Parents will often find excuses not to complete tasks. They seem unable to get the earmold or to ensure that the child wears the hearing aid. What they are acting out is what they are feeling: "I cannot do this" or "I cannot cure that." The clinician can help the parent find fulfillment in carrying out some of the smaller, yet important, activities essential to the child and build up to more critical tasks. Satisfaction leads to a sense of achievement, accomplishment, and power. On the other hand, the clinician does not serve the child or the parent well by forcing activity upon a depressed parent or criticizing inaction. When the parent is ready and able to assume duties, it will happen. A supportive clinician suggests ideas and models activities, allowing the parent to adapt to the child's changing needs and to develop gradually a sense of ability and responsibility.

Anger

When parents feel the frustration of shattered dreams and hopes, when they feel powerless but still sense the need to do something, they might justifiably express anger. The question is, "At whom are they angry?" Themselves? The clinician? The child? Fate? The answer, of course, is all and yet none of these. The danger in anger lies in the responses it may evoke. The most critical situations occur when anger is pointedly directed toward the child, the spouse, or another family member and results in physical or mental abuse.

Despite these negative elements, however, the clinician should recognize that anger is an expression of internal confusion and is actually a coping mechanism. It allows an individual time to reevaluate the unwelcome situation; it also helps develop a sense of focus. Initially, anger may be displayed at everything and everyone, but it will gradually narrow. The fewer the targets for the anger, the more likely a specific constructive action will result. This, of course, reestablishes and redefines competence and leads to further productive action.

The clinician should neither react to anger nor provoke it. Allow expression and help to focus activity effectively. Be aware of the potential for abuse, and have appropriate resources available to help if mistreatment is apparent. Anger is not to be treated; it is to be understood and recognized for what it is. Parents who do not know a clinician well enough to be angry but who nevertheless appear to be so, are probably reacting to their own situation and not to the clinician. Empathy is the appropriate response.

Anxiety

We all have fears about the future. "Will I be healthy?" "Will I have enough money to buy a house?" "How can I ensure that my children are properly clothed and fed?" These are questions we all ask. The parent of a hearing-impaired child has these questions and a host of others. "How can I pay for those hearing aids?" "Will my child learn to talk and go to school?" "Do I have to learn to sign?" "Will I have to give up my own life and activities to take care of this child?" Is it any wonder that such a parent is anxious? Anxiety can lead to frustration and depression. However, as a normal part of a coping process, anxiety forces one to reassess responsibilities and capabilities and to set reasonable goals. Anxiety helps to focus attention on resources (both internal and external) and to move an individual toward rational decisions.

A fundamental role of the clinician is to be a channel to external resources for parents. This does not mean providing the family with a list of things to do and places to go at every session. It does mean having information available as it is requested and being prepared to assist parents in their struggle to clarify issues and learn which questions to ask of whom. Providing the answers to questions not yet asked can be counterproductive. Helping to focus ideas so that questions are asked spontaneously helps to build trust and allows parents to move through the grieving process in a comfortable and positive manner.

COPING

SEVERAL things should occur when parents have adjusted reasonably well to the notion of having a hearing-impaired child. In the newfound acceptance of their offspring, they should restructure the dreams they thought were dashed. Their new dreams should include the hearing-impaired child and should have no less value than the original dreams. They should see a child first, and only then the disability. By containing the effects of the disability, parents learn to recognize and appreciate what their child can do. They come to take pleasure in what is accomplished and not to brood over what might have been achieved "if. . . ."

Parents must also learn to devalue the outward signs of a disability, signs they previously thought were negative. Many parents try to conceal their child's hearing aid or will make excuses for the child's behavior. Recently a parent came to a clinic and refused to put a hearing aid on a child because "It makes her ugly." When appraising her daughter, that parent places great value on physical appearance and sees the hearing aid as destroying that image. She needs to restructure her value system. Until she does so, no clinician is going to convince her to ensure that her daughter wears an aid. Parents who have accepted and adjusted to their child's hearing loss, however, want the hearing aid to be visible so that others recognize that the child may experience difficulty in communication.

It can be quite difficult to comprehend how another person perceives things. Parents know the joy of music and the pleasure of a familiar voice. They often fall into the trap of assuming that because their child does not hear those same sounds, the child does not have as rich a life. It is very hard to grasp the notion that a hearing-impaired child of fifteen years who can read at the level of a ten-year-old can enjoy it more than a normal-hearing child of fifteen who can read like a twenty-year-old but never does. Parents (and clinicians) must realize that utilizing their own values to judge the child's is inappropriate. It is not a question of what you *can* do; it is a question of what you actually *do*! As they begin to understand that their child can derive as much joy from one set of activities as they derive from another, they move toward adjustment and acceptance.

DEVELOPING TRUST AND EMPATHY

TRUST is basic to all relationships; this is no less so in the parent-clinician relationship. Developing trust begins at the first meeting when the clinician is empathetic, understanding, nonjudgmental, and supportive. Sympathy is often equated with pity, but empathy equates with understanding. It is obvious which will be more effective in moving parents through the grieving process. Trustworthiness increases as the parent realizes the clinician promises only what can be delivered—and expects the parent to do the same. The clinician must always be aware of the limitations of time, ability, and motivation and must neither commit nor require more than is possible. Obviously, confidentiality must be maintained. This is true not only for the larger issues but also all those little exchanges, thoughts, and mutterings a grieving parent may utter. The parents must always believe the clinician values them and their child. Critical remarks may appear to lessen that esteem and thus weaken their trust in you or their concept of your trust in them.

This is particularly difficult for the clinician when the parents express unrealistic goals for themselves or their child. Frank responses, diplomatically presented, will go a lot farther than avoidance, small lies, or inappropriate encouragement. Sometimes the parent verbalizes unrealistic objectives and ideas for the sole purpose of eliciting a negative reply. This is not necessarily a test of the clinician's trustworthiness; rather, it may be an attempt by the parents to seek reasonable limits for their new dreams.

The successful clinician utilizes a few simple rules when counseling grieving parents. First, avoid asking the parent "yes" or "no" questions. Open-ended questions are more likely to evoke answers that accurately reflect the parents' thoughts. Second, learn to differentiate between what is said and what is meant. Feelings may or may not be expressed overtly, and real information may be masked by a flood of emotions. Be on the lookout, therefore, for nonverbal clues (e.g., facial expressions, gestures). Third, develop listening skills. Parents cannot express their feelings if they are listening to the clinician pontificate. Finally, avoid forming ideas about the parents before you know the whole story. It is sometimes difficult for young clinicians to accept their own feelings toward a family or child. It is not always possible to believe a parent's grief, attitude, or behavior. Sharing that information with other clinicians is essential to the therapeutic process. Occasionally, it is necessary to transfer a case to another clinician because of certain feelings. This is not failure, nor should it be construed in any negative sense. We all bond with some people and clash with others.

The most significant role the clinician plays is in helping parents to nurture a healthy outlook that includes a sense of control and an acknowledgement of the hearing loss. As the child grows and encounters certain critical stages in life, the parents may require assistance in adjusting to a new perspective. School, puberty, independence, and parental retirement are times of stress and doubt. Will the child succeed? Will the child marry? Will the child always be a financial burden? These are all momentous issues that provide opportunities for the clinician to continue in a strong supportive role.

Moreover, hearing-impaired children may also enter a period of grieving. This occurs most often when they realize that they have a hearing loss, that they are different. It may also occur at such pivotal periods as puberty and independence. At such times, the clinician must maintain a keen awareness of the need to remain available to both parents and child.

Of course, sometimes grief becomes so extreme that sophisticated therapeutic techniques are required. Knowing when and to whom to refer can be the most important step in the counseling process. Very few audiologists are properly trained to do in-depth counseling. Be aware. Get help. Be supportive and remember: Grieving is a part of the natural healing process and is not to be treated. It is to be considered an enriched environment for the growth and development of the family and the child.

REFERENCES

Kubler-Ross, E. 1969. *On death and dying*. New York: Macmillan.

Moses, K.L., and M. Van Hecke-Wulatin. 1981. The socioemotional impact of infant deafness. In *Early management of hearing loss*, ed. G.T Mencher and S.E. Gerber. New York: Grune and Stratton.

14

Pediatric Audiology Service Delivery Models: Systems in Flux

Evelyn Cherow

INTRODUCTION

CHANGE is inevitable. We are on a journey into the twenty-first century. In this context, U.S. policymakers and prognosticators wax polemic about the complex and interrelated issues shaping this country's future: workforce projections and personnel training needs; economic forces and the emerging global economy; healthcare reform, health promotion, and disease prevention. These are bywords symbolizing efforts to streamline healthcare costs while improving the citizenry's physical health and the nation's fiscal health.

The U.S. public education system prepares for major renovation under the rubric of the *Goals 2000* agenda. The term "equal rights" takes on a broader meaning as the multicultural demographic imperative challenges both educational and healthcare system structures and processes. The federal government is insisting that educational and healthcare agencies use innovative ways to measure the outcomes of services. Total quality management (better known as TQM) has leaped from the corporate world and infiltrated the management milieu of schools and hospitals. Third-party payers are paying for best and efficient practices that yield effective outcomes. Last, but certainly not least, savvy "baby boomers" are forging a consumerism movement and demanding greater accountability from service providers as data that reflect the quality and effectiveness of services delivered.

The magnitude and complexity of changes now affecting service delivery models to children at risk for or having hearing loss and the professionals providing these services is probably without precedent in this nation. Consideration of the issues encapsulated in these trends is necessary for the effective planning, conduct, and evaluation of audiology services to children from neonates through

352

adolescence. This chapter explores both trends of consequence to current and future pediatric audiology practice and specific issues of relevance to service providers.

The Broader View

An environmental scanning of issues and consequences affecting professional associations by a "futures think tank" revealed seventeen trends falling into six major categories (Coates and Jarrett 1993). Some of these tendencies have a specific, immediate, or delayed impact on delivery systems (Table 14.1).

A brief discussion of these trend patterns and their interrelatedness and relevance to pediatric service delivery provides a foundation for recommendations to modify and expand audiology service delivery models for children.

Shifting Cultural Patterns and Cultural Diversity

Immigration patterns in the United States over the last twenty-five years have dramatically altered the cultural composition of the U.S. population. Census reports estimated that, in 1990, 25% of the U.S. population consisted of people of color: 12% African-American, 9% Hispanic, 3% Asian-Pacific Americans, and 1% Native Americans and Eskimos. Projections of growth in these populations

Table 14.1.

U.S. Demographics
  The U.S. population is aging and more of our elders will be over 75 years of age;
  Immigration and the growth of minorities drive toward a multi-racial and multi-ethnic society;
  Baby boomers focus on the family through the 1990s and beyond.

Social and Value Changes
  Middle class values become dominant in the U.S.;
  Economics drive family changes and non-traditional families proliferate;
  The white collar and service sectors of the work force continue to lag in productivity, quality, service, and reliability.

Globalization of the American Economy
  Changes in world populations fuel the global economy;
  Regional trading blocs are forming throughout the world;
  New relationships in globalization give rise to certain U.S. policies;
  National standards are increasingly driven by global competition.

Information Technology
  Information networks are drastically modifying all professional relationships;
  Information technology alters the limitations of distance and time.

Science, Technology, and the Environment
  U.S. society is increasingly technology intensive and science dependent.

Government and Regulation
  Proliferation of single issues politics continues;
  Regulation continues as an inevitable growth enterprise;
  States and local government take on new responsibilities and roles.

indicate a 3% rate of population growth for Caucasians compared to 110% for Asian-Pacific Americans, 55% for Hispanics, 38% for Native Americans and Eskimos, and 15% for African-Americans. By the year 2010, people of color should compose one-third of the population of the United States (Battle 1993).

These population estimates have profound assessment and treatment implications for providing appropriate services to pediatric clients and their families or caregivers. Audiologists need to evaluate the instruments used to measure auditory and communication function to determine whether they are appropriately normed for the populations to be tested. New tools are required to accommodate language and cultural differences of these diverse populations. Standardized approaches in the use of foreign language interpreters for interviews and history collection, assessment, and auditory rehabilitation must be generated so that our measures are valid for all clients. Audiologists must develop a knowledge base of the values and beliefs of people from different cultures so that counseling and recommendation strategies are acceptable and effective.

A 1993 demographic profile of the audiology membership of the American Speech-Language-Hearing Association (ASHA) revealed that, of 10,209 certified audiologists, 94.5% were white, 2.08% Asian-Pacific Islander, 1.6% African-American, 1.52% Hispanic, and 0.3% Native American or Alaskan Native. Clearly, despite vigorous recruitment efforts among culturally diverse student populations, the representation of these groups in audiology is inadequate to meet current population trends, much less meet those trends projected for the future.

In 1988, ASHA adopted a definition of bilingual speech-language pathologists and audiologists to guide professionals in serving persons of color:

> Speech-language pathologists or audiologists who present themselves as bilingual for the purposes of providing clinical services must be able to speak (or sign) at least one other language with native or near-native proficiency in lexicon (vocabulary), semantics (meaning), phonology (pronunciation), morphology or syntax (grammar), and pragmatics (uses) during clinical management. . . . (ASHA 1989b, 93)

This definition urges professionals to consider the competence needed to serve populations whose native language is other than standard American English. An opportunity exists to develop unique services for these segments of this country's population and also to offer them to developing nations seeking consultation on audiology program implementation. Efforts by organizations such as the International Society of Audiology, the World Health Organization, Hearing International, and the Pan American Society of Audiology have been instituted to bridge the cultural gaps among nations and provide an essential exchange of science and services for populations at risk for or with hearing impairment.

The Economics of Reform

Economics is concerned with the production, distribution, and consumption of goods and services. Analyses of both educational and healthcare systems in this country over the past decade warn that the outcomes from services in these systems are costly, inefficient, and, in some venues, lag behind those in other industrial countries. For these reasons, the Clinton administration launched an aggressive campaign to overhaul the public educational and healthcare systems in the United States. New models to contain costs and simultaneously define effective and efficient "best practices" or standards of care are evolving. Nationally, statewide, and locally, audiology service providers must take part in efforts to innovate and define new models, or they may find themselves extinct. A discussion of the issues and problems associated with reform efforts will clarify the applications for pediatric service delivery.

HEALTHCARE REFORM

REFORM of the healthcare system takes on a special significance with regard to children. Not only does their good health or lack of it affect them as individuals and their families, but their health status has a multiplier effect on the future productivity and well-being of our democratic society. Changes in the way medical care is provided and financed under a reformed system must not result in a reduction in the quantity or quality of services available to children (Behrman 1993).

On the heels of a period of economic recession and with an estimated 37 million Americans in need of healthcare and without insurance and access to the system, the Clinton administration outlined its proposal for healthcare reform, the *Health Security Act of 1993*. Within this act, coverage for ear exams was discussed only briefly. As a result, ASHA (singly and as part of several coalitions concerned with persons with disabilities) urged that the act and other bills emanating from congressional representatives and senators be expanded to include hearing exams and hearing aids for children. Reassurance forthcoming from the U.S. Department of Health and Human Services (HHS) stipulated that:

> medically necessary or appropriate ear/hearing examinations will be covered under the Health Security Act although they are not explicitly identified in the legislative language. Coverage for ear and hearing examinations under the Health Security Act is provided under the diagnostic services provision. Diagnosis and testing for defects in hearing will be covered under this provision. In addition, routine ear/hearing exams for children are expected to be part of clinician visits at regular intervals.

These visits are fully covered with no cost sharing under the administration proposal. Other ear and hearing examinations determined to be medically necessary or appropriate will receive coverage as well (Ellwood 1993). The fact is that almost two-thirds of all uninsured children have working parents or care-givers without employer insurance coverage for the family or, for 18%, coverage for the children of workers (Marquis and Long 1992).

Children of families living below the poverty level have had access to audiology services and hearing aids through Medicaid law and the Early and Periodic Screening, Diagnosis, and Treatment Program (EPSDT). Revisions in Medicaid law (effective April 1990) through the *1989 Omnibus Budget Reconciliation Act* (OBRA) ensured this coverage through state plans. The Health Care Financing Administration (HCFA) intended, at a minimum, to include diagnosis and treatment (including hearing aids) for defects in hearing. An audiologist who is recognized as a Medicaid provider has been eligible to become a partial EPSDT screening provider.

The 1990 OBRA phase-in would reduce the number of uninsured children by almost one-third through the year 2002 (Marquis and Long 1992). However, with reform of the healthcare system, it is still unclear what will occur with programs funded through Medicaid. Some congressional staff members contend that the basic benefit package cannot afford to provide the scope of services allotted under current EPSDT definitions. For example, the Clinton proposal originally did not provide coverage for outpatient rehabilitation except when related to injury or illness. This stipulation excluded persons with developmental disabilities, and hearing loss is included in federal definitions of the term "developmental disability." Some contend that, whereas the Medicaid provisions are comprehensive, in reality, service access is constrained by low reimbursement rates, complex administrative practices, and a reduced workforce of providers in areas most in need of services (Hill 1992).

One report on the effects of healthcare reform on children's services delineates the major differences between the healthcare needs of children and adults. Most pediatric healthcare emphasizes wellness and preventive care or care for self-limiting acute illnesses and trauma (Behrman 1993). Behrman proposes that the ideal health benefit package for children would encompass the traditional acute medical services and preventive and chronic care services.

Besides the problem of what services will be covered is the debate over which mechanisms are appropriate as delivery models. The contrast between indemnity or fee-for-service models that allow for independent choice of family-preferred providers may be obsolete if the managed care model of primary care-gatekeeper route (to reduce utilization of specialists) dominates reform (see chapter 2). Many employers attempting to reduce healthcare costs are already offering health maintenance organization (HMO) or preferred provider organization (PPO) options for their employees.

Audiologists must consider the forces at work in the healthcare reform movement and provide input to evolving state plans that may interface with federal legal mandates. Pediatric audiology programs need to align with new referral sources to accommodate the changing service delivery patterns. This means providing both wellness model programs for children as well as traditional identification, diagnostic, and treatment services. Contracts with HMOs and PPOs or the formation of a PPO of audiologists should be pursued.

Another critical area of concern (not unique to pediatric audiology service delivery) is the ability of providers to present payers and program administrators with cost effectiveness and cost-benefit data related to outcomes of services. Neither physicians nor other nonphysician providers have created the optimal tools for measuring treatment efficacy. Federal agencies, payers, accrediting agencies, and consumers, however, have demanded that the healthcare delivery process incorporate data collection mechanisms. Early attempts at national collection of clinical outcomes data through the efforts of ASHA bore no fruit as clinical program administrators were unprepared to expend resources on automation (hardware and software) and personnel to input, compile, and analyze such data. As a result, federally funded projects have resulted in development of a functional assessment tool for this purpose.

Audiologists and speech-language pathologists have found that these tools (e.g., the Functional Independence Measure [FIM]) have only limited use for measuring outcomes of treatment of persons with communication and hearing disorders. ASHA is again delineating a plan for gathering the treatment efficacy data necessary to convince federal agencies of the value of providing audiology and speech-language pathology services to persons requiring them.

Audiologists must consider incorporating efficacy measures into the normal course of a business day for the benefit of clients who need access to and coverage for these audiology services. Demand for audiology services is inextricably linked to the perceived value by consumers and payers for such services. Federal and state legislators want to hear both from consumers about the impact of audiology services on their ability to function and from the profession about national efficacy outcomes.

Another cost containment strategy under consideration by the federal government and healthcare institutions is the training and utilization of multiskilled practitioners who can provide services across disciplines and in a support personnel framework. This model has been offered by the American Hospital Association (AHA) and the well-funded Pew Health Professions Commission. The Pew commissioners have developed policy papers on restructuring the nation's healthcare workforce and disseminated these to policy makers with recommendations for accomplishing change. The National Fund for Medical Education (NFME)[1] is initiating a grant program to:

> encourage health professions schools to educate more primary care providers with skills the new healthcare system will require. Through small grants, Primary Care 2000 will help schools in changing curricula, program design, student admissions, and other activities that will influence the nature of education and character of medical, nursing, and other health professional graduates (Pew Health Professions Commission 1994, 1)

---

[1]NFME administers the Pew Commission's grantmaking program.

The Pew Commission is working with the U.S. Bureau of Health Professions to reform allied health education. Several conferences have been held and are planned to outline the workforce needs and provide input to allied health educators on training to prepare practitioners to address system changes. Audiologists must define the efficient and appropriate use of support personnel in providing pediatric audiology services. They must also be clear about professional guidelines for practice with pediatric clients so that critical risk management strategies are ensured and professional liability considerations addressed (ASHA 1994).

EDUCATION REFORM

IN 1990, in response to a study of the nation's schools (*A Nation at Risk* 1983), President Bush and the U.S. governors adopted the America 2000 education strategy, a plan to reform the nation's schools. Six major goals constituted the backbone of the reform plan:

1. All children in America will start school ready to learn;
2. The high school graduation rate will increase to at least 90%;
3. American students will leave grades 4, 8, and 12 having demonstrated competence in challenging subject matter . . . ;
4. U.S. students will be first in the world in science and mathematics achievement;
5. Every adult American will be literate and will possess the knowledge and skills necessary to compete in a global economy and exercise the rights and responsibilities of citizenship;
6. Every school in America will be free of drugs and violence and will offer a disciplined environment conducive to learning.

Report cards, or a public reporting system, were devised to determine how well these goals are met on the local, district, state, and national levels (comparable to attempts to measure healthcare outcomes in the healthcare system). ASHA provided input to the National Education Goals Panel, which was charged with monitoring progress toward meeting the goals. ASHA emphasized the need to consider the receptive and expressive components of language learning and the variables that affect a child's readiness to enter school or achieve competence in subjects. The latter variables include history of chronic middle ear disease, hearing sensitivity, auditory disorders, and multicultural factors.

President Clinton expanded the Bush plan with the enactment of *Goals 2000: Educate America Act of 1993*, seeking to firm up public and private partnerships to effect school reform and to measure the outcome of education efforts in the work world and international competitiveness.

Professionals who have been involved with special education have voiced concerns to policymakers that special education initiatives be considered in this broad context of regular education reform on the federal and state levels. As the *Individuals with Disabilities Education Act* (IDEA) was debated before the responsible committees of the U.S. Congress during reauthorization hearings in 1994, advocates and consumers advocated for reform of special education (The Regional Resource and Federal Center Program 1993).

Considerable debate is underway concerning the interpretation of inclusion (integration of children with disabilities in regular classrooms in neighborhood schools). Certain parties insist that the full continuum of educational placement options be maintained so that families can choose a school setting based on family preferences and individualized assessment. A Policy Guidance issued by the U.S. Department of Education (October 1992) clarified the department's interpretation of free and appropriate public education (FAPE), least restrictive environment (LRE), and the requirements for Individualized Education Program (IEP) development for deaf children. This clarification was issued to ensure appropriate placement decisions for children with hearing loss. The policy guidance was reissued in 1994 to reinforce the Department of Education's commitment to these principles. However, advocates for inclusion are seeking revision of IDEA to mandate neighborhood school placement for all children with disabilities.

Audiologists will be involved with placement decisions, IEP development, and audiology service delivery systems evolving as a result of general reform and IDEA reauthorization. As such, audiologists again will need to demonstrate that student outcomes are enhanced as a result of audiology service delivery and recommendations. The importance of language and communication skill development as fundamental to academic achievement and psychosocial development for children must be emphasized. Measurement and reporting of outcomes of audiology services is critical to ensuring that such services are available to children in need. Audiologists may choose to adapt models for service delivery to be congruent with the collaborative-consultative and curriculum integration models that are emerging.

Access to technology is another critical issue in educating children with hearing loss to meet the goals of school reform. As defined in IDEA, assistive technology devices and services must be provided if required as part of special education, related services, or supplementary aids and services. In response to an inquiry about whether a district is required to buy a hearing aid for a student when the device is on the student's IEP, the Office of Special Education Programs (OSEP) responded that the Department of Education intended that assistive technology devices and services be limited to those situations in which they are required for a child to receive FAPE. OSEP concluded that, when a student's IEP reflects the need for a hearing aid to receive FAPE, the school district is responsible for providing the hearing aid at no cost to the child (letter to Seiler, 20IDELR 1216 [OSEP 1993] *Individuals with Disabilities Education Law Report 1994*). This interpretation has interesting ramifications for delivery of hearing aids to children of school age and reimbursement for the devices.

Policymakers responsible for lawmaking for special education are studying the implications of related services (e.g., audiology, speech-language pathology, occupational and physical therapy) and coverage for these services in the context of definitions for educational versus healthcare or medical services. In either context, audiologists must assume more responsibility for demonstrating enhanced student outcomes related to audiology services.

TRADITIONAL MODELS OF PEDIATRIC AUDIOLOGY SERVICE DELIVERY

AUDIOLOGY services for children evolved in community health departments; community, teaching, and pediatric hospitals; community hearing and speech centers; otolaryngologists' offices; schools; and private practice audiology offices. The 1993 ASHA Membership Update survey data reveal that of the 10,209 certified audiologists who are ASHA members, 10% are employed in schools as their primary employment setting (special, preschool, elementary, or secondary schools). Approximately 73% of ASHA-certified audiologists are employed in healthcare facilities: nonresidential healthcare facilities (48%); hospitals (22%); private physicians' offices (21%); private audiologists' or speech-language pathologists' offices (12%); speech and hearing centers (8%); residential health settings (3%); and home care (1%).

The ASHA membership employment-setting data are not clear as to the number of audiologists who, while employed in healthcare settings, have contracts to provide services to schools. Another critical consideration in pediatric audiology service delivery continues to be access to services, particularly for underserved populations: those who have no insurance coverage. They are estimated at 37 million Americans, including those who live in rural or remote areas of the country (ASHA 1988).

Emphases in pediatric service delivery have traditionally encompassed identification of children at risk or with temporary or permanent hearing loss and provision of intervention (auditory [re]habilitation). Results of studies indicating that both language and cognitive skill development occur during critical periods in the first three to six years of life influenced efforts to produce better hearing assessment tools and systematic mechanisms for finding children at risk for permanent hearing loss. Audiologists have launched hearing conservation programs to teach children and their families to protect their hearing from exposure to loud sounds (e.g., noisy toys, loud music from personal stereos or concerts, appliances, and recreational sources). Primary prevention activities related to noise-induced hearing loss continue to receive media attention as the world becomes a noisier place (ASHA 1991a).

EARLY IDENTIFICATION OF NEONATES AND INFANTS

Joint Committee on Infant Hearing

IN 1969, a group of audiologists, otolaryngologists, pediatricians, and later, nurses formed the Joint Committee on Infant Hearing (JCIH) to urge research on effective methods for screening the hearing of babies (Northern and Downs 1991). Later, the committee recommended the use of a risk register as an effective tool for finding those newborns most at risk for permanent hearing loss in combination with regular hearing testing for those babies who fell within the five risk categories.

This national policy on the need for early identification and intervention for infants with hearing loss based on expanded risk categories served as a standard of care through 1990 (JCIH 1990). Initially, this approach seemed to accommodate cost benefit considerations as well as test sensitivity and specificity concerns. However, subsequent research led the JCIH to modify its stance (JCIH 1994). The JCIH developed a 1994 position statement that calls for the universal detection of all infants with hearing impairment. This change in strategy to target all newborns for screening and follow babies who have risk indicators as well resulted from research indicating that assessment of the risk registry babies missed 50% of those who have or develop hearing loss during critical language learning years (Elssman, Matkin, and Sabo 1987; Mauk et al. 1991; Pappas 1983). The availability of new and more cost effective technologies for screening (automatic auditory brainstem response [ABR] and otoacoustic emissions [OAE]) has paved the way for the advent of universal newborn hearing screening programs to detect infants with conductive, sensorineural, or mixed loss, unilateral or bilateral in nature, and of mild to profound degrees.

The JCIH, in its 1994 position statement, endorsed the goal of universal detection of infants with hearing impairment as early as possible. The committee stated that all infants with hearing impairment should be identified before three months of age and receive intervention by six months of age. JCIH urges a continued use of risk indicators when universal hearing screening is not available or for those infants who require periodic monitoring of hearing. This position statement was reviewed by the policymaking bodies of the component organizations: the American Speech-Language-Hearing Association, the American Academy of Otolaryngology—Head and Neck Surgery, the American Academy of Audiology, the American Academy of Pediatrics, the Council on Education of the Deaf, and the Directors of Speech and Hearing Programs in State Health and Welfare Agencies.

NIH Consensus Development Conference

On March 1–3, 1993, the National Institutes of Health convened a consensus development conference on the topic "Early Identification of Hearing Impairment in Infants and Young Children." These consensus statements are prepared by a nonfederal and nonadvocate panel of experts resulting from presentations of investigators, statements by conference attendees, and panel deliberations. The panel was to address the following issues:

1. Advantages of early identification of hearing impairment and consequences of late identification;

2. Guidelines for deciding which children to screen for hearing impairment and when;

3. Advantages and disadvantages of current screening methods;

4. Guidelines for deciding which model to utilize for hearing screening and follow-up; and

5. Future directions for research in diagnosis and management of hearing impairment in infants and young children.

The panel concluded that:

1. All infants admitted to the neonatal intensive care unit should be screened for hearing loss prior to discharge;

2. Universal screening should be implemented for all infants within the first three months of life;

3. The preferred model for screening should begin with an evoked oto-acoustic emissions (EOAE) test (see chapter 8), followed by an auditory brain-stem response test (see chapter 7) for all infants who fail the EOAE test;

4. Comprehensive intervention and management programs must be an integral part of a universal screening program;

5. Universal neonatal screening should not be a replacement for surveillance throughout infancy and early childhood; and

6. Education of primary caregivers and primary healthcare providers on the early signs of hearing impairment is essential (National Institutes of Health 1993).

The general effect of the NIH consensus statement has been to reinforce the public health agenda for finding babies with hearing loss at as early an age as possible to offset the potential long-term consequences of hearing loss (e.g., delayed language, cognitive and psychosocial development, and academic achievement). In addition, the NIH—through the National Institute on Deafness and Other Communication Disorders (NIDCD)—has funded a critical five-year multisite study to evaluate different assessment protocols and the outcomes of early identification programs. As part of the study, an attempt was made to track the incidence of progressive hearing loss during the first year of life (White and Behrens 1993).

Healthy People 2000

The mission of the United States Public Health Service (PHS) is to focus existing knowledge and resources on the prevention of major chronic illnesses, injuries, and infectious diseases as well as premature mortality and morbidity. To this end, *Healthy People 2000: National Health Promotion and Disease Prevention*, a PHS document, was developed with a set of measurable public health targets to encourage new and increased health promotion and disease prevention activities.The three overriding goals of the enterprise are to (1) increase the span of healthy life for all Americans; (2) reduce health disparities among Americans; and (3) achieve access to preventive services for all Americans (U.S. Department of Health and Human Services, Public Health Service 1991).

The *Healthy People 2000* report contains two targets specific to hearing loss in the section on chronic disabling conditions:

1. Increase to at least 80% the proportion of pediatric primary care providers who routinely refer or screen infants and children for impairments of vision, hearing, speech and language, and assess other developmental milestones as part of well-child care; and

2. Reduce to no more than twelve months the average age at which children with significant hearing impairment are identified.

This public health program is designed to reduce healthcare costs in the United States through widespread prevention efforts. Audiologists can use this document, the NIH consensus report, and the JCIH position statements to prove the need to establish early identification programs.

EARLY IDENTIFICATION PROGRAMS IN STATES

IN July 1992, ASHA chose to survey state health and welfare agencies to assess the status of early identification programs for infants in this country because professionals, consumers, and policymakers had expressed a need for these data (Welsh and Slater 1993). Three types of infant hearing impairment identification programs (IHIIP) were identified: statewide legislatively mandated programs (N=18); statewide programs with no legislative mandate (N=5); and states with individual birthing sites that operate IHIIPs (N=22).

Survey results revealed variety in the approaches used in infant hearing screening, at risk criteria and follow-up mechanisms used, and approaches to collection of data. Welsh and Slater (1993) found that:

1. Various terms had different meanings, depending on the state's specific program;

2. No substantial difference was found between funding sources for legislatively-mandated programs and programs without a legislative mandate;

3. Most states do not operate centrally managed programs;

4. Many states do not have data collection mechanisms; and

5. The purpose of screening programs needed reexamination as follow-up care was not necessarily part of the legal mandate.

PREFERRED PRACTICE PATTERNS, GUIDELINES, AND POLICIES

ASHA has published several practice guidelines and reports that discuss audiological procedures for screening and evaluation of infants and toddlers from birth through age 36 months (ASHA 1989a, 1991a). In addition, preferred practice patterns that outline the critical components of pediatric assessment are available (ASHA 1993). The fitting of FM amplification for infants and pre-school children is addressed in a position statement (ASHA 1991b) that provides a rationale for audiologists to consider both hearing aids and FM systems as necessary technical devices for children with hearing loss.

National Priorities

As the Congress works to carve out a healthcare package that will provide access for all U.S. citizens, ASHA has actively worked with administration and congressional staff to include coverage of audiology services, hearing evaluations, and hearing aids for children. Draft legislation amending the Health Security Act to include audiology services under outpatient rehabilitation and hearing aids for children was reviewed by the U.S. Senate Labor and Human Resources Committee. A similar amendment had been introduced to a bill marked up by the House Education and Labor Subcommittee. It is uncertain how these amendments will fare in the evolution of this controversial piece of legislation.

THE PRESCHOOL THROUGH SECONDARY YEARS

AS Nober discusses in chapter 12, the *Individuals with Disabilities Education Act* (IDEA) Part H Amendments, is the critical legislative initiative affecting service delivery to preschool-aged children with hearing loss. Despite federal legislation, implementation at the state level is dependent on funding and resources available. In addition, because hearing loss is a low incidence disability, program administrators in schools may not be as familiar with the needs of this population as with other disabilities.

For these reasons, the Deaf Education Initiatives Project, funded by the U.S. Department of Education Office of Special Education and Rehabilitative Services (OSERS), and a collaborative effort by the National Association of State Directors of Special Education (NASDSE) and Northern Illinois University, has two major foci. These are: (1) the development of guidelines for educational services to deaf and hard-of-hearing students from identification through secondary level; and (2) training workshops for key personnel with responsibility for planning and implementing educational and related programs for students who are deaf or hard of hearing. The guidelines describe the need for qualified personnel, including audiologists, to provide appropriate services to children in school programs.

A report by the Joint Committee of ASHA and the Council on Education of the Deaf (JCASHA/CED) was developed to outline the roles, knowledge, and experience required by professionals providing services under IDEA-Part H to children who are deaf or hard of hearing, ages birth through 36 months. The report delineates critical professional roles including participation as a multidisciplinary team member; working with families; assessment and diagnosis of hearing loss; assessment of communication competence; assessment of cognitive, motor, and social skills; otologic evaluation; developing and implementing the Individual Family Service Plan; provision of sensory devices; management of sensory devices; maximizing auditory potential; facilitating communication development and cognitive development.

Other program milieus that are appropriate targets for the provision of audiological services include daycare programs and Headstart. The Clinton Administration has designated the Headstart program for increased program development and funding.

The Department of Health and Human Services Agency for Health Care Policy and Research (Stool et al. 1994) has sponsored an expert panel to develop clinical practice guidelines on otitis media with effusion to help healthcare practitioners and consumers in providing a standard of care to this population. The target group is children between 13 and 36 months of age. Audiologists have a significant role to play in assessing the hearing loss associated with chronic or acute middle ear disease and determining the effects on communication.

The ASHA Guidelines for Identification Audiometry (ASHA 1985) presented a philosophy and procedures for identifying children with hearing loss with potential for interfering with communication. The focus group was children age three years through grade three. The authors proposed that the guidelines were appropriate for use with older children as well. Depending on program goals and whether these include the identification of medical conditions requiring medical referral, identification protocols would be altered. No specific guidelines are available that specify the criteria for periodic monitoring of children above grade three. These guidelines and those for screening for middle ear disorders were determined to need updating to reflect current research.

With more exposure to noise in the environment (e.g., music, toys, recreation), children of all ages are at greater risk for noise-induced hearing loss. With the focus on healthcare reform, health promotion, and disease prevention, audiologists can play a key role in the education of children, primary care providers, and educators about the need for hearing conservation programs and auditory monitoring throughout the school years through postsecondary education.

Summary

THIS chapter outlines several general and specific policy-making trends that are influential in determining pediatric audiology service models. Audiologists can make a major contribution to shaping these trends by demonstrating effective and efficient outcomes of audiology services for children at risk for permanent or temporary hearing loss. Automation will be a necessary component of service delivery systems so that professionals can not only capture the types of treatment offered, the populations served, and the effects of different treatment paradigms for children in need of audiology services, but also report meaningful data to consumers and policymakers.

REFERENCES

American Speech-Language-Hearing Association. 1985. Guidelines for identification audiometry. *Asha* 27:49–52.
———. 1988. Utilization and employment of speech-language pathology supportive personnel with underserved populations. *Asha* 30:55–56.
———. 1989a. Audiologic screening of newborn infants who are at risk for hearing impairment. *Asha* 31:89–92.
———. 1989b. Definition: Bilingual speech-language pathologists and audiologists. *Asha* 31:93.
———. 1991a. Guidelines for the audiologic assessment of children from birth through 36 months of age. *Asha* (Suppl. 5) 33:37–43.
———. 1991b. The use of FM amplification instruments for infants and preschool children with hearing impairment. *Asha* (Suppl. 5) 33:1–2.
———. 1993. Preferred practice patterns for the professions of speech-language pathology and audiology. *Asha* (Suppl. 11) 35:1–102.
———. 1994. Professional liability and risk management for the audiology and speech-language pathology professions. *Asha* (Suppl. 12) 36:25–38.
Battle, D.E. 1993. *Communication disorders in multicultural populations*. Boston: Andover Medical Publishers.
Behrman, R.E. 1993. Statement of purpose. In *The future of children*, ed. R.E. Behrman. Los Angeles: David and Lucile Packard Foundation and the Center for the Future of Children.
Coates, J.F., and J. Jarrett. 1993. *Scanning the environment for association implications: Seventeen key trends*. Washington, D.C.: Coates and Jarrett, Inc.
Ellwood, D. Letter to author, 30 November 1993.
Elssman, S., N. Matkin, and M. Sabo. 1987. Early identification of congenital sensorineural hearing impairment. *The Hearing Journal* 13:7–12.
Hill, I.T. 1992. The role of Medicaid and other government programs in providing medical care for children and pregnant women. *The Future of Children* 2:134–153.
Joint Committee of the American Speech-Language-Hearing Association and the Council on Education of the Deaf. n.d. Technical report regarding service provision under the Individuals with Disabilities Education Act (Part H), as amended by IDEA-Part H to children who are deaf and hard of hearing, ages birth to 36 months.
Joint Committee on Infant Hearing. 1991. 1990 position statement. *Asha* (Supplement 5) 33:3–6.
———. 1994 position statement. *Audiology Today* 6:6–9.
Letter to P.J. Seiler, 20 IDELR 1216 OSEP 1993. 1994. Individuals with Disabilities Education Law Report. p. 1216–1217.
Marquis, S.M., and S.H. Long. 1992. Uninsured children and national health care reform. *Journal of the American Medical Association* 268:3473–3477.
Mauk, G.W., K.R. White, L.B. Mortenson, and T.R. Behrens. 1991. The effectiveness of screening programs based on high risk characteristics in early identification of hearing impairment. *Ear and Hearing* 8:217–221.

National Institutes of Health. 1993. Early identification of hearing impairment in infants and young children. *NIH Consensus Statement* 11:1–24. Washington, D.C.: National Institutes of Health.

NFME launches primary care 2000 initiative under new leadership. 1994. *Making progress: Practitioners for 2005.* Pew Health Professions Commission (spring):1.

Northern, J.L., and M.P. Downs. 1991. *Hearing in children.* 4th ed. Baltimore: Williams and Wilkins.

Pappas, D.G. 1983. A study of the high-risk registry for sensorineural hearing impairment. *Journal of Otolaryngology—Head and Neck Surgery* 91:41–4.

Regional Resource and Federal Centers Program. 1993. *Education reforms and special education: The era of change for the future.* Plantation, FL: South Atlantic Regional Resource Center, Florida Atlantic University.

Stool, S.E., A.O. Berg, S. Berman, C.J. Carney, J.R. Cooley, L. Culpepper, R.D. Eavey, L.V. Feagans, T. Finitzo, E.M. Friedman, et al. 1994. Otitis media with effusion in young children. *Clinical Practice Guideline* #12, July. AHCPR Publication No. 94–0622. Rockville, MD: Agency for Health Care Policy and Research, Public Health Service, U.S. Department of Health and Human Services.

U. S. Department of Education. 1992. Deaf students education services: Policy guidance. *Federal Register* (October 30) Vol. 57. No. 211:49274–49276.

U.S. Department of Health and Human Services, Public Health Service. 1991. *Healthy people 2000: National health promotion and disease prevention objectives.* DHHS Publication No. PHS1–50212. Washington, D.C.: Government Printing Office.

U.S. National Commission on Excellence in Education. 1983. *A nation at risk: the imperative for educational reform: a report to the Nation and the Secretary of Education, United States Department of Education.* Washington, D.C.: The Commission.

Welsh, R., and S. Slater. 1993. The state of infant hearing impairment identification programs. *Asha* 35:49–52.

White, K.R., and T.R. Behrens, eds. 1993. The Rhode Island hearing assessment project: Implications for universal newborn hearing screening. *Seminars in Hearing* 14: 1.

Bibliography

Abramovich, S.J., S. Gregory, M. Slemick, and A. Stewart. 1979. Hearing loss in very low birth weight infants treated with neonatal intensive care. *Archives of Disorders of Children* 54:421–426.

Adams, J., E. Courchesne, R. Elmasian, and A. Lincoln. 1987. Increased amplitude of the auditory P2 and P3b components in adolescents with developmental dysphasia. In *Electroencephalography and clinical neurophysiology: Current trends in event-related potential research*, ed. R. Johnson, J.W. Rohrbaugh, and R. Parasuraman. Amsterdam: Elsevier Science Publishers.

Alberti, P.W., and J.F. Jerger. 1974. Probe-tone frequency and the diagnostic value of tympanometry. *Archives of Otolaryngology* 99:206–210.

Alberti, P.W., and R. Kristensen. 1970. The clinical application of impedance audiometry. *Laryngoscope* 80:735–746.

Alberti, P.W., M.L. Hyde, K. Riko, H. Corgin, and S. Ambramovich. 1983. An equivalent of BERA for hearing screening in high-risk neonates. *Laryngoscope* 93:1115–1121.

Alford, B., J.F. Jerger, A. Coats, C. Peterson, and S. Weber. 1973. Neurophysiology of facial nerve testing. *Archives of Otolaryngology* 97:214–217.

Alford, C.A., S. Stagno, and R.F. Pass. 1980. Natural history of perinatal cytomegaloviral infection. In *Perinatal infections*, ed. K. Elliot, M. O'Connor, and J. Whelan. Amsterdam: Excerpta Medica.

Allen, D., I. Rapin, and M. Wiznitzer. 1988. Communication disorders of preschool children: The physician's responsibility. *Developmental and Behavioral Pediatrics* 9:164–170.

Allen, P., F. Wightman, D. Kistler, and T. Dolan. 1989. Frequency resolution in children. *Journal of Speech and Hearing Research* 32:317–322.

Allen, T., and T. Osborn. 1984. Academic integration of hearing-impaired students: Demographic, handicapping, and achievement factors. *American Annals of the Deaf* 129:100–113.

American Academy of Otolaryngology and American Council of Otolaryngology. 1979. *Guide to evaluation of hearing handicap*. 241:2055–2059.

American Psychiatric Association. 1987. *Diagnostic and statistical manual of mental disorders*. 3d ed. Washington, D.C.: American Psychiatric Association.

American Speech-Language-Hearing Association. 1979. Guidelines for acoustic immittance screening of middle ear function. *Asha* 27:49–52.

———. 1985. Guidelines for identification audiometry. *Asha* 27:49–52.

———. 1987. *The short latency auditory evoked potentials*. Rockville, Md.: American Speech-Language-Hearing Association.

———. 1988a. Guidelines for determining threshold level for speech. *Asha* 30:85–89.

———. 1988b. Utilization and employment of speech-language pathology supportive personnel with underserved populations. *Asha* 30:55–56.

———. 1989a. Audiologic screening of newborn infants who are at risk for hearing impairment. *Asha* 31:89–92.

———. 1989b. Definition: Bilingual speech-language pathologists and audiologists. *Asha* 31:93.

———. 1990. Guidelines for screening for hearing impairments and middle ear disorders. *Asha* (Suppl. 2) 32:17–30.

———. 1991a. *Combatting noise in the '90s: A national strategy for the United States.* Rockville, MD: American Speech-Language-Hearing Association.

———. 1991b. Guidelines for the audiologic assessment of children from birth through 36 months of age. *Asha* (Suppl. 5) 33:37–43.

———. 1991c. The use of FM amplification instruments for infants and preschool children with hearing impairment. *Asha* (Suppl. 5) 33:1–2.

———. 1992. *Issues in central auditory processing disorders.* Rockville, Md.: American Speech-Language-Hearing Association.

———. 1993a. Guidelines for audiology services in the schools. *Asha* (Suppl. 10) 35: 24–32.

———. 1993b. Preferred practice patterns for the professions of speech-language pathology and audiology. *Asha* (Suppl. 11) 35:1–102.

———. 1994. Professional liability and risk management for the audiology and speech-language pathology professions. *Asha* (Suppl. 12) 36:25–38.

American Speech-Language-Hearing Association and National Joint Committee on Learning Disabilities. 1993. *Reaction to "full inclusion": A reaffirmation of the rights of students with learning disabilities to a continuum of services* (November):63.

Anderson, H., B. Barr, and E. Wedenberg. 1969. Intra-aural reflexes in retrocochlear lesions. In *Nobel symposium 10: Disorders of the skull base region,* ed. C.A. Hamberger and J. Wersall. Stockholm: Almqvist and Wiksell.

———. 1970. Early diagnosis of VIIIth-nerve tumours by acoustic reflex tests. *Acta Oto-Laryngologica* 262:232–237.

Anonymous. 1989. Early intervention programs for infants and toddlers with handicaps. Final regulations. *Federal Register* 54 119:26306–26348.

Anthony, D.A. 1971. *Seeing essential English.* Anaheim: Anaheim Union High School District.

Aoki, C., and P. Siekevitz. 1988. Plasticity in brain development. *Scientific American* 2596: 56–64.

Arao, H., and H. Niwa. 1991. Auditory brain stem responses in Down's syndrome. *Nippon Jibiinkoka Gakkai Kaiho* 94:1673–82.

Arnold, S. 1985. Objective versus visual detection of the auditory brainstem response. *Ear and Hearing* 6:144–149.

Arnst, D.J., and J. Katz. 1982. *Central auditory assessment: The SSW test—development and clinical use.* San Diego: College-Hill Press.

Audiological Engineering Corporation, 35 Medford Street, Somerville, Mass.

Bader, G.G., I. Witt-Engerstrom, and B. Hagberg. 1989. Neurophysiological findings in the Rett syndrome, II: Visual and auditory brainstem, middle and late evoked responses. *Brain Development* 11:110–114.

Balkany, T.J., S.A. Berman, M.A. Simmons, and B.W. Jafek. 1978. Middle ear effusions in neonates. *Laryngoscope* 88:398–405.

Balkany, T., P.J. Gantz, and J.B. Nadol. 1988. Multichannel cochlear implants in partially ossified cochleas. *Annals of Otology, Rhinology, and Laryngology* (Suppl. 135) 97:3–7.

Baloh, R.W. 1982. Hearing loss. In *Cecil textbook of medicine*, 16th ed., ed. J.B. Wyngarden and L.H. Smith. Philadelphia: W.B. Saunders.

Baran, J.A., and F.E. Musiek. 1991. Behavioral assessment of the central auditory nervous system. In *Hearing assessment*, 2d ed., ed. W.F. Rintelmann. Austin, Texas: Pro-Ed.

Baran, J.A., F.E. Musiek, and A.G. Reeves. 1986. Central auditory function following anterior sectioning of the corpus callosum. *Ear and Hearing* 7:359–362.

Barr, D.F. 1976. *Auditory perceptual disorders.* 2d ed. Springfield, IL: Charles C. Thomas.

Battle, D.E. 1993. *Communication disorders in multicultural populations.* Boston: Andover Medical Publishers.

Bayley, N. 1969. *Bayley scales of infant development.* New York: Psychological Corporation.

Beasley, D.S., and B.A. Freeman. 1977. Time-altered speech as a measure of central auditory processing. In *Central auditory dysfunction*, ed. R.W. Keith. New York: Grune and Stratton.

Beasley, D.S., J.E. Maki, and D.J. Orchik. 1975. Children's perception of time-compressed speech using two measures of speech discrimination. *Journal of Speech and Hearing Disorders* 41:216–225.

Beauchaine, K., and M. Gorga. 1988. Applications of the auditory brainstem response to pediatric hearing aid selection. *Seminars in Hearing* 9:61–74.

Beauchaine, K., M. Gorga, J. Reiland, and L. Larson. 1986. Application of ABRs to the hearing-aid selection process: Preliminary data. *Journal of Speech and Hearing Research* 29:120–128.

Beedle, R.K., and E.R. Harford. 1973. A comparison of acoustic reflex and loudness growth in normal and pathological ears. *Journal of Speech and Hearing Research* 16:271–281.

Behrman, R.E. 1993. Statement of purpose. In *The future of children*, ed. R.E. Behrman. Los Angeles: David and Lucile Packard Foundation and the Center for the Future of Children.

Beijing Institute of Otorhinolaryngology 1992. *Statistics of ototoxic drugs in China.* A report submitted to the World Health Organization. Beijing: Beijing Institute of Otorhinolaryngology.

Beiter, A.L., and J.A. Brimacombe. 1993. Cochlear implants. In *Rehabilitative audiology: Children and adults*, 2d ed., ed. J.G. Alpiner and P.A. McCarthy. Baltimore: Williams and Wilkins.

Bench, J. 1992. *Communication skills in hearing-impaired children.* San Diego: Singular Publishing Group.

Bench, J., and J. Bamford, eds. 1979. *Speech-hearing tests and the spoken language of hearing-impaired children.* London: Academic Press.

Bench, J., Y. Collyer, L. Mentz, and I. Wilson. 1976. Studies in infant behavioral audiometry. I. Neonates. *Audiology* 15:85–105.

Bennett, M. 1984. Impedance concepts relating to the acoustic reflex. In *The acoustic reflex: Basic principles and clinical applications*, ed. S. Silman. New York: Academic Press.

Bennett, M.J., and L.A. Weatherby. 1982a. Multiple probe frequency acoustic reflex measurements. *Scandinavian Audiology* 12:3–9.

———. 1982b. Newborn acoustic reflexes to noise and pure-tone signals. *Journal of Speech and Hearing Research* 25:383–387.

Bentler, R. A. 1993. Amplification for the hearing impaired child. In *Rehabilitative audiology: Children and adults*, 2d ed., ed. J.G. Alpiner and P.A. McCarthy. Baltimore: Williams and Wilkins.

Berg, F. 1986. Classroom acoustics and signal transmission. In *Educational audiology for the hard of hearing child*, ed. F. Berg, J. Blair, S. Viehweg, and A. Wilson-Vlotman. Orlando: Grune and Stratton.

Bergman, B., K. Beauchaine, and M. Gorga. 1992. Application of the auditory brainstem response in pediatric audiology. *The Hearing Journal* 45:19–25.

Bergman, M., H. Costeff, V. Koren, N. Koifman, and A. Reshef. 1984. Auditory perception in early lateralized brain damage. *Cortex* 20:233–242.

Bergstrom, L. 1984. Congenital hearing loss. In *Hearing disorders*, 2d ed., ed. J.L. Northern. Boston: Little, Brown and Co.

Bergstrom, L., M. Neblett, and W. Hemenway. 1972. Otologic manifestations in acrocephalosyndactyly. *Archives of Otolaryngology* 96:117–123.

Berlin, C.I., J.K. Cullen, Jr., L.F. Hughes, H.L. Berlin, S.S. Lowe-Bell, and C.L. Thompson. 1975. Acoustic variables in dichotic listening. In *Proceedings of a symposium on central auditory processing disorders*, ed. M.D. Sullivan. Omaha: University of Nebraska Medical Center.

Berlin, C.I., L.J. Hood, R.P. Cecola, D.F. Jackson, and P. Szabo. 1993. Does type I afferent neuron dysfunction reveal itself through lack of efferent suppression? *Hearing Research* 65:40–50.

Berlin, C.I., L.F. Hughes, S.S. Lowe-Bell, and H.L. Berlin. 1973. Dichotic right ear advantage in children 5 to 13. *Cortex* 9:394–402.

Berlin, C.I., S.S. Lowe-Bell, J.K. Cullen, Jr., S. Thompson, and C. Loovis. 1973. Dichotic speech perception: An interpretation of right-ear advantage and temporal offset effects. *Journal of the Acoustical Society of America* 53:699–709.

Berlin, C.I., S.S. Lowe-Bell, P.J. Jannetta, and D.G. Kline. 1972. Central auditory deficits of temporal lobectomy. *Archives of Otolaryngology* 96:4–10.

Berliner, K.I., and L.S. Eisenberg. 1985. Methods and issues in the cochlear implantation of children: An overview. The cochlear implant: An auditory prosthesis for the profoundly deaf child. *Ear and Hearing* (Suppl. 6) 3:6S–13S.

Bernstein, R.S., and J.S. Gravel. 1992. Orienting as a means of assessing hearing in newly born infants. In *Screening children for auditory function*, ed. F.H. Bess and J.W. Hall III. Nashville: Bill Wilkerson Center Press.

Berrick, J., G. Shubow, M. Schultz, H. Freed, S. Fournier, and J. Hughes. 1984. Auditory processing tests for children: Normative and clinical results on the SSW test. *Journal of Speech and Hearing Disorders* 49:318–325.

Bess, F.H., and J.W. Hall III. 1992. *Screening children for auditory dysfunction*. Nashville: Bill Wilkerson Center Press.

Bess, F.H., A.F. Josey, and L.E. Humes. 1979. Performance intensity functions in cochlear and eighth nerve disorders. *American Journal of Otolaryngology* 1:27–31.

Bess, F.H, and F. McConnell. 1981. *Audiology, education and the hearing impaired child*. St. Louis: C.V. Mosby.

Bess, F.H., and A.M. Tharpe. 1984. Unilateral hearing impairment in children. *Pediatrics* 74:206–216.

Blake, P.E., and J.W. Hall III. 1990. The status of statewide policies for neonatal hearing screening. *Journal of the American Academy of Audiology* 1:67–74.

———. 1992. *Screening children for auditory dysfunction*. Nashville: Bill Wilkerson Center Press.

Blamey, P.J., and G.M. Clark. 1990. Place coding of vowel formants for cochlear implant patients. *Journal of the Acoustical Society of America* 88:667–673.

Blamey, P.J., R.C. Dowell, A.M. Brown, G.M. Clark, and P.M. Seligman. 1987. Vowel and consonant recognition of cochlear implant patients using formant-estimating speech processors. *Journal of the Acoustical Society of America* 82:48–57.

Blamey, P.J., R.C. Dowell, G.M. Clark, and P.M. Seligman. 1987. Acoustic parameters measured by a formant-estimating speech processor for a multiple-channel cochlear implant. *Journal of the Acoustical Society of America* 82:38–47.

Bluestone, C., et al. 1986. Controversies in screening for middle ear disease and hearing loss in children. *Pediatrics* 77:57–70.

Bocca, E. 1958. Clinical aspects of cortical deafness. *Laryngoscope* 68:301–309.

Bocca, E., and C. Calearo. 1963. Central hearing processes. In *Modern developments in audiology*, ed. J. Jerger. New York: Academic Press.

Bocca, E., C. Calearo, and V. Cassinari. 1954. A new method for testing hearing in temporal lobe tumors: Preliminary report. *Acta Oto-Laryngologica* 44:219–221.

Bocca, E., C. Calearo, V. Cassinari, and F. Migliavacca. 1955. Testing "cortical" hearing in temporal lobe tumors. *Acta Oto-Laryngologica* 42:289–304.

Boder, E. 1973. Developmental dyslexia: A diagnostic approach based on three atypical reading-spelling patterns. *Developmental Medicine and Child Neurology* 15:663–687.

Bond, E.K. 1972. Perception of form by the human infant. *Psychological Bulletin* 77:225–245.

Bonfils, P., P. Avan, M. Francois, J. Trotoux, and P. Narcy. 1992. Distortion-product otoacoustic emissions in neonates: Normative data. *Acta Oto-Laryngologica* 112:739–744.

Bonfils, P., A. Dumont, P. Marie, M. Francois, and P. Narcy. 1990. Evoked otoacoustic emissions in new-born hearing screening. *Laryngoscope* 100:186–189.

Bonfils, P., A. Uziel, and R. Pujol. 1988. Screening for auditory dysfunction in infants by evoked oto-acoustic emissions. *Archives of Otolaryngology: Head and Neck Surgery* 114:887–890.

Boothroyd, A. 1968. Developments in speech audiometry. *Sound* 2:3–10.

———. 1984. Auditory perception of speech contrasts by subjects with sensorineural hearing loss. *Journal of Speech and Hearing Research* 27:134–144.

———. 1987. Perception of speech pattern contrasts via cochlear implants and limited hearing. *Annals of Otology, Rhinology, and Laryngology* (Suppl. 128) 96:58–62.

———. 1988. Amplitude compression and profound hearing loss. *Journal of Speech and Hearing Research* 31:362–376.

Boothroyd, A., A.E. Geers, and J.S. Moog. 1991. Practical implications of cochlear implants in children. In *Multichannel cochlear implants in children*, ed. S.J. Staller. *Ear and Hearing* (Suppl. 12) 4:81S–89S.

Bordley, J., and Y.P. Kapur. 1977. Histopathologic changes in the temporal bone resulting from measles infection. *Archives of Otolaryngology* 103:162–168.

Bornstein, M.H., and M.D. Sigman. 1986. Continuity in mental development from infancy. *Child Development* 57:251–274.

Bornstein, S.P., and F.E. Musiek. 1984. Implications of temporal processing for children with learning and language problems, In *Audition in childhood: Methods of study*, ed. D.S. Beasley and T.H. Shriner. San Diego: College-Hill Press.

———. 1992. Recognition of distorted speech in children with and without learning problems. *Journal of the American Academy of Audiology* 3:22–32.

Bradford, L.J. 1975. Respiration audiometry. In *Physiological measures of the audiovestibular system*, ed L.J. Bradford. New York: Academic Press.

Braverman-Callahan, J., and C.K. Radzirwicz. 1989. Hearing impaired children: Language acquisition and remediation. In *Language and communication disorders in children*, ed. D.K. Bernstein and E. Tiegerman. Columbus: Merrill.

Bray, P. 1989. Click-evoked otoacoustic emissions and the development of a clinical otoacoustic hearing test instrument. Ph.D. diss., London University.

Bray, P., and D.T. Kemp. 1987. An advanced cochlear echo technique suitable for infant screening. *British Journal of Audiology* 21:191–204.

Brazelton, T.B. 1973. *Neonatal behavioral assessment scale*. London: William Heinemann.

———. 1984. Neonatal behavioral assessment scale. 2d ed. *Clinics in Developmental Medicine* no. 88. Philadelphia: J.B. Lippincott.

Bricker, D. 1986. *Early education of at-risk and handicapped infants, toddlers, and preschool children*. Glenville, IL: Scott, Foresman.

Brimacombe, J.A., P.L. Arndt, S.J. Staller, and A.L. Beiter. 1993. Multichannel cochlear implantation in adults with severe-to-profound sensorineural hearing loss. Paper presented at the Third International Cochlear Implant Conference, April 4–7. Innsbruck, Austria.

Brimacombe, J.A., and A.L. Beiter. 1994. The application of digital technology to cochlear implants. In *Understanding digitally programmable hearing aids*, ed. R.E. Sandlin. Boston: Allyn and Bacon.

Brivio, L., R. Tornaghi, L. Musetti, P. Marchisio, and N. Principi. 1991. Improvement of auditory brainstem responses after treatment with zidovudine in a child with AIDS. *Pediatric Neurology* 7:53–55.

Brooks, D.N. 1969. The use of the electroacoustic impedance bridge in the assessment of the middle ear function. *International Audiology* 8:563–569.

———. 1971. Electroacoustic impedance bridge studies on normal ears of children. *Journal of Speech and Hearing Research* 14:247–253.

———. 1980. Impedance in screening. In *Clinical impedance audiometry*, 2d ed., ed. J. Jerger and J.L.Northern. Acton, MA: American Electromedics Corporation.

Brooks-Gunn, J., and M. Lewis. 1983. Screening and diagnosing handicapped infants. *Topics in Early Childhood Special Education* 3:14–28.

Brownell, W.E. 1990. Outer hair cell electromotility and oto-acoustic emissions. *Ear and Hearing* 11:82–92.

Brownell, W.E., C.R. Bader, D. Bertrand, and Y. Rabaupierre. 1985. Evoked mechanical responses of isolated outer hair cells. *Science* 227:194–196.

Buchanan, L.H., K.M. Harding, and C.M. Hudner. 1991. Hearing disorder management in Down's syndrome. *Hearing Instruments* 42:12–15.

Burd, L., and W. Fisher. 1986. Central auditory processing disorder or attention deficit disorder? *Journal of Developmental and Behavioral Pediatrics* 7:215–216.

Burns, E.M., K.H. Arehart, and S.L. Campbell. 1992. Prevalence of spontaneous otoacoustic emissions in neonates. *Journal of the Acoustical Society of America* 91:1571–1575.

Calearo, C., and A.R. Antonelli. 1968. Audiometric findings in brainstem lesions. *Acta Oto-Laryngologica* 66:305–319.

Calearo, C., and A. Lazzaroni. 1957. Speech intelligibility in relation to the speed of the message. *Laryngoscope* 67:410–419.

Campbell, T.F., and M.R. McNeil. 1985. Effects of presentation rate and divided attention on auditory comprehension in children with an acquired language disorder. *Journal of Speech and Hearing Research* 28:513–520.

Carey, W.B. 1982. Validity of parental assessments of development and behavior. *American Journal of Diseases of Children* 136:97–99.

Caron, R.F., and A.J. Caron. 1968. The effects of repeated exposure and stimulus complexity on visual fixation in infants. *Psychonomic Science* 10:207–208.

———. 1969. Degree of stimulus complexity on visual fixation in infants. *Psychonomic Science* 14:78–79.

Cassandro, E., F. Mosca, L. Sequino, F. DeFalco, and G. Campanella. 1986. Otoneurological abnormalities in Friedreich's ataxia and other inherited neuropathies. *Audiology* 25:84–91.

Catlin, F.I. 1985. Prevention of hearing impairment from infection and ototoxic drugs. *Archives of Otolaryngology* 111:377–384.

Cavaliere, R., S. Masieri, L. Liberini, R. Proietti, and S.I. Magalini. 1992. Tympanometry for middle-ear effusion in unconscious ICU patients. *European Journal of Anaesthesiology* 9:71–75.

Cevette, M. 1984. Auditory brainstem response testing in an intensive care unit. *Seminars in Hearing* 5:57–69.

Charrow, V.R. 1975. A psycholinguistic analysis of "deaf" English. *Sign Language Studies* 7:139–150.

Chermak, G.D., and M.J. Montgomery. 1992. Form equivalence of the selective auditory attention test administered to 6–year-old children. *Journal of Speech and Hearing Research* 35:661–665.

Chermak, G.D., and F.E. Musiek. 1992. Managing central auditory processing disorders in children and youth. *American Journal of Audiology* 1:61–65.

Chermak, G.D., S.A. O'Neill, and J.A. Seikel. 1992. Criterion validity of the selective auditory attention test. Presented at annual convention of the American Speech-Language-Hearing Association.

Chermak, G.D., M. Vonhof, and R.B. Bendel. 1989. Word identification performance in the presence of competing speech and noise in learning disabled adults. *Ear and Hearing* 10:90–93.

Cherry, R.S. 1980. *Selective auditory attention test (SAAT)*. St. Louis: Auditec.

Christensen, K., and G. Delgado. 1993. *Multicultural issues in deafness*. New York: Longman.

Chuang, K.W., B.R. Vohr, S.J. Norton, and M.D. Lekas. 1993. External and middle ear status related to evoked otoacoustic emission in neonates. *Archives of Otolaryngology—Head and Neck Surgery* 119:276–282.

Chuang, S.W., S.E. Gerber, and A.R.D. Thornton. 1993. Evoked otoacoustic emissions in preterm infants. *International Journal of Pediatric Otorhinolaryngology* 26:39–45.

Churchland, P.S., and T.J. Sejnowski. 1988. Perspectives on cognitive neuroscience. *Science* 242:741–746.

Clark, G.M., P.J. Blamey, A.M. Brown, et al. 1987a. The engineering of the receiver/stimulator and speech processor. In *The University of Melbourne-Nucleus multielectrode cochlear implant*, ed. C.R. Pfaltz. *Advances in Otorhinolaryngology* 38:63–84.

———. The surgery. 1987b. In The University of Melbourne-Nucleus multielectrode cochlear implant, ed. C.R. Pfaltz. *Advances in Otorhinolaryngology* 38:93–112.

Clark, G.M., N.L. Cohen, and R.K. Shepherd. 1991. Surgical safety considerations of multi-channel cochlear implants in children. In *Multichannel cochlear implants in children*, ed. S.J. Staller. *Ear and Hearing* (Suppl. 12) 4:15S–24S.

Clark, G.M., B.K.-H. Franz, B.C. Pyman, and R.L. Webb. 1991. Surgery for multichannel cochlear implantation. In *Cochlear implants: A practical guide*, ed. H. Cooper. London: Whurr Publishers Ltd.

Coates, J.F. 1994. *Managing your future as an association: Thinking about trends and working with their consequences: 1993–2020*. Washington, D.C.: Coates and Jarrett, Inc.

Coates, J.F., and J. Jarrett. 1993. *Scanning the environment for association implications: Seventeen key trends*. Washington, D.C.: Coates and Jarrett, Inc.

Cochlear Corporation. 1986. *Cochlear Corporation/University of Iowa cochlear implant test battery*. Englewood, Colo.: Resource Point.

———. 1990a. *Craig lipreading inventory-word recognition*. Englewood, Colo.: Resource Point.

———. 1990b. *Pediatric test materials and programming kit*. Englewood, Colo.: Resource Point.

Cohen, M., and D. Prasher. 1988. The value of combining auditory brainstem responses and acoustic reflex threshold measurements in neuro-otological diagnosis. *Scandinavian Audiology* 17:153–162.

Cohen, N.L. 1994. The ethics of cochlear implants in young children. *American Journal of Otology* 15:1–2.

Cohen, N.L., and R.A. Hoffman. 1993. Complications of cochlear implant surgery. In *Complications in head and neck surgery*, ed. D.W. Eisele. St Louis: Mosby.

Cohen, O.P., J.E. Fishgrund, and R. Redding. 1990. Deaf children from ethnic, linguistic,and racial minorities backgrounds: An overview. *American Annals of the Deaf* 135:67–73.

Cohen, S.E., and A.H. Parmelee. 1983. Prediction of five-year Stanford-Binet scores in preterm infants. *Child Development* 54:1241–1253.

Cole, R., and J. Jakimik. 1980. A model of speech perception. In *Perception and production of fluent speech*, ed. R. Cole. Hillsdale, N.J.: Lawrence Erlbaum Associates.

Collet, L., D.T. Kemp, E. Veuillet, R. Duclaux, A. Moulin, and A. Morgon. 1990. Effect of contralateral auditory stimuli on active cochlear micromechanical properties in human subjects. *Hearing Research* 43:251–262.

Conrad, R. 1979. *The deaf school child*. London: Harper and Row.

Cook, R.A., and R.W. Teel, Jr. 1979. Negative middle ear pressure and language development. *Clinical Pediatrics* 18:296–297.

Cooper, F.S., P.C. Delattre, A.M. Liberman, J. Borst, and L. Gerstman. 1952. Some experiments on the perception of synthetic speech sounds. *Journal of the Acoustical Society of America* 24:597–606.

Cope, Y., and M.E. Lutman. 1988. Otoacoustic emissions. In *Pediatric audiology 0–5 years*, ed. B. McCormick. London: Taylor and Francis.

Coplan, J. 1993. *Early language milestone scale*. 2d ed. Austin: Pro-Ed.

Coplan J., and J. Gleason. 1982. Validation of early language milestone scale in high-risk population. *Pediatrics* 70:677.

Cornett, O. 1967. Cued speech. *American Annals of the Deaf* 112:3–13.

Council for Exceptional Children. 1993. *The council for exceptional children's draft statement on inclusive schools*. Reprinted in *Masstream* (spring).

Cox, L., M. Hack, and D. Metz. 1981. Brainstem evoked response audiometry in the premature infant population. *International Journal of Pediatric Otorhinolaryngology* 3: 213–224.

Craig, W.N. 1964. Effects of preschool training on the development of reading and lipreading skills of deaf children. *American Annals of Deaf Children* 109:280–296.

Cramer, K.D., and N.P. Erber. 1974. A spondee recognition test for young hearing-impaired children. *Journal of Speech and Hearing Disorders* 39:304–311.

Crandell, C. 1993. Speech recognition in noise by children with minimal degrees of sensorineural hearing loss. *Ear and Hearing* 14:210–216.

Crandell, C., and F. Bess. 1986. Speech recognition of children in a "typical" classroom setting. *Asha* 28:82.

———. 1987. Sound field amplification in the classroom setting. *Asha* 29:87.

Crawford, M. 1991. The effects of sleep stage on the signal to noise ratio of the middle components. Ph.D. diss., Memphis State University.

Cullen, J.K., and C.L. Thompson. 1974. Masking release for speech in subjects with temporal lobe resection. *Archives of Otolaryngology* 100:113–116.

Curati, W.L., M. Graif, D.P.E. Kingsley, T. King, C.L. Scholtz, and R.E. Steiner. 1986. MRI in acoustic neuroma: A review of 35 patients. *Neuroradiology* 28:208–214.

Cutler, A., and D. Norris. 1988. The role of strong syllables in segmentation for lexical access. *Journal of Experimental Psychology: Human Perception and Performance* 14: 113–121.

D'Eugenio, D.B., T.A. Slagle, B.B. Mettelman, and S.J. Gross. 1993. Developmental outcome of preterm infants with transient neuromotor abnormalities. *American Journal of Diseases of Children* 147:570–574.

D'Souza, S.W., E. McCartney, M. Nolan, and I.G. Taylor. 1981. Hearing, speech and language in survivors of severe perinatal asphyxia. *Archives of Diseases in Children* 56: 245–252.

Dalebout, S., N. Nelson, P. Hletko, and B. Frentheway. 1991. Selective auditory attention and children with attention-deficit disorder: Effects of repeated measurement with and without methylphenidate. *Language, Speech, and Hearing Services in Schools* 22:219–227.

Darling, R., and L. Price. 1990. Loudness and auditory brain stem evoked response. *Ear and Hearing* 11:289–295.

Davidson, J., M.L. Hyde, and P.W. Alberti. 1989. Epidemiologic patterns in childhood hearing loss: A review. *International Journal of Pediatric Otorhinolaryngology* 17: 239–266.

Davidson, S., L. Wall, and C. Goodman. 1990. Preliminary studies on the use of ABR amplitude projection procedure for hearing aid selection. *Ear and Hearing* 11:332–338.

Davis, A., and J. Sancho. 1988. Screening for hearing impairment in children: A review of current practice in the United Kingdom. In *International Perspectives on Communication Disorders*, ed. S.E. Gerber and G.T. Mencher. Washington, D.C.: Gallaudet University Press, 1988.

Davis, H. 1976. Principles of electric response audiometry. *Annals of Otology, Rhinology, and Laryngology* (Suppl. 28) 85:1–96.

Davis, H., and S. Onishi. 1969. Maturation of auditory evoked potentials. *International Audiology* 8:24–33.

Davis, H., and S.R. Silverman. 1978. *Hearing and deafness*, 3d ed. New York: Holt, Rhinehart, and Winston.

Davis, H., and S. Zerlin. 1966. Acoustic relations of the human vertex potential. *Journal of the Acoustical Society of America* 39:109–116.

Dayal, V.S., L. Tarantino, and L.P. Swisher. 1966. Neurootologic studies in multiple sclerosis. *Laryngoscope* 76:1798–1809.

De Filippo, C.L., and B.L. Scott. 1978. A method for training and evaluating the reception of ongoing speech. *Journal of the Acoustical Society of America* 63:1186–1192.

DeHirsch K., J. Jansky, and W.S. Langford. 1966. Comparisons between prematurely and maturely born children at three age levels. *American Journal of Orthopsychiatry* 36: 610–628.

Dempsey, C. 1983. Selecting tests of auditory function in children. In *Central auditory processing disorders: Problems of speech, language and learning*, ed. E.Z. Lasky and J. Katz. Baltimore: University Park Press.

Derbyshire, A., and G. McCandless. 1964. Template for EEG response to sound. *Journal of Speech and Hearing Research* 7:96–98.

Dermody, P., R. Katsch, and K. Mackey. 1983. Auditory processing limitations in low verbal children: Evidence from a two-response dichotic listening task. *Ear and Hearing* 4: 272–277.

deVries, L.S., S. Lary, and L.M.S. Dubowitz. 1985. Relationship of serum bilirubin levels to ototoxicity and deafness in high risk low birth weight infants. *Pediatrics* 76:351–354.

Diefendorf, A.O. 1981. An investigation of one aspect of central auditory function in an infant population utilizing a binaural resynthesis fusion task. Ph.D. diss., University of Washington.

Dolnick, E. 1993. Deafness and culture. *Atlantic Monthly* September, 37–53.

Don, M., J. Eggermont, and D. Brackmann. 1979. Reconstruction of the audiogram using brain stem responses and high-pass masking. *Annals of Otology, Rhinology, and Laryngology* (Suppl. 57):1–20.

Don, M., C. Elberling, and M. Waring. 1984. Objective detection of averaged auditory brainstem responses. *Scandinavian Audiology* 13:219–228.

Dorman, M.F., M.T. Hannley, K. Dankowski, L. Smith, and G. McCandless. 1989. Word recognition by 50 patients fitted with the Symbion multichannel cochlear implant. *Ear and Hearing* 10:44–49.

Dowell, R.C., P.M. Seligman, P.J. Blamey, and G.M. Clark. 1987. Speech perception using a two-formant 22-electrode cochlear prosthesis in quiet and in noise. *Acta Oto-Laryngologica* 104:439–446.

Dowell, R.C., L.A. Whitford, P.M. Seligman, B.K.-H. Franz, and G.M. Clark. 1990. Preliminary results with a miniature speech processor for the 22-electrode Melbourne cochlear hearing prosthesis. *Otolaryngology—Head and Neck Surgery* 98:1167–1173.

Downs, M.P. 1976. Early identification of hearing loss: Where are we? Where do we go from here? In *Early identification of hearing loss*, ed. G.T. Mencher. Basel: S. Karger.

Downs, M.P., and G.M. Sterritt. 1964. Identification audiometry for neonates: A preliminary report. *Journal of Auditory Research* 4:69–80.

———. 1967. A guide to newborn and infant hearing screening. *Archives of Otolaryngology* 85:15–22.

Drillien, C.M., A.M. Thompson, and K. Burgoyne. 1980. Low birthweight children at early school age: A longitudinal study. *Developmental Medicine and Child Neurology* 22: 26–47.

Dubowitz, L.M., V. Dubowitz, and C. Goldberg. 1970. Clinical assessment of gestational age in the newborn infant. *Journal of Pediatrics* 77:1–10.

Duffy, F.H. 1982. Topographic display of evoked potentials: Clinical applications of brain electrical activity mapping, BEAM. *Annals of the New York Academy of Science* 388:183–196.

Duffy, F.H., J. Burchfield, and C. Lombroso. 1979. Brain electrical activity mapping. BEAM: A method for extending the clinical utility of EEG and evoked potential data. *Annals of Neurology* 5:309–321.

Duffy, F.H., M.B. Denckla, R.H. Bartell, and G. Sandini. 1980. Dyslexia: Regional differences in brain electrical activity by topographic mapping. *Annals of Neurology* 5:412–420.

Duffy, F.H., and G.B. McAnulty. 1985. Brain electrical activity in mapping. BEAM: The search for a physiology signature of dyslexia. In *Dyslexia: A neuroscientific approach to clinical evaluation*, ed. F.H. Duffy and N. Geschwind. Boston: Little, Brown and Co.

Dunn, L. 1981. *Peabody picture vocabulary test* (Revised). Circle Pines, Minn.: American Guidance Services.

Durieux-Smith, A., T. Picton, C. Edwards, J.T. Goodman, and B. MacMurray. 1985. The crib-o-gram in the NICU: An evaluation based on brain stem electric response audiometry. *Ear and Hearing* 6:20–24.

Durlach, N.I., and H.S. Colburn. 1978. Binaural phenomena. In *Handbook of perception*, Vol. 4., ed. E.C. Carterette and M.F. Friedman. Orlando: Academic Press.

Durrant, J., and R. Hyde. 1993. Observations on temporal aspects of bone-conduction clicks: Real head measurements. *Journal of the American Academy of Audiology* 4:213–219.

Eagney, P. 1987. ASL? English? Which? Comparing comprehension. *American Annals of the Deaf* 132:272–275.

Edwards, C., A. Durieux-Smith, and T. Picton. 1985. Auditory brainstem response audiometry in neonatal hydrocephalus. *Journal of Otolaryngology* (Suppl. 14):40–46.

Eggermont, J.J., C.W. Ponton, S.G. Coupland, and R. Winkelaar. 1991. Frequency dependent maturation of the cochlea and brainstem evoked potentials. *Acta Oto-Laryngologica* 111:220–224.

Eggermont, J.J., and A. Salamy. 1988. Development of ABR parameters in a preterm and a term-born population. *Ear and Hearing* 9:283–289.

Eilers, R.E. 1977. Context-sensitive perception of naturally produced stop and fricative consonants by infants. *Journal of the Acoustical Society of America* 61:1321–1336.

Eilers, R.E., E. Miskiel, O. Ozdamar, R. Urbano, and J.E. Widen. 1991. Optimization of automated hearing test algorithms: Simulations using an infant response model. *Ear and Hearing* 12:191–198.

Eilers, R.E., O. Ozdamar, and M.L. Steffens. 1993. Classification of audiograms by sequential testing: Reliability and validity of an automated behavioral hearing screening algorithm. *Journal of the American Academy of Audiology* 4:172–181.

Eilers, R.E., J.E. Widen, R. Urbano, T.M. Hudson, and L. Gonzales. 1991. Optimization of automated hearing test algorithms: A comparison of data from simulations and young children. *Ear and Hearing* 12:199–214.

Eilers, R.E., W.R. Wilson, and J.M. Moore. 1977. Developmental changes in speech discrimination in infants. *Journal of Speech and Hearing Research* 20:766–780.

Eimas, P.D. 1974. Auditory and linguistic processing of cues for place or articulation by infants. *Perception and Psychophysics* 16:513–521.

Eisenberg, L.S., and W.F. House. 1982. Initial experience with the cochlear implant in children. In *Cochlear implants: Progress and perspectives*, ed. W.F. House and K.I. Berliner. *Annals of Otology, Rhinology, and Laryngology* (Suppl.) 91:67–73.

Eisenberg, L.S., W.M. Luxford, T.S. Becker, and W.F. House. 1984. Electrical stimulation of the auditory system in children deafened by meningitis. *Otolaryngology—Head and Neck Surgery* 92:700–705.

Eisenberg, R.B. 1969. Auditory behavior in the human neonate: Functional properties of sound and their ontogenetic implications. *International Audiology* 8:34–45.

Eisenberg, R.B., E.J. Griffen, D.B. Coursin, and M.A. Hunter. 1964. Auditory behavior in the human neonate: A preliminary report. *Journal of Speech and Hearing Research* 7:245–269.

Elberling, C. 1979. The use of template and cross correlation functions in analysis of brainstem potentials. *Scandinavian Audiology* 8:187–190.

Elberling, C., and M. Don. 1984. Quality estimation of averaged auditory brainstem responses. *Scandinavian Audiology* 13:187–197.

———. 1987. Detection functions for the human auditory brainstem response. *Scandinavian Audiology* 16:89–92.

Elberling, C., and O. Walgreen. 1985. Estimation of the auditory brainstem response (ABR) by means of a Bayesian inference. *Scandinavian Audiology* 14:89–96.

Elliott, L.L. 1979. Performance of children 9 to 17 years on a test of speech intelligibility in noise using sentence material with controlled word predictability. *Journal of the Acoustical Society of America* 66:651–653.

———. 1986. Discrimination and response bias for CV syllables differing in voice onset time among children and adults. *Journal of the Acoustical Society of America* 80:1250–1255.

Elliott, L.L., and M. Hammer. 1988. Longitudinal changes in auditory discrimination in normal children and children with language-learning problems. *Journal of Speech and Hearing Disorders* 53:467–474.

Elliott, L.L., and D. Katz. 1980a. *Development of a new children's test of speech discrimination*. St. Louis: Auditec.

———. 1980b. *Northwestern University children's perception of speech (NU-CHIPS)*. St. Louis: Auditec.

Ellwood, D. personal communication, November 30, 1993.

Elssman, S., N. Matkin, and M. Sabo. 1987. Early identification of congenital sensorineural hearing impairment. *The Hearing Journal* 13:7–12.

Engen, E., and T. Engen. 1983. *Rhode Island test of language structure*. Baltimore: University Park Press.

Erber, N.P. 1979. An approach to evaluating auditory speech perception ability. *The Volta Review* 81:16–24.

———. 1980. Use of the auditory numbers test to evaluate speech perception abilities of hearing impaired children. *Journal of Speech and Hearing Disorders* 45:527–532.

———. 1982. *Auditory training*. Washington, D.C.: A.G. Bell Association.

Erber, N.P., and C.M. Alencewicz. 1976. Audiologic evaluation of deaf children. *Journal of Speech and Hearing Disorders* 41:256–267.

Esbjorner, E., P. Larsson, P. Leissner, and L. Wranne. 1991. The serum reserve albumin concentration for monoacetyldiamino-diphenyl sulphone and auditory evoked responses during neonatal hyperbilirubinaemia. *Acta Paediatrica Scandinavica* 80:406–412.

Evans, L. 1982. *Total communication*. Washington, D.C.: Gallaudet University Press.

Everberg, G. 1957. Deafness in mumps. *Acta Oto-Laryngologica* 48:397–403.

Farrer, S., and R. Keith. 1981. Filtered word testing in the assessment of children's central auditory abilities. *Ear and Hearing* 2:267–269.

Fawer, C., and L. Dubowitz. 1982. Auditory brainstem responses in neurologically normal preterm and fullterm newborn infants. *Neuropediatrics* 13:200–206.

Feagans, L.V., M. Sanyal, F. Henderson, A. Collier, and M. Applebaum. 1987. Relationship of middle ear disease in early childhood to later narrative and additional skills. *Journal of Pediatric Psychology* 12:581–594.

Feinmesser, M., L. Tell, and H. Levi. 1982. Follow-up of 40,000 infants screened for hearing defect. *Audiology* 21:197–203.

Ferre, J.M., and L.A. Wilber. 1986. Normal and learning disabled children's central auditory processing skills: An experimental test battery. *Ear and Hearing* 7:336–343.

Ferry, P.C. 1981. Neurological considerations in children with learning disabilities. In *Central auditory and learning disorders in children*, ed. R.W. Keith. Houston: College-Hill Press.

Field, J., D. DiFranco, P. Dodwell, and D. Muir. 1979. Auditory-visual coordination in two and one-half-month-old infants. *Infant Behavior and Development* 2:113–122.

Field, J., D. Muir, R. Pilon, M. Sinclair, and P. Dodwell. 1980. Infants' orientation to lateral sounds from birth to three months. *Child Development* 51:295–298.

Fiellau-Nikolajsen, M. 1983. Tympanometry and secretory otitis media. *Acta Oto-Laryngologica* (Suppl. 394):1–73.

Fifer, R.C., J.F. Jerger, C.I. Berlin, E.A. Tobey, and J.C. Campbell. 1983. Development of a dichotic sentence identification test for hearing-impaired adults. *Ear and Hearing* 4:300–305.

Finitzo, T., and K.D. Pool. 1987. Brain electrical activity mapping. *Asha* 29:21–25.

Finitzo-Hieber, T. 1981. Classroom acoustics. In *Auditory disorders in school children*, ed. R.J. Roeser and M.P. Downs. New York: Thieme-Stratton.

Finitzo-Hieber, T., and T. Tillman. 1978. Room acoustics effects on monosyllabic word discrimination ability for normal and children with hearing impairments. *Journal of Speech and Hearing Research* 21:440–458.

Fisher, L. 1980. *Fisher's auditory problems checklist*. Cedar Rapids, Iowa: Grant Wood.

Flexer, C., and D.P. Gans. 1985. Comparative evaluation of the auditory responsiveness of normal infants and profoundly multihandicapped children. *Journal of Speech and Hearing Research* 28:163–168.

Forman-Franco, B., G. Karayalin, D. Mandel, and A. Abramson. 1982. The evaluation of auditory function in homozygous sickle cell disease. *Otolaryngology—Head and Neck Surgery* 89:850–856.

Frank, Y., S.M. Vishnubhakat, and S. Pahwa. 1992. Brainstem auditory evoked responses in infants and children with AIDS. *Pediatric Neurology* 8:262–266.

Fraser, G.R. 1976. *The causes of profound deafness in childhood*. Baltimore: Johns Hopkins University Press.

Freeman, B., and D. Beasley. 1978. Performance of reading-impaired and normal reading children on time-compressed monosyllabic and sentential stimuli. Paper presented at annual meeting of the American Speech and Hearing Association.

Friedman, E., N. Luban, G. Herr, and I. Williams. 1980. Sickle cell anemia and hearing. *Annals of Otolaryngology* 89:342–347.

Friel-Patti, S., T. Finitzo-Hieber, G. Conti, and K. Brown. 1982. Language delay in infants associated with middle ear disease and mild fluctuating hearing impairment. *Pediatric Infectious Disease* 1:104–109.

Frumkin, N.L., E.J. Potchen, A.S. Aniskiewicz, J.B. Moore, and P.A. Cooke. 1989. Potential impact of magnetic resonance imaging on the field of communication disorders. *Asha* 31:95–99.

Fujisaki, H., K. Nakamura, and T. Imoto. 1975. Auditory perception of duration of speech and nonspeech stimuli. In *Auditory analysis and perception of speech*, ed. G. Fant and M. Tatham. New York: Academic Press.

Furth, H.G. 1966. A comparison of reading test norms of deaf and hearing children. *American Annals of the Deaf* 111:461–462.

Galaburda, A., G. Sherman, G. Rosen, F. Aboitiz, and N. Geschwind. 1985. Developmental dyslexia: Four consecutive patients with cortical anomalies. *Annals of Neurology* 18: 222–233.

Gans, D.P. 1987. Improving behavior observation audiometry testing and scoring procedures. *Ear and Hearing* 8:92–100.

Gans, D.P., and C. Flexer. 1983. Auditory response behavior of severely handicapped children. *Journal of Auditory Research* 23:137–148.

Gardi, J.N. 1985. Human brain stem and middle latency responses to electrical stimulation: Preliminary observations. In *Cochlear implants*, ed. R.A. Schindler and M. M. Merzenich. New York: Raven Press.

Garstecki, D., C.L. Hutton, M.A. Nerbonne, C.W. Newman, and W.J. Smoski. 1990. Case study examples using self-assessment. *Ear and Hearing* (Suppl.) 11:48S–56S.

Gascon, G.G., R. Johnson, and L. Burd. 1986. Central auditory processing and attention deficit disorders. *Journal of Child Neurology* 1:27–33.

Geers, A.E., and H.S. Lane. 1984. *The CID preschool performance scale.* Chicago: Stoelting.

Geers, A., and J. Moog. 1987. Predicting spoken language acquisition of profoundly hearing impaired children. *Journal of Speech and Hearing Disorders* 52:84–94.

———. 1989. Evaluating speech perception skills: Tools for measuring benefits of cochlear implants, tactile aids, and hearing aids. In *Cochlear implants in young deaf children*, ed. E. Owens and D. Kessler. Boston: College-Hill Press.

———. 1992. The Central Institute for the Deaf cochlear implant study: A progress report. *Journal of Speech-Language Pathology and Audiology* 16:129–140.

Geier, L., J. Gilden, C.M. Luetje, and H.E. Maddox. 1993. Delayed perception of cochlear implant stimulation in children with postmeningitic ossified cochleae. *American Journal of Otolaryngology* 14:556–561.

Gelfand, S.A., N. Piper, and S. Silman. 1983. Effects of hearing levels at the activator and other frequencies upon the expected levels of the acoustic reflex threshold. *Journal of Speech and Hearing Disorders* 48:11–17.

Gerber, S.E. 1969. Auditory behavioral responses of some hearing infants. *Volta Review* 71:340–346.

———. 1982. The use of noise-making toys as audiometric devices. *International Journal of Pediatric Otorhinolaryngology* 4:309–315.

———. 1990. Review of a high risk register for congenital or early-onset deafness. *British Journal of Audiology* 24:347–356.

Gerber, S.E., and M.S. Dobkin. 1984. The effect of noise bandwidth on the auditory arousal response of neonates. *Ear and Hearing* 5:195–198.

Gerber, S.E., C.J. Lynch, and W.S. Gibson, Jr. 1987. The acoustic characteristics of an infant with unilateral vocal fold paralysis. *International Journal of Pediatric Otorhinolaryngology* 13:1–9.

Gerber, S.E., and G.T. Mencher. 1979. Arousal responses of neonates to wide band and narrow band noise. Paper presented at the annual convention of the American Speech-Language-Hearing Association.

Gerber, S.E., M.I. Mendel, and M. Goller. 1979. Progressive hearing loss subsequent to congenital cytomegalovirus infection. Human Communication 4:231–234.

Gerber, S.E., and C.A. Prutting. 1981. Bilingualism: An environment for the deaf infant. In *Early management of hearing loss*, ed. G.T. Mencher and S.E. Gerber. New York: Grune and Stratton.

Gerber, S.E., E. Wile, and N.T. Hamai. 1985. Central auditory dysfunction in deaf children. *Human Communication* 9:39–44.

Gerling, I. 1991. In search of a stringent methodology for using ABR audiometric results. *The Hearing Journal* 44:26–30.

Gersdorff, M.C.H. 1992. Diagnostic value of tympanometry in otitis media with effusion. *Acta Oto-Rhino-Laryngologica Belgica* 46:361–368.

Gibbs, E.D. 1990. Assessment of infant mental ability: Conventional tests and issues of prediction. In *Interdisciplinary assessment of infants: A guide for early intervention professionals*, ed. E.D. Gibbs and D.M. Teti. Baltimore: Paul H. Brookes.

Gillberg, C., U. Rosenhall, and E. Johansson. 1983. Auditory brainstem responses in children. *Journal of Autism and Developmental Disorders* 13:181–195.

Goldstein, P., A. Krumholz, J. Felix, D. Shannon, and R. Carr. 1979. Brainstem evoked responses in neonates. *American Journal of Obstetrics and Gynecology* 135:622–631.

Goodglass, H. 1967. Binaural digit presentation and early lateral brain damage. *Cortex* 3:295–306.

Gorga, M., K. Beauchaine, and J. Reiland. 1987. Comparison of onset and steady-state responses of hearing aids: Implications for use of auditory brainstem response in the selection of hearing aids. *Journal of Speech and Hearing Research* 30:130–136.

Gorga, M., J. Kaminski, K. Beauchaine, W. Jesteadt, and S. Neely. 1989. Auditory brainstem responses from children three months to three years of age: II. Normal patterns of response. *Journal of Speech and Hearing Research* 32:281–288.

Gorga, M., and A.R. Thornton. 1989. The choice of stimuli for ABR measurements. *Ear and Hearing* 10:217–230.

Gormley, K., and A=Ñn Sarachan<Ü•ily. 1987. Evaluating hearing-impaired students: A practical approach. *Volta Review* 89:157–169.

Gottlieb, M.I., P. Zinkus, and A. Thompson. 1979. Chronic middle ear disease and auditory perceptual deficits. *Clinical Pediatrics* 18:725–732.

Gould, H. 1980. Early auditory evoked potentials in infants with craniofacial malformation. *Journal of Auditory Research* 20:244–248.

Gould, H., and D. Caldarelli. 1982. Hearing and otopathology in Apert syndrome. *Archives of Otolaryngology* 108:347–349.

Gould, H., M. Crawford, M. Mendel, and S. Dodson. 1992. Quantification technique for the middle latency response. *Journal of the American Academy of Audiology* 3:153–158.

Gould, H., M. Crawford, W. Smith, N. Beckford, W. Gibson, L. Pettit, and L. Bobo. 1991. Hearing disorders in sickle cell disease: Cochlear and retrocochlear findings. *Ear and Hearing* 12:352–354.

Grandori, F. 1986. Field analysis of auditory evoked brain-stem potentials. *Hearing Research* 21:51–58.

Grass, E. 1978. Electrical safety specifically related to EEG. *Grass Technical Bulletin #X757C78*. Quincy, Mass.: Grass Instrument Co.

Gravel, J.S., ed. 1989. Assessing auditory system integrity in high-risk infants and young children. *Seminars in Hearing* 10:213–292.

Gravel, J.S., and I.F. Wallace. 1992. Listening and language at four years of age: Effects of early otitis media. *Journal of Speech and Hearing Research* 35:588–595.

Green, J., J. Waggener, and B. Kriegsfeld. 1976. Classification and incidence of neoplasms of the central nervous system. In *Advances in neurology*, ed. R. Thompson and J. Green. New York: Raven Press.

Green, M., and J.B. Richmond. 1992. *Pediatric diagnosis: Interpretation of signs and symptoms in different age periods.* 5th ed. Philadelphia: W.B. Saunders.

Greenberg, D.B., W.R. Wilson, J.M. Moore, and G. Thompson. 1978. Visual reinforcement audiometry VRA with young Down's syndrome children. *Journal of Speech and Hearing Disorders* 43:8–458.

Greene, J.C. 1990. *Beginnings for parents of hearing impaired children: A parent manual.* Durham, NC: The Beginnings for Parents of Hearing Impaired Children, Inc.

Greisen, D., and P. Rasmussen. 1970. Stapedius muscle reflexes and otoneurological examinations in brain stem tumors. *Acta Oto-Laryngologica* 70:366–370.

Grellong, B., H.G. Vaughan, Jr., L. Rotkin, et al. 1981. Neonatal performance, cognitive and neurologic outcome to 40 months among low birthweight infants. Presented at Biennial Meeting, Society for Research in Child Development, Boston.

Grundfast, K.M., and A.K. Lalwani. 1992. Practical approach to diagnosis and management of hereditary hearing impairment (HHI). *ENT Journal* 71:479–493.

Gunnarson, A.D., and T. Finitzo. 1991. Conductive hearing loss in infancy: Effects on later auditory brain stem electrophysiology. *Journal of Speech and Hearing Research* 34:1207–1215.

Gupta, A.K., H. Raj, and N.K. Anand. 1990. Auditory brainstem responses (ABR) in neonates with hyperbilirubinemia. *Indian Journal of Pediatrics* 57:705–711.

Gustason, G. 1983. *Teaching and learning signing exact English.* Los Alamitos, Calif.: Modern Signs Press.

Hack, M., J.D. Horbar, M.H. Malloy, J.E. Tyson, E. Wright, and L. Wright. 1991. Very low birth weight outcomes of the National Institute of Child Health and Human Development neonatal network. *Pediatrics* 87:587–597.

Hall, J.W. III. 1992. *Handbook of auditory evoked responses.* Boston: Allyn and Bacon.

Hall, J.W. III, D. Brown, and J. Mackey-Hargadine. 1985. Pediatric applications of serial auditory brainstem and middle-latency evoked response recordings. *International Journal of Pediatric Otorhinolaryngology* 9:201–218.

Hall, J.W. III, and J.H. Grose. 1990. The masking-level difference in children. *Journal of the American Academy of Audiology* 1:81–88.

———. 1991. Notched-noise measures of frequency selectivity in adults and children using fixed-masker-level and fixed-signal-level presentation. *Journal of Speech and Hearing Research* 34:651–660.

Hall, J.W. III, and R. Ruth. 1985. Acoustic reflexes and auditory evoked responses in hearing aid evaluation. *Seminars in Hearing* 6:251–277.

Hall, J.W. III, and T. Weaver. 1979. Impedance audiometry in a young population: The effect of age, sex, and tympanogram abnormalities. *Journal of Otolaryngology* 3:210–221.

Hanson, P., R. Farber, and R. Armstrong. 1970. Distal muscle wasting, nephritis, and deafness. *Neurology* 20:426–434.

Hanson, V.L. 1990. Recall of order information of deaf signers: Phonetic coding in temporal order recall. *Memory and Cognition* 18:604–610.

Hanson,V.L., E.W. Goodell, and C.A. Perfetti. 1991. Tongue-twister effects in the silent reading of hearing and deaf college students. *Journal of Memory and Language* 30: 319–330.

Hardy, J.B., J.F. Drage, and E.C. Jackson. 1979. *The first year of life: The collaborative perinatal project of the National Institute of Neurological and Communication Disorders and Stroke.* Baltimore: Johns Hopkins University Press.

Harford, E.R., and J. Barry. 1965. A rehabilitative approach to the problems of unilateral hearing impairment: The contralateral routing of signals, CROS. *Journal of Speech and Hearing Disorders* 30:121–128.

Harris, F.P., B.L. Lonsbury-Martin, B.B. Stagner, A.C. Coats, and G.K. Martin. 1989. Acoustic distortion products in humans: Systematic changes in amplitude as a function of f_2/f_1 ratio. *Journal of the Acoustical Society of America* 85:220–222.

Harris, F.P., and R. Probst. 1992. Transiently evoked otoacoustic emissions in patients with Ménière's disease. *Acta Oto-Laryngologica* 112:36–44.

Harris, R. 1963. Central auditory functions in children. *Perceptual and Motor Skills* 16: 207–214.

Harris, V., R. Keith, and K. Novak. 1983. Relationship between two dichotic listening tests and the token test for children. *Ear and Hearing* 4:278–282.

Hasenstab, M.S., and J.S. Horner. 1982. *Comprehensive intervention with hearing-impaired infants and preschool children.* Rockville: Aspen Systems.

Haskins, H. 1949a. Kindergarten phonetically balanced word lists (PBK). St Louis: Auditec.
———. 1949b. A phonetically balanced test of speech discrimination for children. Master's thesis, Northwestern University.

Hassmannova, J., J. Myslivecek, and V. Novakova. 1981. Effects of early auditory stimulation on cortical areas. In *Neuronal mechanisms of hearing,* ed. J. Syka and L. Aitkin. New York: Plenum Press.

Hatanaka, T., H. Shuto, A. Yasuhara, and Y. Kobayashi. 1988. Ipsilateral and contralateral recordings of auditory brainstem responses to monaural stimulation. *Pediatric Neurology* 4:354–357.

Hatanaka, T., A. Yasuhara, A. Hori, and Y. Kobayashi. 1990. Auditory brainstem response in newborn infants: Masking effects on ipsi and contralateral recording. *Ear and Hearing* 11:233–236.

Hawkins, D.R. 1982. Overamplification: A well documented case report. *Journal of Speech and Hearing Disorders* 47:382–384.

Health and Human Services. 1991. *Healthy people 2000: National health promotion and disease prevention objectives.* Washington, D.C.: United States Government Printing Office.

Hebert, R., E. Laureau, M. Vanasse, J.E. Richard, J. Morrissette, J. Glorieux, M. Desjardins, J. Letarte, and J.H. Dussault. 1986. Auditory brainstem response audiometry in congenitally hypothyroid children under early replacement therapy. *Pediatric Research* 20: 570–573.

Hecox, K. 1983. Role of auditory brain stem response in the selection of hearing aids. *Ear and Hearing* 4:51–55.

Hecox, K., and R. Galambos. 1974. Brainstem auditory evoked responses in human infants and adults. *Archives of Otolaryngology* 99:30–33.

Hedrick, D., E. Prather, and A. Tobin. 1984. *Sequenced inventory of communication development*. Seattle: University of Washington Press.

Heffernan, H.P., and M.R. Simons. 1979. Temporary increase in sensorineural hearing loss with hearing aid use. *Annals of Otology, Rhinology and Laryngology* 88:86–91.

Heilman, K.M., L.C. Hammer, and B.J. Wilder. 1973. An audiometric defect in temporal lobe dysfunction. *Neurology* 23:384–386.

Henderson, R.H. 1981. Vaccine-preventable diseases: The role of the immunization services. In *Disability prevention: The global challenge*, ed. Sir John Wilson. Oxford: Oxford University Press.

Heward, W., and M. Orlansky. 1992. *Exceptional children: An introductory survey to special education*. 4th ed. Columbus: Merrill.

Hier, D.B., M. LeMay, P.B. Rosenberger, and V.P. Perlo. 1978. Developmental dyslexia: Evidence for a subgroup with a reversal of cerebral asymmetry. *Archives of Neurology* 35:90–92.

Hill, I.T. 1992. The role of Medicaid and other government programs in providing medical care for children and pregnant women. *The Future of Children* 2:134–153.

Himmelfarb, M.Z., E. Shanon, G.R. Popelka, and R.H. Margolis. 1978. Acoustic reflex evaluation in neonates. In *Early diagnosis of hearing loss*, ed. S.E. Gerber and G.T. Mencher. New York: Grune and Stratton.

Hinojosa, R., and M. Marion. 1983. Histopathology of profound sensorineural deafness. In *Cochlear prostheses: An international symposium*, ed. C.W. Parkins and S.W. Anderson. New York: New York Academy of Sciences.

Hirsh, I.J. 1959. Auditory perception of temporal order. *Journal of the Acoustical Society of America* 31:759–767.

———. 1967. Information processing in input channels for speech and language: The significance of serial order of stimuli. In *Brain mechanisms underlying speech and language*, ed. C.H. Millikan and F.L. Darley. New York: Grune and Stratton.

Hirsch, J.E., R.H. Margolis, and J.R. Rykken. 1992. A comparison of acoustic reflex and auditory brain stem response screening of high-risk infants. *Ear and Hearing* 13:181–186.

Hirsh-Pasek, K., and R. Treiman. 1982. Recoding in silent reading: Can the deaf child translate print into a more manageable form? *Volta Review* 84:71–82.

Hodgson, W.R., ed. 1986. *Hearing aid assessment and use in audiologic habilitation*. 3d ed. Baltimore: Williams and Wilkins.

Hoekelman, R., S.B. Friedman, N.M. Nelson, and H.M. Seidel. 1992. *Primary pediatric care*. 2d ed. St. Louis: Mosby Year Book.

Holmes, D.E., and C.M. Woodford. 1977. Acoustic reflex threshold and loudness discomfort level: Relationships in children with profound hearing losses. *Journal of the American Auditory Society* 2:193–196.

Holmquist, J., and J. Miller. 1972. Eustachian tube evaluation using the impedance bridge. In *Mayo Foundation impedance symposium*, ed. D. Rose and L. Keating. Rochester, Minn.: Mayo Foundation.

Holt, J.A., and T. Allen. 1989. The effects of schools and their curricula on the reading and mathematics achievement of hearing impaired students. *International Journal of Educational Research* 13:547–562.

Honzik, M.P. 1976. Value and limitations of infant tests: An overview. In *Origins of intelligence*, ed. M. Lewis. New York: Plenum Press.

House, W.F., and K.I. Berliner. 1991. Cochlear implants: From idea to clinical practice. In *Cochlear implants: A practical guide*, ed. H. Cooper. London: Whurr Publishers Ltd.

House, W.F., W.M. Luxford, and B. Courtney. 1985. Otitis media in children following the cochlear implant. *Ear and Hearing* (Suppl.) 6:24S–26S.

Hubatch, L.M., C.J. Johnson, D.J. Kistler, W.J. Burns, and W. Moneka. 1985. Early language abilities of high-risk infants. *Journal of Speech and Hearing Disorders* 50:195–207.

Hudgins, R., and F. Numbers. 1942. An investigation of intelligibility of speech of the deaf. *Genetic Psychology Monographs* 25:289–392.

Hung, K. 1989. Auditory brainstem responses in patients with neonatal hyperbilirubinemia and bilirubin encephalopathy. *Brain Development* 11:297–301.

Hynd, G.W., J. Obrzut, W. Weed, and C. Hynd. 1979. Development of cerebral dominance: Dichotic listening asymmetry in normal and learning-disabled children. *Journal of Experimental Child Psychology* 28:445–454.

Hynd, G.W., and M. Semrud-Clikeman. 1989. Dyslexia and brain morphology. *Psychological Bulletin* 106:447–482.

Hynd, G.W., M. Semrud-Clikeman, A.R. Lorys, E.S. Novey, and D. Eliopulos. 1990. Brain morphology in developmental dyslexia, attention deficit disorder/hyperactivity. *Archives of Neurology* 47:919–926.

Hynd, G.W., M. Semrud-Clikeman, and H. Lyytinen. 1991. Brain imaging in learning disabilities. In *Neuropsychological foundations of learning disabilities*, ed. J.E. Obrzut and G.W. Hynd. San Diego: Academic Press.

Iinuma, K., K. Haginoya, I. Handa, A. Kojima, N. Fueki, J. Aikawa, M. Ito, J. Hatazawa, and T. Ido. 1989. Computed tomography, magnetic resonance imaging, positron emission tomography, and evoked potential at early stage of adrenoleuko-dystrophy. *Tohuku Journal of Experimental Medicine* 159:195–203.

Inagaki, M., Y. Tomita, S. Takashima, K. Ohtani, G. Andoh, and K. Takeshita. 1987. Functional and morphometrical maturation of the brainstem auditory pathway. *Brain Development* 9:597–601.

Indian Council of Medical Research. 1983. *Collaborative study on prevalence and etiology of hearing impairment*. New Delhi: Indian Council of Medical Research.

Jackler, R.K., W.M. Luxford, and W.F. House. 1987. Congenital malformations of the inner ear: A classification based on embryogenesis. *Laryngoscope* (Suppl. 40) 90:2–14.

Jacobson, J.T., and C.R. Morehouse. 1984. A comparison of auditory brainstem response and behavioral screening in high risk and normal newborn infants. *Ear and Hearing* 5: 247–253.

Jacobson, J.T., C.R. Morehouse, and M. Johnson. 1982. Strategies for infant auditory brainstem response assessment. *Ear and Hearing* 3:263–270.

Jaroff, L. 1992. *The new genetics*. Knoxville, Tenn.: Whittle Communications.

Jeffers, J., and M. Barley. 1977. *Speech reading: "Lipreading."* Springfield, Ill.: Charles C. Thomas.

Jepsen, O. 1963. Middle ear muscle reflexes in man. In *Modern developments in audiology*, ed. J.F. Jerger. New York: Academic Press.

Jerger, J. 1960a. Audiological manifestations of lesions in the auditory nervous system. *Laryngoscope* 70:417–425.

———. 1960b. Observations on auditory behavior in lesions of the central auditory pathways. *Archives of Otolaryngology* 71:797–806.

———. 1970. Clinical experience with impedance audiometry. *Archives of Otolaryngology* 92:311–324.

———. 1975. Diagnostic use of impedance measures. In *Handbook of clinical impedance audiometry*, ed. J. Jerger. Dobbs Ferry, N.Y.: American Electromedics Corp.

Jerger, J., L. Anthony, S. Jerger, and L. Mauldin. 1974. Studies in impedance audiometry: Middle ear disorders. *Archives of Otolaryngology* 99:165–171.

Jerger, J., P. Burney, L. Mauldin, and B. Crump. 1974. Predicting hearing loss from the acoustic reflex. *Journal of Speech and Hearing Disorders* 39:11–22.

Jerger, J., E. Harford, J. Clemis, and B. Alford. 1974. The acoustic reflex in eighth nerve disorders. *Archives of Otolaryngology* 99:409–413.

Jerger, J., and D. Hayes. 1977. Diagnostic speech audiometry. *Archives of Otolaryngology* 103:216–222.

Jerger, J., and S. Jerger. 1971. Diagnostic significance of PB word function. *Archives of Otolaryngology* 93:573–580.

———. 1974. Auditory findings in brain stem disorders. *Archives of Otolaryngology* 99:342–350.

———. 1975. Clinical validity of central auditory tests. *Scandinavian Audiology* 4:147–163.

———. 1977. Diagnostic value of crossed versus uncrossed acoustic reflexes: Eighth nerve and brainstem disorders. *Archives of Otolaryngology* 103:445–450.

Jerger, J., S. Jerger, and L. Mauldin. 1972. Studies in impedance audiometry: I. Normal and sensorineural ears. *Archives of Otolaryngology* 96:513–523.

Jerger, J., K. Johnson, S. Jerger, N. Coker, F. Pirozzolo, and L. Gray. 1991. Central auditory processing disorder: A case study. *Journal of the American Academy of Audiology* 2:36–54.

Jerger, J., and J.L. Northern. 1980. *Clinical impedance audiometry*. Acton, Mass.: American Electromedics Corp.

Jerger, J., C. Speaks, and J. Trammel. 1968. A new approach to speech audiometry. *Journal of Speech and Hearing Disorders* 33:318–328.

Jerger, J., N. Weikers, F. Sharbrough, and S. Jerger. 1969. Bilateral lesions of the temporal lobe: A case study. *Acta Oto-Laryngologica* (Suppl.) 258:1–51.

Jerger, S. 1980. Evaluation of central auditory function in children. In *Central auditory and language disorders in children*, ed. R.W. Keith. Houston: College-Hill Press.

———. 1983. Decision matrix and information theory analyses in the evaluation of neuro-audiological tests. *Seminars in Hearing* 4:121–132.

———. 1987. Validation of the pediatric speech intelligibility test in children with central nervous system lesions. *Audiology* 26:298–311.

Jerger, S., and J. Jerger. 1982. Pediatric speech intelligibility test: Performance-intensity characteristics. *Ear and Hearing* 3:325–333.

———. 1983. Evaluation of diagnostic audiometric tests. *Audiology* 22:144–161.

———. 1984. *Pediatric speech intelligibility test: Manual for administration*. St. Louis: Auditec.

Jerger, S., J. Jerger, and S. Abrams. 1983. Speech audiometry in the young child. *Ear and Hearing* 4:56–66.

Jerger, S., J. Jerger, B.R. Alford, and S. Abrams. 1983. Development of speech intelligibility in children with recurrent otitis media. *Ear and Hearing* 4:138–145.

Jerger, S., J. Jerger, L. Mauldin, and P. Segal. 1974. Studies in impedance audiometry: II. Children less than 6 years old. *Archives of Otolaryngology* 99:1–9.

Jerger, S., K. Johnson, and L. Loiselle. 1988. Pediatric central auditory dysfunction: Comparison of children with confirmed lesions versus suspected processing disorders. *American Journal of Otology* 9:63–71.

Jerger, S., R. Martin, and J. Jerger. 1987. Specific auditory perceptual dysfunction in a learning disabled child. *Ear and Hearing* 8:78–86.

Jerger, S., and R. Zeller. 1989. Dichotic listening in a child with a cerebral lesion: The "paradoxical" ipsilateral ear deficit. *Ear and Hearing* 10:167–172.

Jirsa, R.E. 1992. The clinical utility of the P3 AERP in children with auditory processing disorders. *Journal of Speech and Hearing Research* 35:903–912.

Jirsa, R.E., and K.B. Clontz. 1990. Long latency auditory event-related potentials from children with auditory processing disorders. *Ear and Hearing* 11:222–232.

Johnson, J.L., G.W. Mauk, K.M. Takekawa, P.R. Simon, C.C.J. Sia, and P.M. Blackwell. 1993. Implementing a statewide system of services for infants and toddlers with hearing disabilities. *Seminars in Hearing* 14:105–119.

Johnsen, N.J., P. Bagi, and C. Elberling. 1983. Evoked acoustic emissions from the human ear. III. Findings in neonates. *Scandinavian Audiology* 12:17–24.

Johnsen, N.J., P. Bagi, J. Parbo, and C. Elberling. 1988. Evoked acoustic emissions from the human ear. IV. Final results in 100 neonates. *Scandinavian Audiology* 17:27–34.

Johnsen, N.J., J. Parbo, and C. Elberling. 1989. Evoked acoustic emissions from the human ear. V. Developmental changes. *Scandinavian Audiology* 18:59–62.

Johnson, D., M. Enfield, and R. Sherman. 1981. The use of the staggered spondaic word test and the competing environmental sounds test in the evaluation of central auditory function in hearing disabled children. *Ear and Hearing* 2:70–77.

Johnson, S.J., H. Hosford-Dunn, S. Paryani, A. Yeager, and N. Malachowski. 1986. Prevalence of sensorineural hearing loss in premature and sick term infants with perinatally acquired cytomegalovirus infection. *Ear and Hearing* 7:325–327.

Joint Committee of the American Speech-Language-Hearing Association and the Council on Education of the Deaf. n.d. Technical report regarding service provision under the Individuals with Disabilities Education Act (Part H), as amended by IDEA-Part H to children who are deaf and hard of hearing, ages birth to 36 months.

Joint Committee on Infant Hearing. 1972. Supplementary statement on infant hearing screening. *Asha* 16:160.

———. 1991. 1990 position statement. *AAO-HNS Bulletin.* (March):15–18.

———. 1991. 1990 position statement. *Asha* (Supplement 5) 33:3–6.

———. 1994. 1993 position statement. *Asha.*

———. 1994. 1994 position statement. *Audiology Today* 6:6–9.

Kaga, K., and R. Marsh. 1986. Auditory brainstem responses in young children with Down's syndrome. *International Journal of Pediatric Otorhinolaryngology* 11:29–38.

Kalil, R.E. 1989. Synapse formation in the developing brain. *Scientific American* 2616:76–85.

Kampfe, C.M., and A.G. Turecheck. 1987. Reading achievement of prelingually deaf students and its relationship to parental method of communication: A review of the literature. *American Annals of the Deaf* 132:11–15.

Kamuro, K., M. Inagaki, and Y. Tomita. 1992. Correlation between morphological abnormalities of Chiari malformation and evoked potentials. *No-To-Hattatsu* 24:554–558.

Kankkunen, A. 1982. Preschool children with impaired hearing in Göteborg. 1964–1980. *Acta Oto-Laryngologica* (Suppl. 391) 14:1–124.

Kaplan, G.J., J.K. Fleshman, T.R. Bender, C. Baum, and P.S. Clark. 1973. Long term effects of otitis media: A ten-year cohort study of Alaskan Eskimo children. *Pediatrics* 52:577–585.

Kapur, Y.P. 1983. The principal causes of acute conditions: Deafness. In *Disability prevention: The global challenge*, ed. Sir John Wilson. Oxford: Oxford University Press.

Katz, J. 1962. The use of staggered spondaic words for assessing the integrity of the central auditory system. *Journal of Auditory Research* 2:327–337.

———. 1970. Audiologic diagnosis: Cochlea to cortex. *Menorah Medical Journal* 1:25–38.

———. 1983. Phonemic synthesis. In *Central auditory processing disorders: Problems of speech, language, and learning*, ed. E.Z. Lasky and J. Katz. Baltimore: University Park Press.

———. 1992. Classification of auditory processing disorders. In *Central auditory processing: A transdisciplinary view*, ed. J. Katz, N.A. Stecker, and D. Henderson. St. Louis: Mosby Year Book.

———. 1994. *Handbook of clinical audiology*. 4th ed. Baltimore: Williams and Wilkins.

Katz, J., R.A. Basil, and J.M. Smith. 1963. A staggered spondaic word test for detecting central auditory lesions. *Annals of Otology, Rhinology, and Laryngology* 72:906–917.

Katz, J., and R. Illmer. 1972. Auditory perception in children with learning disabilities. In *Handbook of clinical audiology*, ed. J. Katz. Baltimore: Williams and Wilkins.

Katz, J., D. Kushner, and G. Pack. 1975. The use of competing speech SSW and environmental sounds: CES tests for localizing brain lesions. Presented at annual convention of the American Speech and Hearing Association.

Katz, J., and L. Wilde. 1985. Auditory perceptual disorders in children. In *Handbook of clinical audiology*, 3d ed., ed. J. Katz. Baltimore: Williams and Wilkins.

Kaufman, N.L. 1980. Review of research on reversal errors. *Perceptual and Motor Skills* 51:55–79.

Kavanagh, K., and W. Domico. 1986. High-pass digital filtration of the 40–Hz. response and its relationship to the spectral content of the middle latency and 40–Hz. responses. *Ear and Hearing* 7:93–99.

Keith, R.W. 1979. Loudness and the acoustic reflex: Cochlear-impaired listeners. *Journal of the American Auditory Society* 5:65–70.

———. 1981a. Audiological and auditory-language tests of central auditory function. In *Central auditory and language disorders in children*, ed. R.W. Keith. Houston: College-Hill Press.

———. 1981b. Tests of central auditory function. In *Auditory disorders in school children*, ed. R.J. Roeser and M.P. Downs. New York: Thieme-Stratton, Inc.

———. 1983. Interpretation of the staggered spondee word (SSW) test. *Ear and Hearing* 4:287–292.

———. 1986. *SCAN: A screening test for auditory processing disorders*. San Antonio: Psychological Corp.

———. 1988. Central auditory tests. In *Handbook of speech–language pathology, and audiology*, ed. N.J. Lass, L.V. McReynolds, and J.L. Northern. Philadelphia: B.C. Decker.

Keith, R.W., ed. 1977. *Central auditory dysfunction*. New York: Grune and Stratton.

Keith, R.W., and P. Engineer. 1991. Effects of methylphenidate on the auditory processing abilities of children with attention deficit-hyperactivity disorder. *Journal of Learning Disabilities* 24:630–636.

Keith, R.W., and S. Jerger. 1991. Central auditory disorders. In *Diagnostic audiology*, ed. J.T. Jacobson and J.L. Northern. Austin, Texas: Pro-Ed.

Keith, R.W., J. Rudy, P.A. Donahue, and B. Katbamna. 1989. Comparison of SCAN results with other auditory and language measures in a clinical population. *Ear and Hearing* 10:382–386.

Keller, W.D. 1992. Auditory processing disorder or attention-deficit disorder? In *Central auditory processing: A transdisciplinary view*, ed. J. Katz, N.A. Stecker, and D. Henderson. St. Louis: Mosby Year Book.

Kemp, D.T. 1978. Stimulated acoustic emissions from within the human auditory system. *Journal of the Acoustical Society of America* 64:1386–1391.

Kemp, D.T., P. Bray, L. Alexander, and A.M. Brown. 1986. Acoustic emission cochleography: Practical aspects. *Scandinavian Audiology Supplementum* 25:71–96.

Kemp, D.T., and S. Ryan. 1993. The use of transient evoked otoacoustic emissions in neonatal hearing screening program. *Seminars in Hearing* 14:30–45.

Kemp, D.T., S. Ryan, and P. Bray. 1990. A guide to the effective use of otoacoustic emissions. *Ear and Hearing* 11:93–105.

Kennedy, C.R., L. Kimm, D.C. Dees, P.I.P. Evans, M. Hunter, S. Lenton, and A.R.D. Thornton. 1991. Otoacoustic emissions and auditory brainstem responses in the newborn. *Archives of Disease in Childhood* 66:1124–1129.

Ketten, D.R. 1994. Differences in postmeningitic inner ear occlusions in children vs. adults. Paper presented at the Fifth Symposium on Cochlear Implants in Children, February 4–5. New York.

Kiessling, J. 1982. Hearing aid selection by brainstem audiometry. *Scandinavian Audiology* 11:269–275.

Kileny, P. 1982. Auditory brainstem responses as indicators of hearing aid performance. *Annals of Otolaryngology* 9:61–64.

———. 1991. Use of electrophysiologic measures in the management of children with cochlear implants: Brainstem, middle latency, and cognitive (P300) responses. In *Cochlear implants in children,* ed. R.T. Miyamoto and M.J. Osberger. *American Journal of Otolaryngology* (Suppl.) 12: 37–42.

———. 1994. Objective measures: Evoked potentials as indicators of auditory electrical excitability. Paper presented at the Fifth Symposium on Cochlear Implants in Children, February 4–5. New York.

Kileny, P., and J.L. Kemink. 1987. Electrically evoked middle-latency auditory potentials in cochlear implant candidates. *Archives of Otolaryngology—Head and Neck Surgery.* 113:1072–1077.

Kimura, D. 1961a. Cerebral dominance and the perception of verbal stimuli. *Canadian Journal of Psychology* 15:166–171.

———. 1961b. Some effects of temporal lobe damage on auditory perception. *Canadian Journal of Psychology* 15:157–165.

———. 1964. Left-right differences in the perception of melodies. *Quarterly Journal of Experimental Psychology* 14:355–358.

King, C., and S. Quigley. 1985. *Reading and deafness.* San Diego: College-Hill Press.

Kinsbourne, M. 1973. Minimal brain dysfunction as a neurodevelopmental lag. *Annals of the New York Academy of Sciences* 205:268–273.

Koch, H., and N.J. Dennison. 1974. *Office visits to pediatricians.* Washington, D.C.: National Center for Health Statistics.

Kodama, S., K. Tanaka, H. Konishi, K. Momota, H. Nakasako, S. Nakayama, J. Yagi, and K. Koderasawa. 1989. Supplementary thyroxine therapy in patients with hypothyroidism induced by long term anticonvulsant therapy. *Acta Paediatrica Japan* 31:555–562.

Kok, M.R., G.A. van Zanten, and M.P. Brocaar. 1992. Growth of evoked otoacoustic emissions during the first days postpartum. *Audiology* 31:140–149.

———. 1993. Aspects of spontaneous otoacoustic emissions in healthy newborns. *Hearing Research* 69:115–123.

Kok, M.R., G.A. van Zanten, M.P. Brocaar, and H.C.S. Wallenburg. 1993. Click-evoked otoacoustic emissions in 1036 ears of healthy newborns. *Audiology* 32:213–224.

Konigsmark, B.W. 1969. Hereditary deafness in man. *New England Journal of Medicine* 281:713–720, 774–778, 827–832.

Konigsmark, B., and R. Gorlin. 1976. *Genetic and metabolic deafness.* Philadelphia: W.B. Saunders.

Kraus, N., P. Kileny, and T. McGee. 1994. Middle latency auditory evoked potentials. In *Handbook of clinical audiology*, 4th ed., ed. J. Katz. Baltimore: Williams and Wilkins.

Kraus, N., and T. McGee. 1988. Color imaging of the human middle latency response. *Ear and Hearing* 9:159–167.

Kraus, N., T. McGee, A. Micco, A. Sharma, T. Carrell, and T. Nicol. 1993. Mismatch negativity in school-age children to speech stimuli that are just perceptibly different. *Electroencephalography and Clinical Neurophysiology* 88:123–130.

Kraus, N., T. McGee, A. Sharma, T. Carrell, and T. Nicol. 1992. Mismatch negativity event-related potential elicited by speech stimuli. *Ear and Hearing* 13:158–164.

Kraus, N., O. Ozdamar, L. Stein, and N. Reed. 1984. Absent auditory brain stem response: Peripheral hearing loss or brain stem dysfunction? *Laryngoscope* 94:400–406.

Kraus, N., N. Reed, I. Smith, L. Stein, and C. Cartee. 1987. High-pass filter settings affect the detectability of MLRs in humans. *Electroencephalography and Clinical Neurophysiology* 68:234–236.

Kretschmer, R., and L. Kretschmer. 1978. *Language development and intervention with the hearing impaired.* Baltimore: University Park Press.

Kreul, J., J. Nixon, K. Kryter, D. Bell, S. Lang, and E. Schubert. 1968. A proposed clinical test of speech discrimination. *Journal of Speech and Hearing Research* 11:536–552.

Kubler-Ross, E. 1969. *On death and dying.* New York: Macmillan.

———. 1974. *Questions and answers on death and dying.* New York: Collier Books.

Kuhl, P.K., and J.D. Miller. 1975. Speech perception in early infancy: Discrimination of speech-sound changes. *Journal of the Acoustical Society of America* (Suppl. 1) 58:566.

Kurdziel, S., D. Noffsinger, and W. Olsen. 1976. Performance by cortical lesion patients on 40% and 60% time-compressed materials. *Journal of the American Audiological Society* 2:3–7.

Kurtzberg, D., H.G. Vaughan, Jr., C.M. McCarton-Daum, B.A. Grellong, S. Albin, and L. Rotkin. 1979. Neurobehavioral performance of low birth weight infants at 40 weeks conceptional age: Comparison with normal full-term infants. *Developmental Medicine and Child Neurology* 21:590–607.

Kutnik, L. 1993. *Surviving the '90s: A primer.* AAP conference, La Jolla, Calif.

Kyle, J., and B. Woll. 1985. *Sign language: The study of deaf people and their language.* Cambridge: Cambridge University Press.

Lafrenière, D., M.D. Jung, J. Smurzynski, G. Leonard, D.O. Kim, and J. Sasek. 1991. Distortion-product and click-evoked otoacoustic emissions in healthy newborns. *Archives of Otolaryngology: Head and Neck Surgery* 117:1382–1389.

Lane, H. 1988. Is there a "psychology of the deaf"? *Exceptional Children* 55:7–19.

————. 1992. *The mask of benevolence.* New York: Alfred A. Knopf.

Lane, H., B. Brauer, L. Fleischer, J. Groode, N. Marbury, and M. Schwartz. 1991. Cochlear implants in children: A position paper of the National Association of the Deaf. *NAD Broadcaster* (March).

Lane, R., M. Mendel, G. Kupperman, M. Vivion, L. Buchanan, and R. Goldstein. 1974. Phase distortion of the AER imposed by analog filtering. *Archives of Otolaryngology* 99:428–432.

Langford, S.E., and W.L. Faires. 1973. Objective evaluation of monaural vs. binaural amplification for congenitally hard-of-hearing children. *Journal of Auditory Research* 13:263–267.

Lary, S., G. Briassoulis, L. deVries, L. Dubowitz, and V. Dubowitz. 1985. Hearing threshold in preterm and term infants by auditory brainstem response. *Journal of Pediatrics* 107:593–599.

Lashley, K.S. 1951. The problem of serial order in behavior. In *Cerebral mechanisms in behavior,* ed. L.A. Jeffress. New York: Wiley.

Lasky, E.Z., and J. Katz, eds. 1983. *Central auditory processing disorders.* Baltimore: University Park Press.

Lasky, E.Z., and H. Tobin. 1973. Linguistic and nonlinguistic competing message effects. *Journal of Learning Disabilities* 6:243–250.

Lasky, R., J. Perlman, and K. Hecox. 1992. Distortion-product otoacoustic emissions in human newborns and adults. *Ear and Hearing* 13:430–441.

Laureau, E., M. Vanasse, R. Hebert, J. Letarte, J. Glorieux, M. Desjardins, and J. Dussault. 1986. Somatosensory evoked potentials and auditory brain-stem responses in congenital hypothyroidism. I: A longitudinal study before and after treatment in six infants detected in the neonatal period. *Electroencephalography and Clinical Neurophysiology* 64:501–510.

Lemieux, G., and J. Neemeh. 1967. Charcot-Marie-Tooth disease and nephritis. *Canadian Medical Association Journal* 97:1193–1198.

Letter to P.J. Seiler, 20 IDELR 1216 OSEP 1993. 1994. Individuals with Disabilities Education Law Report. p. 1216–1217.

Levine, E. 1960. *The psychology of deafness: Techniques of appraisal for rehabilitation.* New York: Columbia University Press.

————. 1981. *The ecology of early deafness: Guides to fashioning environments and psychological assessment.* New York: Columbia University Press.

Levine, M.D., W.B. Carey, and A.C. Crocker. 1992. *Developmental-behavioral pediatrics.* Philadelphia: W.B. Saunders.

Levitt, H. 1989. Speech and hearing in communication. In *The handbook of special education: Research and practice.* Vol. 3, ed. M. Wang, M. Reynolds, and H. Waldberg. Oxford: Pergamon Press.

Lewis, M., and S. Goldberg. 1969. The acquisition and violation of expectancy: An experimental paradigm. *Journal of Experimental Psychology* 1:75–86.

Liberman, A. 1970. The grammars of speech and language. *Cognitive Psychology* 1:301.

Lidén, G., and E.R. Harford. 1985. The pediatric audiologist: From magician to clinician. *Ear and Hearing* 6:6–9.

Lidén, G., and A. Kankkunen. 1969. Visual reinforcement audiometry. *Acta Oto-Laryngologica* 67:281–292.

Linden, A. 1964. Distorted speech and binaural speech resynthesis tests. *Acta Oto-Laryngologica* 58:32–48.

Lindsay, J., F. Black, and W. Donnelly. 1975. Acrocephalo-syndactyly Apert's syndrome: Temporal bone findings. *Annals of Otolaryngology* 84:174–178.

Lindsay, J.R., and W.G. Hemenway. 1954. Inner ear pathology due to measles. *Annals of Otology, Rhinology, and Laryngology* 263:754–771.

Ling, D. 1976. *Speech and the hearing impaired child: Theory and practice.* Washington, D.C.: Alexander Graham Bell Association.

———. 1978. Auditory coding and recoding: An analysis of auditory training procedures for hearing impaired children. In *Auditory management of hearing impaired children*, ed. M. Ross and T. Giolas. Baltimore: University Park Press.

———., ed. 1984. *Early intervention of hearing impaired children: Total communication options.* San Diego: College-Hill Press.

Lipsitt, L.P., and J.S. Werner. 1981. The infancy of human learning processes. In *Developmental plasticity: Behavioral and biological aspects of variations in development*, ed. E.S. Gollin. New York: Academic Press.

Lochner, J., and J. Burger. 1961. The intelligibility of speech under reverberant conditions. *Acustica* 11:195–200.

Locke, J.L. 1978. Phonemic effects in the silent reading of hearing and deaf students. *Cognition* 6:185–187.

Lonsbury-Martin, B.L., F.P. Harris, B.B. Stagner, M.D. Hawkins, and G.K. Martin. 1990. Distortion-product emissions in humans: II. Relations to stimulated and spontaneous emissions and acoustic immittance in normally hearing subjects. *Annals of Otology, Rhinology, and Laryngology* (Suppl. 147) 99:14–28.

Lonsbury-Martin, B.L., G.K. Martin, M.J. McCoy, and M.L. Whitehead. 1994. Otoacoustic emissions testing in young children: Middle-ear influences. *American Journal of Otology* (Suppl. 1) 15:13–20.

Los Angeles County, Office of the Los Angeles County Superintendent of Schools, Audiology Services, and Southwest School for the Hearing Impaired. 1980. *Test of auditory comprehension.* North Hollywood: Forworks.

Lubert, N. 1981. Auditory perceptual impairments in children with specific language disorders. *Journal of Speech and Hearing Disorders* 46:3–9.

Luce, P. 1986. Neighborhoods of words in the mental lexicon: Research on speech perception. Technical Report no. 6. Bloomington: Indiana University Department of Psychology, Speech Research Laboratory.

Lukas, R.A., and J. Guenchur-Lukas. 1985. Spondaic word tests. In *Handbook of clinical audiology*, 3d ed., ed. J. Katz. Baltimore: Williams and Wilkins.

Lurquin, P., P. Magera, S. Hassid, and D. Hennebert. 1989. Evolution du seuil auditif durant les premiers mois de la vie liee aux modifications de la physiologie du conduit auditif externe. [Development of the auditory threshold during the first months of life related to modifications of the physiology of the external auditory canal]. *Acta Otorhinolaryngologica Belgica* 43:417–426.

Luterman, D. 1984. *Counseling the communicatively disordered and their families.* Boston: Little, Brown and Co.

———. 1987. *Deafness in the family.* Boston: Little, Brown and Co.

Luxford, W.M., and D.E. Brackmann. 1985. The history of cochlear implants. In *Cochlear implants*, ed. R.F. Gray. San Diego: College-Hill Press.

Luxford, W.M., and W.F. House. 1985. Cochlear implants in children: Medical and surgical considerations. *Ear and Hearing* (Suppl) 6:20S–23S.

Lynn, G.E., and J. Gilroy. 1972. Neuroaudiological abnormalities in patients with temporal lobe tumors. *Journal of Neurological Sciences* 17:167–184.

———. 1975. Effects of brain lesions on the perception of monotic and dichotic speech stimuli. In *Proceedings of symposium on central auditory processing disorders*, ed. H. Sullivan. Omaha: University of Nebraska Medical Center.

———. 1977. Evaluation of central auditory dysfunction in patients with neurological disorders. In *Central auditory dysfunction*, ed. R.W. Keith. New York: Grune and Stratton.

Lynn, G.E., J. Gilroy, P.C. Taylor, and R.P. Leiser. 1981. Binaural masking-level differences in neurological disorders. *Archives of Otolaryngology* 107:357–362.

Madell, J.R. 1990. Audiological evaluation. In *Hearing-impaired children in the mainstream*, ed. M.Ross. Parkton, Md.: York Press.

———. 1992a. FM systems as primary amplification for children with profound hearing loss. *Ear and Hearing* 13: 102–107.

———. 1992b. FM systems for children birth to age five. In *FM auditory training systems: Characteristics, selections, and use*, ed. M.A.Ross. Timonium, Md.: York Press.

Mangham, C.A., W.M. Luxford, T.J. Balkany, F.O. Black, N.L. Cohen, B.J. Gantz, M.S. Hirshorn, J.L. House, S.A. Martinez, R.E. Mischke, R.T. Miyamoto, M. Novak, and J.J. Shea. 1986. Cochlear prosthesis surgery in children. In *Cochlear implants in children*, ed. D.J. Mecklenburg. *Seminars in Hearing* 7:361–369.

Manning, W., K. Johnston, and D. Beasley. 1977. The performance of children with auditory perceptual disorders on a time-compressed speech discrimination measure. *Journal of Speech and Hearing Disorders* 42:77–84.

Margolis, R.H., and J.W. Heller. 1987. Screening tympanometry: Criteria for medical referral. *Audiology* 26:197–208.

Margolis, R.H., and J.E. Shanks. 1985. Tympanometry. In *Handbook of clinical audiology*, 2d ed., ed. J. Katz. Baltimore: Williams and Wilkins.

Marquis, S.M., and S.H. Long. 1992. Uninsured children and national health care reform. *Journal of the American Medical Association* 268:3473–3477.

Marslen-Wilson, W.D. 1987. Functional parallelism in spoken word-recognition. *Cognition* 25:71–102.

Martin, F.N., and G.W. Brunette. 1980. Loudness and the acoustic reflex. *Ear and Hearing* 1:106–108.

Martin, F.N., and J.G. Clark. 1977. Audiologic detection of auditory processing disorders in children. *Journal of the American Audiology Society* 3:140–146.

Martin, J.A.M. 1982. Aetiological factors relating to childhood deafness in the European community. *Audiology* 21:149–158.

Massaro, D.W. 1987. *Speech perception by ear and eye: A paradigm for psychological inquiry*. Hillsdale, N.J.: Lawrence Erlbaum.

Matkin, N.D. 1984. Early recognition and referral of hearing impaired children. *Pediatrics in Review* 6:151–156.

Matkin, N.D., and P.E. Hook. 1983. A multidisciplinary approach to central auditory evaluations. In *Central auditory processing disorders: Problems of speech, language, and learning*, ed. E.Z. Lasky and J. Katz. Baltimore: University Park Press.

Matkin, N.D., and J. Thomas. 1972. The utilization of CROS hearing aids in children. *Maico Audiological Library Series* 10:8.

Matzker, J. 1959. Two methods for the assessment of central auditory functions in cases of brain disease. *Annals of Otology, Rhinology, and Laryngology* 68:1155–1197.

———. 1962. The binaural test. *International Audiology* 1:209–211.

Mauk, G.W., K.R. White, L.B. Mortenson, and T.R. Behrens. 1991. The effectiveness of screening programs based on high risk characteristics in early identification of hearing impairment. *Ear and Hearing* 8:217–221.

Maurizi, M., G. Almadori, L. Cagini, E. Molini, F. Ottaviani, G. Paludetti, and F. Pierri. 1986. Auditory brainstem responses in the full-term newborn: Changes in the first 58 hours of life. *Audiology* 25:239–247.

Maurizi, M., F. Ottaviani, G. Paludetti, and S. Lungarotti. 1985. Audiological findings in Down's children. *International Journal of Pediatric Otorhinolaryngology* 9:227–232.

Maxon, A.B. 1981. Binaural amplification of young children: A clinical application of Ross's theory. *Ear and Hearing* 2:215–219.

Maxon, A.B., and I. Hochberg. 1982. Development of psychoacoustic behavior: Sensitivity and discrimination. *Ear and Hearing* 3:301–308.

McAfee, M.C., J.F. Kelly, and V.J. Samar. 1990. Spoken and written English errors of post-secondary students with severe hearing impairment. *Journal of Speech and Hearing Disorders* 55:528–634.

McCall, R.B. 1983. A conceptual approach to early mental development. In *Origins of intelligence*, ed. M. Lewis. New York: Plenum Press.

McClelland, J.L., and J.L. Elman. 1986. The TRACE model of speech perception. *Cognitive Psychology* 18:1–86.

McClellend, R., and B. Sayers. 1984. Evaluation of the cross correlation method for detection of auditory threshold for brainstem auditory evoked potentials. In *Evoked potentials II*, The Second International Evoked Potentials Symposium, ed. R.H. Nodar and C. Barber. Boston: Butterworth.

McConnell, P., and M. Berry. 1981. The effect of refeeding after neonatal starvation on Purkinje cell dendritic growth in the rat. *Journal of Comparative Neurology* 178:759–772.

McCormick, B. 1993. Behavioural hearing tests 6 months to 3; 6 years. In *Paediatric audiology, 0–5 years*, ed. B. McCormick. 2d ed. London: Whurr Publishers, Ltd.

McCormick, B., ed. 1993. *Paediatric audiology: 0–5 years*, 2d ed. London: Whurr Publishers, Ltd.

McDermott, H.J., C.M. McKay, and A.E. Vandali. 1992. A new portable sound processor for the University of Melbourne-Nucleus limited multielectrode cochlear implant. *Journal of the Acoustical Society of America* 91:3367–3371.

McFarland, W., M. Vivion, and R. Goldstein. 1977. Middle components of the AER to tone-pips in normal-hearing and hearing-impaired subjects. *Journal of Speech and Hearing Research* 20:781–798.

McKay, C.M., and H.J. McDermott. 1993. Perceptual performance of subjects with cochlear implants using the spectral maxima sound processor (SMSP) and the mini speech processor (MSP). *Ear and Hearing* 14:350–367.

McKay, C.M., H.J. McDermott, A.E. Vandali, and G.M. Clark. 1991. Preliminary results with a six spectral maxima sound processor for the University of Melbourne-Nucleus multiple-electrode cochlear implant. *Journal of the Otolaryngological Society of Australia* 6:354–359.

McKay, C.M., H.J. McDermott, A.E. Vandali, and G.M. Clark. 1992. A comparison of speech perception of cochlear implantees using the spectral maxima sound processor (SMSP) and the MSP (MULTIPEAK) processor. *Acta Otolaryngologica* 112:752–761.

McMillan, P.M., M.J. Bennett, C.D. Marchant, and P. Shurin. 1985. Ipsilateral and contralateral acoustic reflexes in neonates. *Ear and Hearing* 6:320–324.

McPherson, B., and C.A. Holborow. 1985. A study of deafness in West Africa: The Gambian hearing health project. *International Journal of Pediatric Otorhinolaryngology* 10:115–135.

McPherson, D., R. Amlie, and E. Foltz. 1985. Auditory brainstem response in infant hydrocephalus. *Child's Nervous System* 1:70–76.

McPherson, D., and N. Clark. 1983. ABR in hearing aid utilization: Simulated deafness. *Hearing Instruments* 34:12–15, 66.

McRandle, C., M. Smith, and R. Goldstein. 1974. Early averaged electroencephalic responses to clicks in neonates. *Annals of Otology, Rhinology, and Laryngology* 83:695–702.

Meadow-Orlans, K. 1990. Research in developmental aspects of deafness. In *Educational and developmental aspects of deafness*, ed. D. Moores and K. Meadow-Orlans. Washington, D.C.: Gallaudet University Press.

Mecklenburg, D.J., M.E. Demorest, and S.J. Staller. 1991. Scope and design of the clinical trial of the Nucleus multichannel cochlear implant in children. In *Multichannel cochlear implants in children*, ed. S.J. Staller. *Ear and Hearing* (Suppl) 12(4):10S–14S.

Mecklenburg, D.J., and E. Lehnhardt. 1991. The development of cochlear implants in Europe, Asia, and Australia. In *Cochlear implants: A practical guide*, ed. H. Cooper. London: Whurr Publishers Ltd.

Mecklenburg, D.J., and J.K. Shallop. 1988. Cochlear implants. In *Handbook of speech-language pathology and audiology*, ed. N.J. Lass, L.V. McReynolds, J.L. Northern, and D.E. Yoder. Toronto: B.C. Decker.

Mencher, G.T. 1985. Hearing screening programs and identification of central auditory disorders. *Human Communication* 9:45–49.

Mencher, G.T., B. McCullouch, A.J. Derbyshire, and R. Dethlefs. 1977. Observer bias as a factor in neonatal hearing screening. *Journal of Speech and Hearing Research* 20:27–34.

Mendel, M. 1985. Middle and late auditory evoked potentials. In *Handbook of clinical audiology*, 3d ed., ed. J. Katz. Baltimore: Williams and Wilkins.

Mendel, M., C. Adkinson, and L. Harker. 1977. Middle components of the evoked potentials in infants. *Annals of Otology, Rhinology, and Laryngology* 86:293–300.

Mendel, M., and R. Goldstein. 1971. Early components of the averaged electroencephalic response to constant level clicks during all-night sleep. *Journal of Speech and Hearing Research* 14:829–840.

Mendelson, T., and A. Salamy. 1981. Maturational effects on the middle components of the averaged electroencephalic response. *Journal of Speech and Hearing Research* 24:140–144.

Metz, O. 1946. The acoustic impedance measured on normal and pathologic ears. *Acta Oto-Laryngologica* (Suppl. 63):1–254.

Meyerhoff, W.L., and S.L. Liston. 1991. Metabolic hearing loss. In *Otolaryngology*, 3d ed., ed. M.M. Paparella et al. Philadelphia: W.B. Saunders.

Mikhael, M.A., I.S. Ciric, and A.P. Wolff. 1987. MR diagnosis of acoustic neuromas. *Journal of Computer Assisted Tomography* 11:232–235.

Milner, B., S. Taylor, and R. Sperry. 1968. Lateralized suppression of dichotically presented digits after commissural section in man. *Science* 161:184–185.

Miyamoto, R.T., M.J. Osberger, S.L. Todd, and A.M. Robbins. 1993. Speech perception skills of children with multichannel cochlear implants. Paper presented at the Third International Cochlear Implant Conference, April 4–7. Innsbruck, Austria.

Moog, J., and A. Geers. 1979. *Grammatical analysis of elicited language: Simple sentence level.* St. Louis: Central Institute for the Deaf.

———. 1980. *Grammatical analysis of elicited language: Complex sentence level.* St. Louis: Central Institute for the Deaf.

———. 1990. *Early speech perception test for profoundly hearing-impaired children.* St. Louis: Central Institute for the Deaf.

Moore, E. 1983. *Bases of auditory brain-stem evoked responses.* New York: Grune and Stratton.

Moore, J.M., G. Thompson, and M. Thompson. 1975. Auditory localization of infants as a function of reinforcement conditions. *Journal of Speech and Hearing Disorders* 40:29–34.

Moore, J.M., W.R. Wilson, and G. Thompson. 1977. Visual reinforcement of head-turn responses in infants under 12 months of age. *Journal of Speech and Hearing Disorders* 42:328–334.

Moores, D.F. 1987. *Educating the deaf: Psychology, principles, and practices.* 3d ed. Boston: Houghton Mifflin.

———. 1991. The great debate: Where, how and what to teach deaf children. *American Annals of the Deaf* 135:35–37.

Moores, D.F., B. Cerney, and M. Garcia. 1990. School placement and least restrictive environment. In *Educational and developmental aspects of deafness*, ed. D.F. Moores and K. Meadow-Orlans. Washington, D.C.: Gallaudet University Press.

Morales-García, C., and J.O. Poole. 1972. Masked speech audiometry in central deafness. *Acta Oto-Laryngologica* 74:307–316.

Morest, D.K. 1983. Degeneration in the brain following noise exposure. In *New perspectives in noise induced hearing loss*, ed. R.P. Hammernik, D. Henderson, and R.J. Salvi. New York: Raven Press.

Morgan, D., M. Zimmerman, and J. Dubno. 1987. Auditory brainstem evoked response characteristics in the full-term newborn. *Annals of Otology, Rhinology, and Laryngology* 96:142–151.

Morse, P.A. 1972. The discrimination of speech and non-speech stimuli in early infancy. *Journal of Experimental Child Psychology* 14:477–492.

Moses, K.L. 1985. Infant deafness and parental grief: Psychosocial early intervention. In *Education of the hearing-impaired child*, ed. F. Powell, T. Fenitzo-Hieber, S.F. Friel-Patti, and D. Henderson. San Diego: College-Hill Press.

Moses, K.L., and M. Van Hecke-Wulatin. 1981. The socioemotional impact of infant deafness. In *Early management of hearing loss*, ed. G.T Mencher and S.E. Gerber. New York: Grune and Stratton.

Mott, J.B., S.T. Norton, S.T. Neely, and B. Warr. 1989. Changes in spontaneous otoacoustic emissions produced by acoustic stimulation of the contralateral ear. *Hearing Research* 38:229–242.

Moulin, A., L. Collet, and R. Duclaux. 1993. Contralateral auditory stimulation alters acoustic distortion products in humans. *Hearing Research* 65:193–210.

Mueller, H.G. 1986. Binaural amplification: Attitudinal factors. *The Hearing Journal* 39:7–10.

Mueller, H.G., W.G. Beck, and R.K. Sedge. 1987. Comparison of the efficiency of cortical level speech tests. *Seminars in Hearing* 8:279–298.

Mueller, H.G., and D.B. Hawkins. 1990. Three important considerations in hearing aid selection. In *Handbook of hearing aid amplification*, ed. R. Sandlin. Boston: College-Hill Press.

Mueller, H.G., D. Hawkins, and J. Northern. 1992. *Probe microphone measurements: Hearing aid selection and assessment*. San Diego: Singular Publishing Group.

Muir, D., W. Abraham, B. Forbes, and L. Harris. 1979. The ontogenesis of an auditory localization response from birth to four months of age. *Canadian Journal of Psychology* 33: 320–333.

Muir, D., and J. Field. 1979. Newborn infants orient to sounds. *Child Development* 50: 431–436.

Musiek, F.E. 1983a. Assessment of central auditory dysfunction: The dichotic digit test revisited. *Ear and Hearing* 4:79–83.

———. 1983b. The evaluation of brainstem disorders using ABR and central auditory tests. *Monographs in Contemporary Audiology* 4:1–24.

———. 1983c. The results of three dichotic speech tests on subjects with intracranial lesions. *Ear and Hearing* 4:318–323.

———. 1989. Probing brain function with acoustic stimuli. *Asha* 31: 100–108.

Musiek, F.E., and J.A. Baran. 1987. Central auditory assessment: Thirty years of challenge and change. *Ear and Hearing* 8:22–35.

Musiek, F.E., J.A. Baran, and M.L. Pinheiro. 1990. Duration pattern recognition in normal subjects and patients with cerebral and cochlear lesions. *Audiology* 29:304–313.

———. 1992. P300 results in patients with lesions of the auditory areas of the cerebrum. *Journal of the American Academy of Audiology* 3:5–15.

Musiek, F.E., and G.D. Chermak. 1994. Three commonly asked questions about central auditory processing disorders: Assessment. *American Journal of Audiology* 3:23–27.

———. 1995. Three commonly asked questions about central auditory processing disorders: Management. *American Journal of Audiology* 4:15–18.

Musiek, F.E., and N.A. Geurkink. 1980. Auditory perceptual problems in children: Considerations for the otolaryngologist and audiologist. *Laryngoscope* 90:962–971.

———. 1982. Auditory brainstem response (ABR) and central auditory test (CAT) findings for patients with brainstem lesions: A preliminary report. *Laryngoscope* 92:891–900.

Musiek, F.E., N.A. Geurkink, and S. Keitel. 1982. Test battery assessment of auditory perceptual dysfunction in children. *Laryngoscope* 92:251–257.

Musiek, F.E., and K.M. Gollegly. 1988. Maturational considerations in the neuroauditory evaluation of children. In *Hearing impairment in children*, ed. F.H. Bess. Parkton, Md.: York Press.

Musiek, F.E., K.M. Gollegly, and J.A. Baran. 1984a. Myelination of the corpus callosum and auditory processing problems in learning disabled children: Theoretical and clinical correlates. *Seminars in Hearing* 5:219–242.

———. 1984b. Myelination of the corpus callosum in learning disabled children: Theoretical and clinical correlates. *Seminars in Hearing* 5:219–229.

Musiek, F.E., K.M. Gollegly, and M.K. Ross. 1985. Profiles of types of central auditory processing disorders in children with learning disabilities. *Journal of Childhood Communication Disorders* 9:43–61.

Musiek, F.E., and K. Kibbe. 1984. Audiologic test results in patients with commissurotomy. In *Epilepsy and the corpus callosum*, ed. A.G. Reeves. New York: Plenum Press.

Musiek, F.E., S. Lenz, and K. Gollegly. 1991. Neuroaudiologic correlates to anatomical changes of the brain. *American Journal of Audiology* 1:19–24.

Musiek, F.E., D. Noffsinger, R. Wilson, S. Bornstein, and C. Martinez. 1992. Tonal and speech materials for central auditory assessment. Presented at annual convention of the American Speech-Language-Hearing Association. San Antonio, Texas.

Musiek, F.E., and M.L. Pinheiro. 1985. Dichotic speech tests in the detection of central auditory dysfunction. In *Assessment of central auditory dysfunction: Foundations and clinical correlates*, ed. M.L. Pinheiro and F.E. Musiek. Baltimore: Williams and Wilkins.

———. 1987. Frequency patterns in cochlear, brainstem and cerebral lesions. *Audiology* 26:79–88.

Musiek, F.E., M.L. Pinheiro, and D.H. Wilson. 1980. Auditory pattern perception in "split brain" patients. *Archives of Otolaryngology* 106:610–612.

Musiek, F.E., S.B. Verkest, and K.M. Gollegly. 1988. Effects of neuromaturation on auditory-evoked potentials. In *Seminars in hearing*, ed. D.W. Worthington. New York: Thieme Medical Publishers.

Musiek, F.E., D.J. Weider, and R.J. Mueller. 1983. Reversible audiologic results in a patient with an extra-axial brain stem tumor. *Ear and Hearing* 4:169–172.

Musiek, F.E., and D.H. Wilson. 1979. SSW and dichotic digit results pre- and postcommissurotomy: A case report. *Journal of Speech and Hearing Disorders* 44:528–533.

Musiek, F.E., D.H. Wilson, and M.L. Pinheiro. 1979. Audiological manifestations in split-brain patients. *Journal of the American Auditory Society* 5:25–29.

Musket, C.H. 1988. Maintenance of personal hearing aids. In *Auditory disorders in school children*, 2d ed., ed. R. Roeser and M. Downs. New York: Thieme Medical Publishers.

Myklebust, H. 1964. *The psychology of deafness: Sensory deprivation, learning, and adjustment.* 2d ed. New York: Grune and Stratton.

Näätänen, R. 1992. *Attention and brain function.* Hillsdale, NJ: Lawrence Erlbaum and Associates.

Nabalek, A., and L. Robinette. 1978. Influences of the precedence effect on word identification by normally hearing and hearing impaired subjects. *Journal of the Acoustical Society of America* 63:187–194.

Nadol, J.B. 1980. Hearing loss as a sequela of meningitis. *Laryngoscope* 88:739–755.

Nass, R. 1984. Case report: Recovery and reorganization after congenital unilateral brain damage. *Perceptual and Motor Skills* 59:867–874.

National Institutes of Health. 1993. Early identification of hearing impairment in infants and young children. *NIH Consensus Statement* 11:1–24. Washington, D.C.: National Institutes of Health.

Neff, W.D. 1964. Temporal pattern discrimination in lower animals and its relation to language perception in man. In *Disorders of language*, ed. A.V.S. deRueck and M. O'Connor. Boston: Little, Brown and Co.

Nevins, M.E., R.E. Kretschmer, P.M. Chute, S.A. Hellman, and S.C. Parisier. 1991. The role of an educational consultant in a pediatric cochlear implant program. *Volta Review* 93: 197–204.

Newhoff, M., M.J. Cohen, G.W. Hynd, J.J. Gonzalez, and C.A. Riccio. 1992. Etiological, educational and behavioral correlates of ADHD and language disabilities. Presented at annual convention of the American Speech-Language-Hearing Association, San Antonio, Texas.

Newton, V.E. 1985. Etiology of sensorineural hearing loss in young children. *Journal of Otology and Laryngology* (Suppl. 10):1–57.

NFME. 1994. NFME launches primary care 2000 initiative under new leadership. *Making progress: Practitioners for 2005*. Pew Health Professions Commission (spring): 1.

Niccum, N., A. Rubens, and C. Speaks. 1981. Effects of stimulus material on the dichotic listening performance of aphasic patients. *Journal of Speech and Hearing Research* 24: 526–534.

Niedermeyer, E., and F. Lopes da Silva. 1987. *Electroencephalography: Basic principles, clinical applications, and related fields*. 2d ed. Baltimore: Urban and Schwarzenberg.

Niemoeller, A. 1981. Physical concepts of speech communication in classrooms for the deaf. In *Amplification in education*, ed. F. Bess, B. Freeman, and J. Sinclair. Washington, D.C.: A.G. Bell Association for the Deaf.

Nix, G.W. 1983. How total is total communication? *Journal of the British Association of Teachers of the Deaf* 7:177–181.

Nober, E.H. 1967. Articulation of the deaf. *Exceptional Children* 33:611–621.

———. 1993. *Section IV. P.L. 99–457 and its effects on educational management of hearing impaired children*. Presented to in-service, training, research, and assistive warning device programs for the hearing impaired in Australia and New Zealand. Durham, N.H.: University of New Hampshire, International Exchange of Experts and Information in Rehabilitation.

Nober, E.H., and L.W. Nober. 1962. Speech reception thresholds and discrimination scores as a function of method of presentation and frequency response. *Journal of Auditory Research* 2:1–4.

———. 1977. Effects of hearing loss on speech and language in the post-babbling stage. In *Hearing loss in children*, ed. B. Jaffe. Baltimore: University Park Press.

Nodar, R.H., J. Hahn, and H.L. Levine. 1980. Brain stem auditory evoked potentials in determining site of lesion of brain stem gliomas in children. *Laryngoscope* 90:258–266.

Noffsinger, D. 1982. Clinical application of selected binaural effects. *Scandinavian Audiology Supplement* 15:157–165.

Noffsinger, D., C.D. Martinez, and A.B. Schaefer. 1982. Auditory brainstem responses and masking level differences from persons with brainstem lesions. *Scandinavian Audiology Supplement* 15:81–93.

Noffsinger, D., W.O. Olsen, R. Carhart, C.W. Hart, and V. Sahgal. 1972. Auditory and vestibular aberrations in multiple sclerosis. *Acta Oto-Laryngologica* (Suppl.) 303:1–63.

Norris, T.W., P.G. Stelmachowicz, and D.J. Taylor. 1974. Acoustic reflex relaxation to identify sensorineural hearing impairment. *Archives of Otolaryngology* 99:197.

Northern, J.L. 1981. Impedance measurement in infants. In *Early management of hearing loss*, ed. G.T. Mencher and S.E. Gerber. New York: Grune and Stratton.

Northern J.L., F.O. Black, J.A. Brimacombe, N.L. Cohen, L.S. Eisenberg, S.V. Kuprenas, S.A. Martinez, and R.E. Mischke. 1986. Selection of children for cochlear implantation. In *Cochlear implants in children*, ed. D.J. Mecklenburg. *Seminars in Hearing* 7:341–347.

Northern, J.L., and M.P. Downs. 1991. *Hearing in children*. 4th ed. Baltimore: Williams and Wilkins.

Northern, J.L., S.A. Gabbard, and D.L. Kinder. 1990. Pediatric consideration in selecting and fitting hearing aids. In *Handbook of hearing aid amplification*, vol. II, ed. R.E. Sandlin. Boston: College-Hill Press.

Norton, S.J. 1993. Application of transient evoked otoacoustic emissions to pediatric populations. *Ear and Hearing* 14:64–73.

———. 1994. Emerging role of evoked otoacoustic emissions in neonatal hearing screening. *American Journal of Otology* (Suppl. 1) 15:4–12.

Norton, S.J., and J.E. Widen. 1990. Evoked otoacoustic emissions in normal-hearing infants and children: Emerging data and issues. *Ear and Hearing* 11:121–127.

Nozza, R.J., C.D. Bluestone, D. Kardatzke, and R. Bachman. 1992. Toward the validation of aural acoustic immittance measures for diagnosis of middle ear effusion in children. *Ear and Hearing* 13:442–453.

Obrzut, J., G. Hynd, A. Obrzut, and F. Pirozzolo. 1981. Effects of directed attention on cerebral asymmetries in normal and learning-disabled children. *Developmental Psychology* 17:118–125.

Obrzut, J., W. Weed, and C. Hynd. 1979. Development of cerebral dominance: Dichotic listening asymmetry in normal and learning-disabled children. *Journal of Experimental Child Psychology* 28:445–454.

O'Donoghue, G.M., R.K. Jackler, W.M. Jenkins, and R.A. Schindler. 1986. Cochlear implantation in children: The problem of head growth. *Otolaryngology—Head and Neck Surgery* 94:78–81.

Ohta, F., R. Hayashi, and M. Morimoto. 1967. Differential diagnosis of retrocochlear deafness: Binaural fusion test and binaural separation test. *International Audiology* 6:58–62.

Oller, D.K., H. Jensen, and R. Lafayette. 1978. The relatedness of phonological processes of a hearing-impaired child. *Journal of Communication Disorders* 11:97–105.

Olsen, W. 1981. The effects of noise and reverberation on speech intelligibility. In *Amplification in education*, ed. F. Bess, B. Freeman, and J. Sinclair. Washington, D.C.: A.G. Bell Association for the Deaf.

Olsen, W.O., and D. Noffsinger. 1976. Masking level differences for cochlear and brain stem lesions. *Annals of Otology, Rhinology, and Laryngology* 85:820–825.

Olsen, W.O., D. Noffsinger, and R. Carhart. 1976. Masking level differences encountered in clinical populations. *Audiology* 15:287–301.

Olsen, W.O., D. Noffsinger, and S. Kurdziel. 1975a. Acoustic reflex and reflex decay: Occurrence in patients with cochlear and eighth nerve lesions. *Archives of Otolaryngology* 101:622–625.

———. 1975b. Speech discrimination in quiet and in white noise by patients with peripheral and central lesions. *Acta Oto-Laryngologica* 80:375–382.

Osberger, M.J. 1994. Auditory perception and speech production results. Paper presented at the Fifth Symposium on Cochlear Implants in Children, April 4–5, New York.

Osberger, M.J., A.M. Robbins, R.T. Miyamoto, S.W. Berry, W.A. Myres, K.S. Kessler, and M.L. Pope. 1991. Speech perception abilities of children with cochlear implants, tactile aids, or hearing aids. In *Cochlear implants in children*, ed. R.T. Miyamoto and M.J. Osberger. *American Journal of Otology* (Suppl.) 12:105–115.

Osterhammel, D., and P. Osterhammel. 1979. Age and sex variations for the normal stapedial reflex thresholds and tympanometric compliance values. *Scandinavian Audiology* 8:153–158.

Otte, J., H.F. Schuknecht, and A.G. Kerr. 1978. Ganglion cell populations in normal and pathological human cochlea: Implications for cochlear implantation. *Laryngoscope* 88: 1231–1246.

Ovesen, T., P.B. Paaske, and O. Elbrond. 1993. Accuracy of an automatic impedance apparatus in a population with secretory otitis media: Principles in the evaluation of tympanometrical findings. *American Journal of Otolaryngology* 1:100–104.

Owens, E., D.K. Kessler, M.W. Raggio, and E.D. Schubert. 1985. Analysis and revision of the minimal auditory capabilities (MAC) battery. *Ear and Hearing* 6:280–290.

Owens, J.J., M.J. McCoy, B.L. Lonsbury-Martin, and G.K. Martin. 1992. Influence of otitis media on evoked otoacoustic emissions in children. *Seminars in Hearing* 13:63–66.

———. 1993. Otoacoustic emissions in children with normal ears, middle-ear dysfunction, and ventilating tubes. *American Journal of Otology* 14:34–40.

Ozdamar, O., and N. Kraus. 1983. Auditory middle-latency responses in humans. *Audiology* 22:34–49.

Pal, J., H.L. Bhatia, B.G. Prasad, D. Dyal, and P.C. Jain. 1974. Deafness among the urban community: An epidemiological study at Lucknow UP, India. *Indian Journal of Medical Research* 62:857–868.

Palmer, C., A. Derbyshire, and A. Lee. 1966. A method for analyzing individual cortical responses to auditory stimuli. *Electroencephalography and Clinical Neurophysiology* 20: 204–206.

Pappas, D.G. 1983. A study of the high-risk registry for sensorineural hearing impairment. *Journal of Otolaryngology—Head and Neck Surgery* 91:41–4.

Paradise, J.L., C.G. Smith, and C.D. Bluestone. 1976. Tympanometric detection of middle ear effusion in infants and young children. *Pediatrics* 58:198–210.

Parke, R. 1974. *Father-infant interaction in maternal attachment and mothering disorders: A roundtable.* Sausalito, CA: Johnson and Johnson Co.

Parving, A. 1983. Epidemiology of hearing loss and aetiological diagnosis of hearing impairment in childhood. *International Journal of Pediatric Otorhinolaryngology* 5:151–165.

———. 1984. Early detection and identification of congenital/early acquired disability. Who takes the initiative? *International Journal of Pediatric Otorhinolaryngology* 7:107–117.

———. 1991. Detection of infants with congenitally acquired hearing disability. *Acta Oto-Laryngologica* (Suppl. 482):111–116.

———. 1992. Pediatric audiologic medicine: A strategy for a regular department. *Journal of Audiological Medicine* 1:99–111.

Patrick, J.F., and G.M. Clark. 1991. The Nucleus 22–channel cochlear implant system. In *Multichannel cochlear implants in children*, ed. S.J. Staller. *Ear and Hearing* (Suppl.) 12(4):3S–9S.

Paul, P., and D. Jackson. 1993. *Toward a psychology of deafness.* Boston: Allyn and Bacon.

Paul, P., and S. Quigley. 1990. *Education and deafness.* New York: Longman.

Pelson, R.O., and S.S. Budden. 1987. Auditory brainstem response findings in Rett syndrome. *Brain Development* 9:514–516.

Perez, H., J. Vilchez, T. Sevilla, and L. Martinez. 1988. Audiologic evaluation in Charcot-Marie-Tooth disease. *Scandinavian Audiology* (Suppl. 30):211–213.

Peterson, J.L., and G. Lidén. 1972. Some static characteristics of the stapedial muscle reflex. *Audiology* 11:94–114.

Pickles, J.O. 1982. *An introduction to the physiology of hearing.* New York: Academic Press.

Picton, T.W., S.A. Hillyard, H.J. Kraus, and R. Galambos. 1974. Human auditory evoked potentials, I: Evaluation of components. *Electroencephalography and Clinical Neurophysiology* 36:179–190.

Picton, T., R. Linden, G. Hamel, and J. Maru. 1983. Aspects of averaging. *Seminars in Hearing* 4:327–341.

Picton, T., K. Oulette, G. Hamel, and A. Smith. 1979. Brainstem evoked potential to tone pips in notched noise. *Journal of Otolaryngology* 8:289–314.

Picton, T.W., D.L. Woods, J. Baribeau-Braun, and T.L. Healey. 1977. Evoked potential audiometry. *Journal of Otolaryngology* 6:90–119.

Pinheiro, M.L. 1977. Tests of central auditory function in children with learning disabilities. In *Central auditory dysfunction*, ed. R.W. Keith. New York: Grune and Stratton.

Pinheiro, M.L., G.P. Jacobson, and F. Boller. 1982. Auditory dysfunction following a gunshot wound of the pons. *Journal of Speech and Hearing Disorders* 47:296–300.

Pinheiro, M.L., and F.E. Musiek. 1985. Sequencing and temporal ordering in the auditory system. In *Assessment of central auditory dysfunction: Foundations and clinical correlates*, ed. M. Pinheiro and F. Musiek. Baltimore: Williams and Wilkins.

Pinheiro, M.L., and F.E. Musiek, eds. 1985. *Assessment of central auditory dysfunction*. Baltimore: Williams and Wilkins.

Pintner, R., and D. Patterson. 1916. A measurement of the language ability of deaf children. *Psychological Review* 23:413–436.

Plinkert, P.K., G. Sesterhenn, R. Arold, and H.P. Zenner. 1990. Evaluation of otoacoustic emissions in high-risk infants by using an easy and rapid objective auditory screening method. *European Archives of Otorhinology* 247:356–360.

Plotnick, C.H., and J.G. Leppler. 1986. Infant hearing assessment: A program for identification and habilitation within four months of age. *The Hearing Journal* 39:23–25.

Pohl, P. 1979. Dichotic listening in a child recovering from acquired aphasia. *Brain and Language* 8:372–379.

Pollack, D. 1985. *Educational audiology for the limited-hearing infant and preschooler*. 2d ed. Springfield: Charles C. Thomas.

Pollack, M.C., ed. 1988. *Amplification for the hearing-impaired*. 3d ed. New York: Grune and Stratton.

Popelka, R.G., ed. 1981. *Hearing assessment with the acoustic reflex*. New York: Grune and Stratton.

Popelka, G.R., R.H. Margolis, and T.L. Wiley. 1976. Effect of activating signal bandwidth on acoustic reflex thresholds. *Journal of the Acoustical Society of America* 59:153–159.

Porter, T.A. 1974. Otoadmittance measurements in a residential deaf population. *American Annals of the Deaf* 119:47–52.

Preus, M., and G.C. Fraser. 1971. Genetics of hereditary nephropathy with deafness: Alport's syndrome. *Clinical Genetics* 2:331–333.

Prevec, T., K. Ribaric, K., and D. Butinar. 1984. Contingent negative variation audiometry in children. *Audiology* 23:114–126.

Prieve, B.A. 1992. Otoacoustic emissions in infants and children: Basic characteristics and clinical application. *Seminars in Hearing* 13:37–52.

Prieve, B.A., M.P. Gorga, A. Schmidt, S.T. Neelym, J. Peters, L. Schultes, and W. Jesteadt. 1993. Analysis of transient-evoked otoacoustic emissions in normal-hearing and hearing-impaired ears. *Journal of the Acoustical Society of America* 93:3308–3319.

Primus, M.A., and G. Thompson. 1985. Response strength of young children in operant audiometry. *Journal of Speech and Hearing Research* 28:539–547.

Probst, R., B.L. Lonsbury-Martin, and G.K. Martin. 1991. A review of otoacoustic emissions. *Journal of the Acoustical Society of America* 89:2027–2067.

Prosser, S., E. Arslan, G. Conti, and S. Michelini. 1983. Evaluation of the monaurally evoked brainstem response in the diagnosis of sensorineural hearing loss. *Scandinavian Audiology* 12:103–106.

Protti, E. 1983. Brainstem auditory pathways and auditory processing disorders: Diagnostic implications of subjective and objective tests. In *Central auditory processing disorders*, ed. E. Lasky and J. Katz. Baltimore: University Park Press.

Quenin, C.S., and I. Blood. 1989. A national survery of cued speech programs. *Volta Review* 91:283–289.

Quigley, S. 1969. *The influence of fingerspelling on the development of language, communication and educational achievement in deaf children.* Urbana: University of Illinois, Institute for Research on Exceptional Children.

Quigley S., and R. Kretschmer. 1982. *The education of deaf children: Issues, theory and practice.* Austin: Pro-Ed.

Quigley, S., and P. Paul. 1984. *Language and deafness.* San Diego: College-Hill Press.

Rackliffe, L., and F.E. Musiek. 1983. An introduction to ABR in hearing aid evaluation. *Hearing Instruments* 34:9–10.

Rapin, I. 1983. The child neurologist's contribution to the care of children with hearing loss. In *The Multiply Handicapped Hearing Impaired Child*, ed. G.T. Mencher and S.E. Gerber. New York: Grune and Stratton.

Rauschecker, J.P., and P. Marler. 1987. Cortical plasticity and imprinting: Behavioral and physiological contrasts and parallels. In *Imprinting and cortical plasticity*, ed. J.P. Rauschecker and P. Marler. New York: John Wiley.

Rayner, K., and A. Pollatsek. 1989. *The psychology of reading.* Englewood Cliffs, N.J.: Prentice-Hall.

Reagan, T. 1990. Cultural considerations in the education of deaf children. In *Educational and developmental aspects of deafness*, ed. D. Moores and K. Meadow-Orlans. Washington, D.C.: Gallaudet University Press.

Regional Resource and Federal Centers Program. 1993. *Education reforms and special education: The era of change for the future.* Plantation, Fla.: South Atlantic Regional Resource Center, Florida Atlantic University.

Rickards, F.W., S.J. Dettman, P.A. Busby, R.L. Webb, R.C. Dowell, S.E. Dennehy, and T.G. Nienhuys. 1990. Preoperative evaluation and selection of children and teenagers. In *Cochlear prostheses*, ed. G.M. Clark, Y.C. Tong, and J.F. Patrick. Edinburgh: Churchill Livingstone.

Rintelmann, W.F., and F.H. Bess. 1988. High-level amplification and potential hearing loss in children. In *Hearing impairment in children*, ed. F.H. Bess. Parkton, Md.: York Press.

Rintelmann, W.F., and G.E. Lynn. 1983. Speech stimuli for assessment of central auditory disorders. In *Principles of speech audiometry*, ed. D.F. Konkle and W.F. Rintelmann. Baltimore: University Park Press.

Robb, M., and J. Saxman. 1985. Developmental trends in vocal fundamental frequency of young children. *Journal of Speech and Hearing Research* 28:421–427.

Roberts, J.E., M.R. Burchinal, B.P. Davis, A.M. Collier, and F.W. Henderson. 1991. Otitis media in early childhood and later language. *Journal of Speech and Hearing Research* 34:1158–1168.

Robertson, D., and D.R.F. Irvine. 1989. Plasticity of frequency organization in auditory cortex of guinea pigs with partial unilateral deafness. *Journal of Comparative Neurology* 282:456–471.

Robertson, P.O., J.L. Peterson, and L.E. Lamb. 1968. Relative impedance measurements in young children. *Archives of Otolaryngology* 88:162–168.

Rodier, P.M. 1980. Chronology of neuron development: Animal studies and their clinical implications. *Developmental Medicine and Child Neurology* 22:525–545.

Roeser, R., and M. Downs. 1988. Maintenance of personal hearing aids. In *Auditory disorders in school children*, eds. R. Roeser and M. Downs. 2d ed. New York: Thieme Medical Publishers.

Roeser, R., K. Millay, and J. Morrow. 1983. Dichotic consonant-vowel (cv) perception in normal and learning-impaired children. *Ear and Hearing* 4:293–299.

Rosenberger, P., and D. Hier. 1980. Cerebral asymmetry and verbal intellectual deficits. *Annals of Neurology* 8:300–304.

Ross, M.A., ed. 1992. *FM auditory training systems: Characteristics, selections, and use.* Timonium, Md.: York Press.

Ross, M., D. Brackett, and A. Maxon. 1982. *Hard of hearing children in the regular schools.* Englewood Cliffs, N.J.: Prentice-Hall.

———. 1991. *Assessment and management of mainstreamed hearing impaired children.* Austin: Pro-Ed.

Ross, M., and T. Giolas. 1971. Effects of three classroom listening conditions on speech intelligibility. *American Annals of the Deaf* 116:580–584.

———. 1978. *Auditory management of hearing-impaired children: Principles and prerequisites for intervention.* Baltimore: University Park Press.

Ross, M., and J. Lerman. 1970. A picture identification test for hearing-impaired children. *Journal of Speech and Hearing Research* 13:44–53.

———. 1971. *Word intelligibility by picture identification.* Pittsburgh: Stanwix House.

Ross, M., and K. Randolph. 1990. A test of the auditory perception of alphabet letters for hearing impaired children: The APAL test. *The Volta Review* 92:237–244.

Roush, J., A. Drake, and J.E. Sexton. 1992. Identification of middle ear dysfunction in young children: A comparison of tympanometric screening procedures. *Ear and Hearing* 13:63–69.

Roush, J., and C.A. Tait. 1984. Binaural fusion, masking level differences, and auditory brain stem responses in children with language-learning disabilities. *Ear and Hearing* 5:37–41.

Rubel, E., D. Born, J. Deitch, and D. Durham. 1984. Recent advances toward understanding auditory system development. In *Hearing science*, ed. C. Berlin. San Diego: College-Hill Press.

Ruben, R.J. 1983. Diseases of the inner ear and sensorineural deafness. In *Pediatric otolaryngology*, vol. 1, ed. C.D. Bluestone and S.E. Stool. Philadelphia: W.B. Saunders.

———. 1991. Language screening as a factor in the management of the pediatric otolaryngic patient. *Archives of Otolaryngology—Head and Neck Surgery* 117:1021–1025.

Ruben, R.J., and I. Rapin. 1988. Management of the hearing-impaired deaf infant and child. In *Otologic medicine and surgery*, ed. P.W. Alberti and R.J. Ruben. New York: Churchill Livingstone.

Ruben, R.J., and D.L. Rozycki. 1970. Clinical aspects of genetic deafness. *Annals of Otology, Rhinology, and Laryngology* 80:255–263.

Ruben, R.J., and S.M. Yankelowitz. 1989. Spontaneous perilymphatic fistula in children. *American Journal of Otology* 10:198–207.

Rybak, L.P., and G.J. Matz. 1988. Ototoxicity. In *Otologic medicine and surgery*, ed. P.W. Alberti and R.J. Ruben. New York: Churchill Livingstone.

Sakashita, T., Y. Minowa, K. Hachikawa, T. Kubo, and Y. Nakai. 1991. Evoked otoacoustic emissions from ears with idiopathic sudden deafness. *Acta Oto-Laryngologica* (Suppl. 486):66–72.

Salamy, A., L. Eldridge, J. Anderson, and D. Bull. 1990. Brainstem transmission time in infants exposed to cocaine in utero. *The Journal of Pediatrics* 117:627–629.

Salomon, G., B. Anthonisen, J. Groth, and P.P. Thomsen. 1992. Otoacoustic hearing screening in newborns: Optimization. In *Screening children for auditory function*, ed. F.H. Bess and J.W. Hall III. Nashville: Bill Wilkerson Center Press.

Salvia, J., and J.E. Ysseldyke. 1981. *Assessment in special and remedial education*. 2d ed. Boston: Houghton Mifflin.

Sanders, D. 1965. Noise conditions in normal school classrooms. *Exceptional Children* 31:-344–353.

Sanderson-Leepa, M.E., and W.F. Rintelmann. 1976. Articulation functions and test-retest performance of normal-hearing children on three speech discrimination tests: WIPI, PBL-50, and NU Auditory Test no. 6. *Journal of Speech and Hearing Disorders* 41:503–519.

Sando, I., S. Suehiro, and R.P. Wood. 1983. Congenital anomalies of the external and middle ear. In *Pediatric otolaryngology*, ed. C.D. Bluestone and S.E. Stool. Philadelphia: W.B. Saunders.

Scarr, S., and M.L.Williams. 1971. The assessment of neonatal and later status of low birthweight infants. Presented at meeting of the Society for Research in Child Development, Minneapolis.

Schain, R. 1977. *Neurology of childhood learning disorders*. 2d ed. Baltimore: Williams and Wilkins.

Schein, J.D., and M.T. Delk. 1974. *The deaf population of the United States*. Washington, D.C.: National Association of the Deaf.

Schimmel, H. 1967. The + − reference: Accuracy of estimated mean components in average response studies. *Science* 157:92–93.

Schimmel, H., I. Rapin, and M. Cohen. 1974. Improving evoked response audiometry. *Audiology* 13:33–65.

Schindler, R.A., and D.K. Kessler. 1993. Clarion cochlear implant: Phase I investigational results. *American Journal of Otology* 14:263–272.

Schlaggar, B.L., and D.D.M. O'Leary. 1991. Potential of visual cortex to develop an array of functional units unique to somatosensory cortex. *Science* 252:1556–1560.

Schlesinger, H. 1972. A developmental model applied to problems of deafness. In *Sound and sign: Childhood deafness and mental health*, ed. H. Schlesinger and K. Meadow. Berkeley: University of California Press.

Schmitt, B.D. 1975. The minimal brain dysfunction myth. *American Journal of Diseases of Children* 129:1313–1318.

Schneider, P.K., J.A. Rich, and C. Bazell. 1989. The effect of SSPL setting on gain measurement in the soundfield in children: A pilot study. Poster session presented at MSHA Annual Conference, March.

Schulman, C.A. 1973. Heart rate audiometry. Part I. An evaluation of heart rate response to auditory stimuli in newborn hearing screening. *Neuropaediatrie* 4:362–374.

Schuyler, V., N. Rushmer, R. Arpan, A. Melum, J. Sowers, and N. Kennedy. 1985. *Parent-*

infant communication: A program of clinical and home training for parents and hearing-impaired infants. Portland, Oreg.: Infant Hearing Resource Publications.

Schwartz, S., ed. 1987. *Choices in deafness: A parent's guide*. Kensington, Md.: Woodbine House.

Schuyler, V., and N. Rushmer. 1987. *Parent-infant habilitation*. Portland: IHR Publications.

Selters, W., and D. Brackman. 1977. Acoustic tumor detection with brainstem electric response audiometry. *Archives of Otolaryngology* 103:181–187.

Shallop, J.K., A.L. Beiter, D.W. Goin, and R.E. Mischke. 1990. Electrically evoked auditory brain stem responses (EABR) and middle latency responses (EMLR) obtained from patients with the Nucleus multichannel cochlear implant. *Ear and Hearing* 11:5–15.

Shallop, J.K., and D. J. Mecklenburg. 1987. Technical aspects of cochlear implants. In *Handbook of hearing aid amplification*, ed. R.E. Sandlin. San Diego: College-Hill Press.

Shanks, J.E. 1984. Tympanometry. *Ear and Hearing* 5:268–280.

Shanks, J.E., and R.H. Wilson. 1986. Effects of direction and rate of ear-canal pressure changes on tympanometric measures. *Journal of Speech and Hearing Research* 29: 11–19.

Sharp, M., and D. Orchick. 1978. Auditory function in sickle cell anemia. *Archives of Otolaryngology* 104:322–324.

Shih, L., B. Cone-Wesson, and B. Reddix. 1988. Effects of maternal cocaine abuse on the neonatal auditory system. *International Journal of Pediatric Otorhinolaryngology* 15: 245–251.

Shimizu, H. 1992. Carhart Memorial Lecture: 1991. Childhood hearing impairment: Issues and thoughts on diagnostic approaches. *American Auditory Society Bulletin* 17: 15–37.

Shimizu, H., and F. Brown. 1981. ABR in children with MBD. Presented at annual convention of the American Speech-Language-Hearing Association, Los Angeles.

Shimizu, H., H. Moser, and S. Naidu. 1989. Auditory brainstem response and audiologic findings in adrenoleukodystrophy: Its variant and carrier. *Otolaryngology—Head and Neck Surgery* 98:215–220.

Siegenthaler, B., and G. Haspiel. 1966. *Development of two standardized measures of hearing for speech by children*. Cooperative research program project #2372. Washington, D.C.: United States Office of Education.

Silman, S. 1976. The growth function of the stapedius reflex in normal ears and ears with hearing loss due to cochlear dysfunction. Ph.D. diss., New York University, New York.

———. 1988. The applicability of the modified bivariate plotting procedure to subjects with functional hearing loss. *Scandinavian Audiology* 17:125–127.

———. 1990. Detection of middle-ear effusion. Short course presented at Annual Convention of the American Speech-Language-Hearing Association, Seattle.

Silman, S., and S.A. Gelfand. 1979. The effects of aging on the acoustic reflex thresholds. *Journal of the Acoustical Society of America* 66:735–738.

———. 1981. The relationship between magnitude of hearing loss and acoustic reflex threshold levels. *Journal of Speech and Hearing Disorders* 46:312–316.

Silman, S., S.A. Gelfand, and T.H. Chun. 1978. Some observations in a case of acoustic neuroma. *Journal of Speech and Hearing Disorders* 43:459–466.

Silman, S., S.A. Gelfand, J.C. Howard, and T.J. Showers. 1982. Clinical application of the bivariate plotting procedure in the prediction of hearing loss with the bivariate plotting procedure. *Journal of Speech and Hearing Research* 27:12–19.

Silman, S., S.A. Gelfand, N. Piper, C.A. Silverman, and L. Van Frank. 1984. Prediction of hearing loss from the acoustic reflex threshold. In *The acoustic reflex: Basic principles and clinical applications*, ed. S. Silman. New York: Academic Press.

Silman, S., G.R. Popelka, and S.A. Gelfand. 1978. Effect of sensorineural hearing loss on acoustic stapedius reflex growth functions. *Journal of the Acoustical Society of America* 64:1406–1411.

Silman, S., and C.A. Silverman. 1991. *Auditory diagnosis: Principles and applications*. San Diego: Academic Press.

Silman, S., C.A. Silverman, and D.S. Arick. 1992. Acoustic-immittance screening for detection of middle-ear effusion in children. *Journal of the American Academy of Audiology* 3:262–268.

———. 1994. Pure-tone assessment and screening of children with middle-ear effusion. *Journal of the American Academy of Audiology*. 5:173–182.

Silman, S., C.A. Silverman, S.A. Gelfand, J. Lutolf, and D.J. Lynne. 1988. Ipsilateral acoustic-reflex adaptation testing for detection of facial-nerve pathology: Three case studies. *Journal of Speech and Hearing Disorders* 53:378–382.

Silman, S., C.A. Silverman, T.J. Showers, and S.A. Gelfand. 1984. The effect of age on prediction of hearing loss with the bivariate plotting procedure. *Journal of Speech and Hearing Research* 27:12–19.

Silverman, C.A., S. Silman, and M.H. Miller. 1983. The acoustic reflex threshold in aging ears. *Journal of the Acoustical Society of America* 73:248–255.

Simmons, F.B. 1966. Electrical stimulation of the auditory nerve in man. *Archives of Otolaryngology* 84:2–54.

Sininger, Y. 1993. Auditory brain stem response for objective measures of hearing. *Ear and Hearing* 14:23–30.

Skinner, M.W. 1988. *Hearing aid evaluation*. Englewood Cliffs, N.J.: Prentice Hall.

Skinner, M.W., G.M. Clark, L.A. Whitford, P.M. Seligman, S.J. Staller, D.B. Shipp, J.K. Shallop, C. Everingham, C.M. Menapace, P.L. Arndt, T. Antogenelli, J.A. Brimacombe, S. Pijl, P. Daniels, C.R. George, H.J. McDermott, and A.L. Beiter. 1994. Evaluation of a new spectral peak coding strategy for the Nucleus 22 channel cochlear implant system. *American Journal of Otolaryngology* 15 (Suppl. 2): 15–27.

Skinner, M.W., L.K. Holden, T.A. Holden, R.C. Dowell, P.M. Seligman, J.A. Brimacombe, and A.L. Beiter. 1991. Performance of postlinguistically deaf adults with the wearable speech processor (WSPIII) and mini speech processor (MSP) of the Nucleus multielectrode cochlear implant. *Ear and Hearing* 12:3–22.

Sloan, C. 1980a. Auditory processing disorders and language development. In *Auditory processing and language: Clinical and research perspectives*, ed. P.J. Levinson and C. Sloan, 101–115. New York: Grune and Stratton.

———. 1980b. Auditory processing disorders in children: Diagnosis and treatment. In *Auditory processing and language: Clinical and research perspectives*, ed. P.J. Levinson and C. Sloan 117–133. New York: Grune and Stratton.

Smith, D.W. 1981. *Recognizable patterns of human deformation*. Philadelphia: W.B. Saunders.

Smith, G.A., and R.A. Gussen. 1976. Inner ear pathology following mumps infection: Report of a case in an adult. *Archives of Otolaryngology* 102:108–111.

Smith, P.S.U., T.L. Wiley, and G.M. Pyle. 1993. Efficacy of ASHA guidelines for screening middle-ear function in children. Poster session presented at the Annual Convention of the American Speech-Language-Hearing Association. November, Anaheim.

Smoski, W.J. 1990. Use of CHAPPS in a children's audiology clinic. *Ear and Hearing* (Suppl.) 11:53–56.

Smoski, W.J., M.A. Brunt, and C. Tannahill. 1992. Listening characteristics of children with central auditory processing disorders. *Language, Speech, and Hearing Services in Schools* 23:145–152.

Smurzynski, J., M.D. Jung, D. Lafrenière, D.O. Kim, M.V. Kamath, J.C. Rowe, M.C. Holman, and G. Leonard. 1993. Distortion-product and click-evoked otoacoustic emissions of preterm and full-term infants. *Ear and Hearing* 14:258–274.

Sobhy, O. 1993. Frequency specificity of the auditory middle latency response. Ph.D. diss., Memphis State University.

Sobhy, O., and H. Gould. 1993. Interaural attenuation using insert earphones: Electrocochleographic approach. *Journal of the American Academy of Audiology* 4:76–79.

Sohmer, H., and M. Student. 1978. Auditory nerve and brainstem evoked responses in normal, autistic, minimal brain dysfunction and psychomotor retarded children. *Electroencephalography and clinical neurophysiology* 44:380–388.

Solnit, S. 1961. Mourning and the birth of a defective child. *Psychoanalytic Study of the Child,* Monograph #16.

Sommers, R.K., and M.L. Taylor. 1972. Cerebral speech dominance in language-disordered and normal children. *Cortex* 8:224–232.

Sparks, R., and N. Geschwind. 1968. Dichotic listening in man after section of neocortical commissures. *Cortex* 4:3–16.

Speaks, C., T. Gray, J. Miller, and A. Rubens. 1975. Central auditory deficits and temporal-lobe lesions. *Journal of Speech and Hearing Disorders* 40:192–205.

Speaks, C., and J. Jerger. 1965. Method for measurement of speech identification. *Journal of Speech and Hearing Research* 8:185–194.

Speaks, C., N. Niccum, and D. van Tassel. 1985. Effects of stimulus material on the dichotic listening performance of patients with sensorineural hearing loss. *Journal of Speech and Hearing Research* 18:16–25.

Spektor, Z., G. Leonard, D.O. Kim, M.D. Jung, and J. Smurzynski. 1991. Otoacoustic emissions in normal and hearing-impaired children and normal adults. *Laryngoscope* 101: 965–976.

Sprague, B.H., T.L. Wiley, and R. Goldstein. 1985. Tympanometric and acoustic reflex studies in neonates. *Journal of Speech and Hearing Research* 28:265–272.

Squires, K., and K. Hecox. 1983. Electrophysiological evaluation of higher level auditory processing. *Seminars in Hearing* 4:415–432.

Stach, B.A. 1992. Controversies in the screening of central auditory processing disorders. In *Screening children for auditory function,* ed. F.H. Bess and J.W. Hall III. Nashville: Bill Wilkerson Center Press.

Stach, B.A., L.H. Loiselle, and J.F. Jerger. 1988. Auditory evoked potential abnormalities in children with central auditory disorder. *Asha* 30:133 (abstract).

Stach, B., W. Stoner, S. Smith, and J. Jerger. 1994. Auditory evoked potentials in Rett syndrome. *Journal of the American Academy of Audiology* 5:226–230.

Staller, S.J. 1985. Cochlear implant characteristics: A review of current technology. In *Cochlear implants,* ed. G.A. McCandless. *Seminars in Hearing* 23–32.

Staller, S.J., A.L. Beiter, and J.A. Brimacombe. 1991. Children and multichannel cochlear implants. In *Cochlear implants: A practical guide,* ed. H. Cooper. London: Whurr Publishers Ltd.

Staller, S.J., R.C. Dowell, A.L. Beiter, and J.A. Brimacombe. 1991. Perceptual abilities of children with the Nucleus 22-channel cochlear implant. In *Multichannel cochlear implants in children*, ed. S.J. Staller. *Seminars in Hearing* (Suppl.) 12(4): 34S–47S.

Steele, M.W. 1981. Genetics of congenital deafness. *Pediatric Clinics of North America* 28: 973–980.

Stein, L., S. Clark, and N. Kraus. 1983. The hearing-impaired infant: Patterns of identification and habilitation. *Ear and Hearing* 4:232–236.

Stein, L., T. Jabaley, R. Spitz, D. Stoakley, and T. McGee. 1990. The hearing-impaired infant: Patterns of identification and habilitation revisited. *Ear and Hearing* 11:128–133.

Stephens, S., and A. Thornton. 1976. Subjective and electrophysiologic tests in brainstem lesions. *Archives of Otolaryngology* 102:608–613.

Stevens, J.C., H.D. Webb, J. Hutchinson, J. Connell, M.F. Smith, and J.T. Buffin. 1989. Click evoked otoacoustic emissions compared with brain stem electric response. *Archives of Disease in Childhood* 64:1105–1111.

———. 1990. Click evoked oto-acoustic emissions in neonatal screening. *Ear and Hearing* 11:128–133.

———. 1991. Evaluation of click-evoked oto-acoustic emissions in the newborn. *British Journal of Audiology* 25:11–14.

Stevens, J.C., H.D. Webb, M.F. Smith, J.T. Buffin, and H. Ruddy. 1987. A comparison of otoacoustic emissions and brain stem electric response audiometry in the normal newborn and babies admitted to a special care baby unit. *Clinical Physical and Physiological Measurement* 8:95–104.

Stockard, J.E., J.J. Stockard, and R. Coen. 1983. Auditory brain stem response variability in infants. *Ear and Hearing* 4:11–23.

Stokoe, W. 1960. Sign language structure: An outline of the visual communication systems of the American deaf. *Studies in Linguistics.* Occasional Papers no. 8. Buffalo: State University of New York at Buffalo Department of Anthropology and Linguistics.

———. 1975. The use of sign language in teaching English. *American Annals of the Deaf* 120:417–421.

Stool, S.E., A.O. Berg, S. Berman, C.J. Carney, J.R. Cooley, L. Culpepper, R.D. Eavey, L.V. Feagans, T. Finitzo, E.M. Friedman, et al. 1994. Otitis media with effusion in young children. *Clinical Practice Guideline* #12, July. AHCPR Publication No. 94–0622. Rockville, MD: Agency for Health Care Policy and Research, Public Health Service, U.S. Department of Health and Human Services.

Strickland, E.A., E.M. Burns, and A. Tubis. 1985. Incidence of spontaneous otoacoustic emissions in children and infants. *Journal of the Acoustical Society of America* 78:931–935.

Stubblefield, J., and C. Young. 1975. Central auditory dysfunction in learning-disabled children. *Journal of Learning Disabilities* 8:32–37.

Sugimoto, T., A. Yasuhara, T. Ohta, N. Nishida, S. Saitoh, J. Hamabe, and N. Niikawa. 1992. Angelman syndrome in three siblings: Characteristic epileptic seizures and EEG abnormalities. *Epilepsia* 33:1078–1082.

Sussman, J.E. 1991. Stimulus ratio effects on speech discrimination by children and adults. *Journal of Speech and Hearing Research* 34:671–678.

Suzuki, T., and Y. Ogiba. 1960. A technique of pure-tone audiometry for children under three years of age: Conditioned orientation reflex (COR) audiometry. *Revue de Laryngologie, Otologie, Rhinologie* 81:33–45.

Sweetow, R., and R. Reddell. 1978. The use of masking level differences in the identification of children with perceptual problems. *Journal of the American Auditory Society* 4: 52–56.

Swisher, L., and I. Hirsh. 1972. Brain damage and the ordering of two temporally successive stimuli. *Neuropsychologia* 10:137–152.

Tallal, P. 1985. Neuropsychological research approaches to the study of central auditory processing. *Human Communication* 9 (Part 1):17–22.

Tallal, P., and M. Piercy. 1973. Developmental aphasia: Impaired rate of nonverbal processing as a function of sensory modality. *Neuropsychologia* 11:389–398.

———. 1974. Developmental aphasia: Rate of auditory processing and selective impairment of consonant perception. *Neuropsychologia* 12:83–94.

———. 1975. Developmental aphasia: The perception of brief vowels and extended consonants. *Neuropsychologia* 13:69–74.

Taylor, M., W. Chan-Lui, and W. Logan. 1985. Longitudinal evoked potential studies in hereditary ataxias. *Canadian Journal of Neuroscience* 12:100–105.

Teatini, G.P. 1970. Sensitized speech tests: Results in normal subjects. In *Speech audiometry*, ed. C. Rojskjaer. Odense: Danavox.

Teele, D.W., J.O. Klein, B.A. Rosner, et al. 1980. Epidemiology of otitis media in children. *Annals of Otology, Rhinology, and Laryngology* (Suppl. 68) 89:5–6.

———. 1984. Otitis media with effusion during the first three years of life and development of speech and language. *Pediatrics* 74:282–287.

Terkildsen, K. 1964. Clinical application of impedance measurements with a fixed frequency technique. *International Audiology* 3:123–128.

Tharpe, A.M., and D.H. Ashmend. 1993. Computer simulation technique for assessing pediatric auditory test protocols. *Journal of the American Academy of Audiology* 4:80–90.

Thielemeir, M.A. 1982. *Discrimination after training test*. Los Angeles: House Ear Institute.

———. 1984. *The discrimination after training test*. Los Angeles: House Ear Institute.

Thielemeir, M.A., L.L. Tonokawa, B. Petersen, and L.S. Eisenberg. 1985. Audiological results in children with a cochlear implant. *Ear and Hearing* (Suppl.) 6:27S–35S.

Thoman, E.B., and P.T. Becker. 1979. Issues in assessment and prediction for the infant born at risk. In *Infants born at risk*, ed. T. Field. Jamaica, N.Y.: Spectrum.

Thompson, G., and R.C. Folsom. 1984. A comparison of two conditioning procedures in the use of visual reinforcement audiometry (VRA). *Journal of Speech and Hearing Disorders* 49:241–245.

Thompson, G., and B.A. Weber. 1974. Responses of infants and young children to behavior observation audiometry (BOA). *Journal of Speech and Hearing Disorders* 39:140–147.

Thompson, G., W.R. Wilson, and J.M. Moore. 1979. Application of visual reinforcement audiometry (VRA) to low-functioning children. *Journal of Speech and Hearing Disorders* 44:80–90.

Thompson, M., and G. Thompson. 1972. Response of infants and young children as a function of auditory stimuli and test method. *Journal of Speech and Hearing Research* 15: 699–707.

Thornton, A., M. Mendel, and C. Anderson. 1977. Effects of stimulus frequency and intensity on the middle components of the averaged auditory electroencephalic response. *Journal of Speech and Hearing Research* 20:81–94.

Thornton, A.R.D., G. Farrell, and E. McSporran. 1989. Clinical methods for the objective estimation of loudness discomfort level (LDL) using auditory brainstem responses in patients. *Scandinavian Audiology* 18:225–230.

Thornton, A.R.D., L. Yardley, and G. Farrell. 1987. The objective estimation of loudness discomfort level using auditory brainstem evoked responses. *Scandinavian Audiology* 16: 219–225.

Thringer, K., A. Kankkunen, G. Lidén, and A. Niklasson. 1984. Perinatal risk factors in the etiology of hearing loss in preschool children. *Developmental Medicine and Child Neurology* 26:799–807.

Tillman, T.W., and R. Carhart. 1966. An expanded test for speech discrimination utilizing CNC monosyllabic words (Northwestern University auditory test no. 6). Technical report, SAM-TR-66–55, USAF School of Aerospace Medicine. Aerospace Medical Division (AFSC), Brooks Air Force Base, Texas.

Tillman, T., R. Carhart, and W. Olsen. 1970. Hearing aid efficiency in a competing speech situation. *Journal of Speech and Hearing Research* 13:789–811.

Tobey, E.A., and J.K. Cullen, Jr. 1984. Temporal integration of tone glides by children with auditory-memory and reading problems. *Journal of Speech and Hearing Research* 27: 527–533.

Tobey, E.A., and M.S. Hasenstab. 1991. Effects of a Nucleus multichannel cochlear implant upon speech production in children. In *Multichannel cochlear implants in children*, ed. S.J. Staller. *Ear and Hearing* (Suppl.) 12:48S–54S.

Tokioka, A.B., D.H. Crowell, and J.W. Pierce. 1987. Electrophysiological investigation of cognition in infants. In *Thinking across cultures: The third international conference on thinking*, ed. D.M. Topping, D.C. Crowell, and V.N. Kobayashi. Hillsdale, N.J.: Lawrence Erlbaum Associates.

Tong, Y.C., R.C. Black, G.M. Clark, I.C. Forster, J.B. Millar, B.J. O'Loughlin, and J.F. Patrick. 1979. A preliminary report on a multiple-channel cochlear implant operation. *Journal of Laryngology and Otology* 93:7:679–695.

Tong, Y.C., G.M. Clark, P.J. Blamey, P.A. Busby, and R.C. Dowell. 1982. Psychophysical studies for two multiple-channel cochlear implant patients. *Journal of the Acoustical Society of America* 71:153–160.

Tong, Y.C., G.M. Clark, P.M. Seligman, and J.F. Patrick. 1980. Speech processing for a multiple-electrode cochlear implant prosthesis. *Journal of the Acoustical Society of America* 68:1897–1899.

Trine, M.B., J.E. Hirsch, and R.H. Margolis. 1993. The effect of compensatory ear-canal pressure on otoacoustic emissions. *Ear and Hearing* 14:401–407.

Turner, R.G., and D.W. Nielsen. 1984. Application of clinical decision analysis to audiological tests. *Ear and Hearing* 5:125–133.

Tye-Murray, N. 1987. Effects of vowel context on the articulatory closure postures of deaf speakers. *Journal of Speech and Hearing Research* 30:99–104.

Tye-Murray, N., M. Lowder, and R.S. Tyler. 1990. Comparison of the F_0F_2 and $F_0F_1F_2$ processing strategies for the Cochlear Corporation cochlear implant. *Ear and Hearing* 11: 195–200.

Tyler, R.S., J. Preece, and M. Lowder. 1983. *The Iowa cochlear implant tests*. Iowa City: University of Iowa, Department of Otolaryngology, Head and Neck Surgery.

Tyler, R.S., and N. Tye-Murray. 1991. Cochlear implant signal-processing strategies and patient perception of speech and environmental sounds. In *Cochlear implants: A practical guide*, ed. H. Cooper. London: Whurr Publishers Ltd.

U. S. Department of Education. 1992. *Deaf students education services: Policy guidance*. *Federal Register* (October 30) Vol. 57. No. 211:49274–49276.

———. 1992. *To assure the free appropriate education of all handicapped children.* Fourteenth annual report to Congress on the implementation of P.L. 94–142: The education for all handicapped children act. Washington, D.C.: U.S. Government Printing Office.

U.S. Department of Health and Human Services, Public Health Service. 1990. *Healthy people 2000: National health promotion and disease prevention objectives.* Washington, D.C.: U.S. Government Printing Office.

———. 1991. *Healthy people 2000: National health promotion and disease prevention objectives.* DHHS Publication No. PHS1–50212. Washington, D.C.: Government Printing Office.

U.S. Department of Health and Human Services, Agency for Health Care Policy and Research. 1994. *Clinical practice guideline: Otitis media with effusion in young children.* Washington, D.C.: Public Health Service.

U.S. National Commission on Excellence in Education. 1993. *A nation at risk: the imperative for educational reform: a report to the Nation and the Secretary of Education, United States Department of Education.* Washington, D.C.: The Commission.

Upfold, L.J., and J. Isepy. 1982. Childhood deafness in Australia. *Medical Journal of Australia* 2:323–326.

Uziel, A., and J.P. Piron. 1991. Evoked otoacoustic emissions from normal newborns and babies admitted to an intensive care baby unit. *Acta Oto-Laryngologica* (Suppl. 482): 85–91.

Van Camp, K.J., R.H. Margolis, R.H. Wilson, W.L. Creten, and J.E. Shanks. 1986. Principles of tympanometry. *ASHA* Monograph no. 24. Rockville, Md.: American Speech-Language-Hearing Association.

Vanhuyse, V.J., W.L. Creten, and K.J. Van Camp. 1975. On the W-notching of tympanograms. *Scandinavian Audiology* 4:45–50.

von Wallenberg, E.L., and R.D. Battmer. 1991. Comparative speech recognition results in eight subjects using two different coding strategies with the Nucleus 22–channel cochlear implant. *British Journal of Audiology* 25:371–380.

Waldstein, R. 1990. Effects of postlingual deafness on speech production: Implications for the role of auditory feedback. *Journal of the Acoustical Society of America* 88: 2099–2114.

Wallace, I.F., S.K. Escalona, C.M. McCarton-Daum, and H.G. Vaughan. 1982. Neonatal precursors of cognitive development in low birth weight children. *Seminars in Perinatology* 6:327–333.

Wallace, I.F., J.S. Gravel, C.M. McCarton, and R.J. Ruben. 1988. Otitis media and language development at 1 year of age. *Journal of Speech and Hearing Disorders* 54:245–251.

Wallace, S.P., C.A. Prutting, and S.E. Gerber. 1990. Degeneration of speech, language, and hearing in a patient with mucopolysaccharidosis VII. *International Journal of Pediatric Otolaryngology* 19:97–107.

Waring, M.D., M. Don, and J.A. Brimacombe. 1985. ABR assessment of stimulation in induction coil implant patients. In *Cochlear implants,* ed. R.A. Schindler and M.M. Merzenich. New York: Raven Press.

Warren, R.M. 1983. Multiple meanings of "phoneme": Articulatory, acoustic, perceptual, graphemic, and their confusions. In *Speech and language: Advances in basic research and practice,* vol. 9, ed. N.J. Lass. New York: Academic Press.

Weatherby, L., and M. Bennett. 1980. The neonatal acoustic reflex. *Scandinavian Audiology* 9:103–110.

Webb, J.D., and J.C. Stevens. 1991. Auditory screening in high risk neonates: Selection of a test protocol. *Clinical Physical and Physiological Measurement* 12:75–76.

Webb, R.L., B.C. Pyman, B.K.-H. Franz, and G.M. Clark. 1990. The surgery of cochlear implantation. In *Cochlear prostheses*, ed. G.M. Clark, Y.C. Tong, and J.F. Patrick. Edinburgh: Churchill Livingstone.

Weber, B.A. 1969. Validation of observer judgements in behavioral observation audiometry. *Journal of Speech and Hearing Disorders* 34:350–355.

———. 1982. Comparison of auditory brain stem response latency norms for premature infants. *Ear and Hearing* 3:257–262.

———. 1994. Auditory brainstem response: Threshold estimation and auditory screening. In *Handbook of clinical audiology*, 4th ed., ed. J. Katz. Baltimore: Williams and Wilkins.

Webster, A., and J. Elwood. 1985. *The hearing impaired child in the ordinary school.* London: Croom Helm.

Webster, D.B., and M. Webster. 1977. Neonatal sound deprivation affects brainstem auditory nuclei. *Archives of Otolaryngology* 103:392–396.

Wechsler, D. 1967. *Wechsler primary and preschool intelligence scale.* New York: Psychological Corp.

———. 1974. *Wechsler intelligence scale for children* (Revised). New York: Psychological Corp.

Weisenberger, J.M., and L. Kozma-Spytek. 1991. Evaluating tactile aids for speech perception and production by hearing-impaired adults and children. In *Cochlear implants in children*, ed. R.T. Miyamoto and M.J. Osberger. *American Journal of Otolaryngology* (Suppl.) 12:188–200.

Welsh, R., and S. Slater. 1993. The state of infant hearing impairment identification programs. *Asha* 35:49–52.

Werner, L.A. 1992. Interpreting developmental psychoacoustics. In *Developmental psychoacoustics*, ed. L.A. Werner and E.W. Rubel. Washington, D.C.: American Psychological Association.

White, E.J. 1977. Children's performance on the SSW test and Willeford battery: Interim clinical data. In *Central auditory dysfunction*, ed. R.W. Keith. New York: Grune and Stratton.

White, K.R., and T.R. Behrens, eds. 1993. The Rhode Island infant hearing assessment project: Implications for universal newborn hearing screening. *Seminars in Hearing* 14:1.

White, K.R., A.B. Maxon, T.R. Behrens, P.M. Blackwell, and B.R. Vohr. 1992. Neonatal screening using evoked otoacoustic emissions: The Rhode Island hearing assessment project. In *Screening children for auditory function*, ed. F.H. Bess and J.W. Hall III. Nashville: Bill Wilkerson Center Press.

White, K.R., B.R. Vohr, and T.R. Behrens. 1993. Universal newborn hearing screening using transient evoked otoacoustic emissions: Results of the Rhode Island hearing assessment project. *Seminars in Hearing* 14:18–29.

Widen, J.E. 1990. Behavioral screening of high-risk infants using visual reinforcement audiometry. *Seminars in Hearing* 11:342–356.

———. 1993. Adding objectivity to infant behavioral audiometry. *Ear and Hearing*, 14:49–57.

Wilcox, S. 1988. Introduction: Academic acceptance of American Sign Language. *Sign Language Studies* 59:101–108.

———. 1990. The structure of signed and spoken languages. *Sign Language Studies* 67:141–151.

Wiley, T.L., D.L. Oviatt, and M.G. Block. 1987. Acoustic immittance measures in normal ears. *Journal of Speech and Hearing Research* 30:161–170.

Willeford, J.A. 1976. Differential diagnosis of central auditory dysfunction. In *Audiology: An audio journal for continuing education*, vol. 2, ed. L. Bradford. New York: Grune and Stratton.

———. 1977. Assessing central auditory behavior in children: A test battery approach. In *Central auditory dysfunction*, ed. R.W. Keith. New York: Grune and Stratton.

———. 1978. Sentence tests of central auditory function. In *Handbook of clinical audiology*, 2d ed., ed. J. Katz. Baltimore: Williams and Wilkins.

———. 1980. Central auditory behaviors in learning disabled children. *Seminars in Speech Language and Hearing* 1:127–140.

———. 1985. Assessment of central auditory disorders in children. In *Assessment of central auditory dysfunction: Foundations and clinical correlates*, ed. M.L. Pinheiro and F.E. Musiek. Baltimore: Williams and Wilkins.

Willeford, J.A., and J.M. Billger. 1985. Auditory perception in children with learning disabilities. In *Handbook of clinical audiology*, 3d ed., ed. J. Katz. Baltimore: Williams and Wilkins.

Willeford, J.A., and J.M. Burleigh. 1985. *Handbook of central auditory processing disorders in children*. Orlando: Grune and Stratton.

Willott, J.F., R.M. Demuth, and S.M. Lu. 1984. Excitability of auditory neurons in the dorsal and ventral cochlear nuclei of DBA/2 and C57BL/6 mice. *Experimental Neurology* 83:495–506.

Willows, D.M., J.R. Kershner, and E. Corcos. 1986. Visual processing and visual memory in reading and writing disabilities: A rationale for reopening a "closed case." Paper presented at symposium, The Role of Visual Processing and Visual Memory in Reading and Writing. Annual meeting of the American Educational Research Association, April, San Francisco.

Wilson, B.S., C.C. Finley, D.T. Lawson, R.D. Wolford, D.K. Eddington, and W.M. Rabinowitz. 1991. Better speech recognition with cochlear implants. *Nature* 352:236–238.

Wilson, C.B., J.S. Remington, S. Stagno, and D.W. Reynolds. 1980. Development of adverse sequelae in children born with subclinical congenital toxoplasma infection. *Pediatrics* 66:767–774.

Wilson, R.H., J.E. Shanks, and D.J. Lilly. 1984. Acoustic-reflex adaptation. In *The acoustic reflex: Basic principles and clinical applications,* ed. S. Silman. New York: Academic Press.

Wilson, W.R. 1978. Behavioral assessment of auditory function in infants. In *Communicative and cognitive abilities: Early behavioral assessment*, ed. F.D. Minifie and L.L. Lloyd. Baltimore: University Park Press.

Wilson, W.R., and J.M. Moore. 1978. Pure-tone earphone thresholds of infants utilizing visual reinforcement audiometry (VRA). Paper presented at the American Speech and Hearing Association Annual Convention, San Francisco.

Wilson, W.R., J.M. Moore, and G. Thompson. 1976. Sound-field auditory thresholds of infants utilizing visual reinforcement audiometry (VRA). Paper presented at American Speech and Hearing Association Annual Convention, Houston.

Wilson, W.R., and G. Thompson. 1984. Behavioral audiometry. In *Pediatric audiology: Current trends*, ed. J. Jerger. San Diego: College-Hill Press.

Witkin, B.R. 1971. Auditory perception: Implications for language development. *Language, Speech, and Hearing Services in Schools* 4:31–52.

Wong, P., and R. Bickford. 1980. Brain stem auditory evoked potentials: The use of noise estimate. *Electroencephalography and Clinical Neurophysiology* 50:25–34.

World Health Organization. 1971. *Mass health examinations.* Public Health Papers no. 45:81–82. Geneva: World Health Organization.

———. 1985. WHA39-19.

———. 1986. *Prevention of deafness and hearing impairment.* Report by the Director General of the 79th Session, EB 79/10. Geneva: World Health Organization.

———. 1991. *Report of the informal working group on prevention of deafness and hearing impairment programme planning.* Geneva: World Health Organization.

Worthington, D. 1981. ABR in special populations. Paper presented at ABR workshop, Cleveland, Ohio.

Wright, F., R. Schain, W. Weinberg, and R. Ischelle. 1982. Learning disabilities and associated conditions. In *The practice of pediatric neurology*, ed. K. Swaiman and F. Wright. St. Louis: C.V. Mosby.

Yang, E.Y., A.L. Rupert, and G. Moushegian. 1987. A developmental study of bone conduction auditory brain stem response in infants. *Ear and Hearing* 8:244–251.

Yellin, M.W., J.F. Jerger, and R.C. Fifer. 1983. Norms for disproportionate loss in speech intelligibility. Presented at American Speech-Language-Hearing Association convention, Cincinnati.

Yune, H.Y., R.T. Miyamoto, and M.E. Yune. 1991. Medical imaging in cochlear implant candidates. In *Cochlear implants in children,* ed. R.T. Miyamoto and M.J. Osberger. *American Journal of Otolaryngology* (Suppl.) 12:11–17.

Zapala, D. 1993. Statistical quantification of auditory brain-stem response waveshape quality and its relation to peak latency measurement accuracy. Ph.D. diss., Memphis State University.

Zorowka, P.G. 1993 Otoacoustic emissions: A new method to diagnose hearing impairment in children. *European Journal of Pediatrics* 152:626–634.

Author Index

Subject Index

on central auditory processing, 208–209, 233, 237–238
on middle latency response morphology, 155
on otoacoustic emissions, 184–186
on static-acoustic immittance, 115–117
on tympanometric amplitude and shape, 117
on tympanometric gradient and width, 118
on tympanometric peak pressure, 117
MCL (most comfortable loudness level), 164, 263
ME (Manual English), 330
Measles, as cause of postnatal hearing loss, 9
Medial olivocochlear bundle pathway, 174
Medicaid, 356
Memory, and cerebral metabolism, 31
Ménière's disease, 173
Meningitis
as cause of hearing loss, 8, 20, 21, 28, 39, 42, 284
influence on acoustic immittance, 134
and risk of hearing loss, 187
Meningococcal meningitis. See Meningitis
Meningomyelocele, 160
Mensa Society, 31
Mental retardation, 7, 26, 73, 317, 318, 333
Metabolic problems, as cause of hearing loss, 7, 19
Metalinguistic skills, 210–211, 219, 237
Michelson, R., 277
Middle ear, acoustic reactance of, 104
Middle-ear effusion (MEE)
and acoustic immittance, 126–129, 135–137
in children, 27, 28, 29, 126–129
detection of, 135–137
in developmentally disabled children, 28
influence on tympanic membrane, 47
and language acquisition, 27, 29
in neonates, 113, 129
and tympanosclerosis, 125
Middle-ear pathology
and acoustic immittance, 124–125
assessment of, 286
hearing loss associated with, 27, 28
influence on measurement of otoacoustic emissions, 183–184, 189, 195, 197–200
malformations associated with Apert syndrome, 159
in neonates, 28, 183–184, 189
prevalence in young-patient populations, 183–184
and reading skills, 31
and speech regression, 29–30
Middle latency (evoked) response (MLR), 146–148, 149, 153, 155–158, 214, 215, 223, 228, 285–286
Mines, Art, 271

Minimal Auditory Capabilities (MAC) Battery, 95, 97, 298
Minimal Pairs test, 298
Minimum auditory response level (MRL), 63
Mismatched negativity (MMN) response, 148
MLD (masking level differences), 215, 216, 218, 219, 234–235
MLR (middle latency response), 146–148, 149, 153, 155–158, 214, 215, 223, 228, 285–286
Model Secondary School for the Deaf Act (PL 89-694), 317
Monaural functioning, evaluation of, 98
Monaural hearing aids, 257–258
Monaural low-redundancy speech tests, 216, 229–230
Mondini dysplasia, 285
Monoacetyldiaminodiphenyl sulphone (MADDS), 162
Monosyllable, Trochee, Spondee (MTS) test, 96, 294–295, 297, 299–300
Morphogenesis, 26
Most comfortable loudness level (MCL), 164, 263
Mothers, influence on intrauterine development, 20–21, 22, 24, 40, 211
Motor skills, problems with, 28, 42
Mouth, assessment of, 38, 53–54
MPEAK (Multipeak) coding strategy, 281–282, 307
MRI (magnetic resonance imaging), 52, 214, 284
MRL (minimum auditory response level), 63
MTS (Monosyllable, Trochee, Spondee) test, 96, 294–295, 297, 299–300
Mucopolysaccharides diseases (MPS), 19
Multiculturalism, 316, 336–338, 352, 353–354
Multipeak (MPEAK) coding strategy, 281–282, 307
Multiple dysmorphic abnormalities, 28
Mumps, as cause of postnatal hearing loss, 9
Musculoskeletal system, assessment of, 37, 38
Mutagenic agents, exposure to, 19
Myelomeningocele, infected, 21
Myopia (nearsightedness), 30

NAD (National Association for the Deaf), 305–306
NAL-R formula, for ear measurement, 263
Narcotics, influence on intrauterine development, 22
Nasal aspiration, 29
NASDSE (National Association of State Directors of Special Education), 364
National Association for the Deaf (NAD), 305–306
National Association of State Directors of Special Education (NASDSE), 364
National Button-Battery Ingestion Hotline, 275